Shared Mass Trauma in Social Work

IØ131Ø56

This edited volume looks at the phenomenon of shared trauma and how it affects social workers and their clients alike. Bringing together established voices from the field of social work, *Shared Mass Trauma in Social Work* presents ideas of how to provide resilient care and practice while social workers and their clients are both experiencing the same mass trauma.

Social workers are often on the front line when community trauma occurs, and the boundary between their experiences and those of clients can become blurred. In this timely resource, Ann Goelitz and the contributors aim to share both their findings and evidence-based tools to help professionals look after themselves and their clients in times of turmoil. Beginning by setting a conceptual framework for shared trauma and reviewing related research, the contributors discuss the concept as it relates to events such as the coronavirus pandemic, climate change and natural disasters, police brutality and racism, and war and terrorism. Filled with case studies that bring the text to life, chapters then move to the modalities of psychotherapy, group work, and community organizing, before concluding with reflections and lessons learnt for future practice. The glossary of terms, sample syllabus, and practical exercises to support training social workers are a bonus for educators.

Shared Mass Trauma in Social Work incorporates specific implications, trauma-informed care, social work principles, and practical tips to support training and established clinicians working in unprecedented circumstances.

Ann Goelitz, PhD, LCSW, is a psychotherapist and author of *From Trauma to Healing: A Social Worker's Guide to Working with Survivors*, now in its 2nd edition (Routledge). She has also taught at Columbia University and Hunter College, US, presented extensively, and written numerous academic articles.

"I cannot think of a book more timely than *Shared Mass Trauma in Social Work*. With the systemic insight that defines social work scholarship and practice, Dr. Goelitz has assembled both a research and practice-informed volume that is a critical resource for human services professionals who are still wondering which end is up after the global pandemic. Her attention to the scourge of police brutality, systemic racism, and other unrest is also critical, bringing in contributions from scholars with first-hand connections to the matters discussed. I highly recommend this work for all who seek to be the change moving forward."

Jamie Marich, PhD, LPCC-S, LICDC-CS, REAT, RYT-500, *Founder of The Institute for Creative Mindfulness, author of* Trauma and the 12 Steps *and* Healing Addiction with EMDR Therapy: A Trauma-Focused Guide, *and many other volumes on trauma recovery*

"*Shared Mass Trauma in Social Work* is extremely timely and pertinent, especially in today's climate with mass trauma permeating our lives. This guidebook shares ways to effectively help ourselves and those we work with. I feel so fortunate to have come across it when I can really use its wisdom, guidance, and treatment suggestions. I am impressed by the variety of trauma related topics and top-tier authors, researchers and clinicians who offered their insights and perspectives. Thank you Dr. Goelitz for offering this pearl of wisdom to the field."

Michelle Maidenberg, PhD, MPH, LCSW-R, CGP, *Author of* Free Your Child from Overeating: 53 Mind-Body Strategies for Lifelong Health, *upcoming book* ACE Your Life: Unleash Your Best Self and the Life You Want to Be Living, *Psychology Today blogger*

Shared Mass Trauma in Social Work

Implications and Strategies for Resilient Practice

Edited by
Ann Goelitz

Routledge
Taylor & Francis Group

NEW YORK AND LONDON

Cover image: Getty

First published 2023
by Routledge
605 Third Avenue, New York, NY 10158

and by Routledge
4 Park Square, Milton Park, Abingdon, Oxon OX14 4RN

Routledge is an imprint of the Taylor & Francis Group, an informa business

Library of Congress Cataloging-in-Publication Data
A catalog record for this title has been requested

ISBN: 978-1-032-00676-5 (hbk)
ISBN: 978-1-032-01062-5 (pbk)
ISBN: 978-1-003-17694-7 (ebk)

DOI: 10.4324/9781003176947

Typeset in Times New Roman
by Taylor & Francis Books

This book is dedicated to those who lost lives and hearts to the two pandemics of COVID-19 and racism.

Contents

Acknowledgements

First and foremost I'd like to thank Heather Evans, the best editor ever. It was in a conversation with you, just after finishing the 2nd edition of *From Trauma to Healing*, that this book was birthed. We were tossing around ideas for future books and it turned out you were looking for edited books for social workers. This was at the beginning of COVID-19 so it was no mistake that the topic of shared trauma came to my mind. You liked the idea and offered support along the way, making me feel more like a comrade than client, while also staying professional and prodding me along so I didn't get too far off track. Thank you for helping make this happen. I don't think you'll be sorry. It's an amazing book, if I don't say so myself.

Of course I'd be nowhere without those of you who contributed by writing book chapters. Carol, you were the first I approached. Thank you for your support, suggestions (including other possible contributors), and for jumping on board immediately. Having you at my back helped get other contributors and added immensely to the book since you are **the** expert on shared trauma. Shari, Julian, Alana, Rachel, Aimee, Tina, Tiong, Orit, Johanna, Jonathan, Carolyn, Alex, Ozy, and JaLisa—without you, this could never have happened. I'm so grateful you said yes as well, writing in such an authentic, yet professional, manner and getting the message across so beautifully. Some of you came into the process late. Others struggled with their topics, with how they fit with shared trauma, and at times with my edits. Thank you for hanging in there and making this happen. It was so worth the effort. I know many social workers will be helped by this book.

Other contributors include Kevin, who wrote such a heartfelt and powerful foreword for the book, and the endorsers on the back cover—Michelle and Jamie. Thank you for your support of the book and for lending your names to it in order to help it get out to as many as possible who can be helped by it. I appreciate you being a part of this as well.

I also want to send out a shout of appreciation to all who wanted to contribute but couldn't. Almost without fail, those who said no wanted to be a part of the project but were unable to for various reasons. The encouraging way you said no added to my conviction. Thank you for that.

Last, but certainly not least, I want to thank my friends and family who supported me throughout this effort, putting up with unanswered calls and not seeing me often. I love you all. Carol, you, in particular, were a big part of the book. You're my personal cheerleader, reader and often my editor when I write. Even when I sent you my final chapter on Thanksgiving eve for a look-see, you said yes. You are truly the best. I hope you know how much you mean to me.

My mother, Syd, served a similar role when she was alive. Thank you, Syd. I so appreciate your support and love. This book would probably never have come to pass if you had not instilled in me the love of books. Thank you for that. You are my mentor and guide as I write and I love you for that.

Finally, *you're probably saying*, thank you to the love of my life with whom I've built such a magical life, my darling Mike. We've certainly had a year of it—COVID-19 and building a home together—as I wrote this book. How the heck did we do it? Without your patience and love it wouldn't have happened. Thank you for that. I saved you, the best, for last.

I am grateful.

Contributors

Ozy Aloziem, MSW, is an award-winning Igbo social worker committed to collective liberation and racial justice. Originally raised on Omaha land, she has been a visitor on Arapaho, Cheyenne, and Ute territories since 2015. Ozy is the Denver Public Library's first Equity, Diversity & Inclusion Manager. She is a nationally recognized facilitator, speaker, and racial equity consultant. Ozy prioritizes racial and gender equity in her scholarship and activism. She uses this focus to amplify voices of marginalized communities that are left on the fringes of research, public policy, and global conversation. Presently, Ozy's research is centered around radical healing and radical imagination.

Johanna E. Barry, PhD, LCSW/LICSW, is an Assistant Professor of Social Work at Augsburg University in Minneapolis, MN. Dr Barry received her Master of Social Work from the University of Chicago and her PhD from Loyola University Chicago. As a licensed clinical social worker, she has had the privilege to work with both children and adults over the last decade who seek healing from issues stemming from complex trauma including adverse childhood experiences, community violence, intimate partner and family violence, war trauma or genocide, cultural dislocation, and sexual exploitation and trafficking. Her current research lies at the intersection of intimate partner violence and child welfare.

Shari Bloomberg, DSW, LCSW, is an adjunct professor at NYU Silver School of Social Work. She also speaks on trauma, emphasizing domestic violence, both locally and nationally, and maintains a private practice in New Jersey.

Julian Cohen-Serrins, LCSW, is a PhD student at New York University's Silver School of Social Work. He received his MSW from the University of Pennsylvania's School of Social Policy and Practice. His clinical career has spanned across various mental health organizations in both clinical and leadership roles, from large state-run inpatient psychiatric centers to wellness clinics, homeless shelters, and partial hospital programs. Julian's research area relates to workplace mental health and especially its intersection with organizational and policy-level approaches. His current research focuses on discerning and implementing optimal burnout reduction interventions and its intersections with organizational justice and support.

Rachel Dekel, PhD, is a Full Professor at the Louis and Gabi Weisfeld School of Social Work at Bar-Ilan University and was the school's Director from 2012–2016. Since 2018 she has served as the academic head of the International School. Her research focuses on coping with traumatic events such as war, terror, and family violence, especially its additional effects on families. She has published more than 150 articles and book chapters. Professor Dekel is also the founder of the Bar-Ilan Clinic for conjoint intervention for couples in which one partner suffers from PTSD. More information can be found at www.RachelDekel.com.

Alex Gitterman, Professor of Social Work at the University of Connecticut School of Social Work, has published numerous cutting-edge books and articles on social work practice, group work, resilience, field instruction, supervision, organizational behavior, and teaching. He serves as the Editor of a series for Columbia University Press about Helping Empower the Powerless. Currently he serves on the editorial boards of the following journals: *Clinical Social Work, Clinical Journal of Supervision; Journal of Human Behavior in the Social Environment; Social Work with Groups; Social Work in Health Care; Reflections: Narratives of Professional Helping,* and *Teaching in Social Work.*

Ann Goelitz is a writer and a scholar with a wide scope of clinical experience. For the past ten plus years, she has specialized in her private psychotherapy practice on EMDR, hypnosis, and cognitive behavioral therapy, helping clients heal from trauma and loss. A seasoned educator, she has done extensive public speaking, published numerous articles, and co-authored an award-winning resource directory for caregivers. Her book, *From Trauma to Healing: A Social Worker's Guide to Working with Survivors,* now in its second edition, has received endorsement and accolades. She has taught at Columbia University and Hunter College.

Aimee Jette is a Clinical Art Therapist and Licensed Professional Counselor who has found that art has the ability to transcend the barriers of language, assisting trauma work with clients. Aimee pursued her MA in Creative Arts Therapy Counseling from Hofstra University after working with resettled refugees conducting art workshops for women from Uganda, Tanzania, and the Democratic Republic of Congo. She has a private practice in Ridgefield, CT. Additionally, she is the founder of Art in Common, a community outreach non-profit whose mission is to increase community awareness around important social issues and engender connection through the creative process.

Carolyn Knight, MSW, PhD, has more than 30 years of experience working with adult survivors of childhood trauma. She has written about and presented workshops on trauma-informed practice and supervision and is the author of *Introduction to Working with Adult Survivors of Childhood Trauma* and co-editor of *Trauma-informed Supervision in a Global Context* (with L.D. Borders). Dr Knight is co-author, with Alex Gitterman and Carel Germain, of the 2021 social work practice text, *The Life Model of Social Work Practice*, 4th ed. and co-editor of *Group Work with Populations at Risk*, 4th ed (with G. Greif).

Orit Nuttman-Shwartz, PhD, MSW, GA, is a Full Professor at the School of Social Work at Sapir College in Israel. She was the founder and first head of the school and Past Chairperson of the Israel National Social Work Council. Her research deals with the effects of continuous and shared exposure to threats on individuals and communities, and on clients and social workers. She has published more than 80 articles and book chapters. Nuttman-Shwartz was awarded the Katan Prize and the Israeli parliament Award for Academic Scholarship in Social Work. She can be contacted at orits@sapir.ac.il.

Tina Sacks is an associate professor at UC Berkeley's School of Social Welfare. Her fields of interest include racial inequities in health, social determinants of health, and poverty and inequality. Professor Sacks focuses on how macro-structural forces, including structural discrimination and immigration, affect women's health. Her current work investigates the persistence of racial and gender discrimination in health care settings among racial/ethnic minorities who are not poor. She published a book on this subject entitled *Invisible Visits: Black Middle-Class Women in the American Healthcare System* (2019).

Alana Siegel, PsyD, is an instructor at Tel Aviv University and a psychologist in private practice in Tel Aviv. She completed her undergraduate degree with Honors in Human Development at Cornell University and graduated with a Master's degree in International Affairs from the Institut d'Etudes Politiques (Sciences Po) in Paris. Dr Siegel earned her doctorate in Clinical and School Child Psychology at Yeshiva University. She completed postdoctoral research fellowships at Bar-Ilan University and at Tel Aviv University. Her research focuses on secondary traumatic stress, posttraumatic stress disorder, and resilience. Dr Siegel can be contacted at www.DrAlanaSiegel.com or at DrAlanaSiegel@gmail.com.

Jonathan B. Singer, PhD, LCSW, is Associate Professor of Social Work at Loyola University Chicago, President of the American Association of Suicidology, co-lead of the Social Work Grand Challenge "Harness Technology for Social Good," founder and host of the award-winning Social Work Podcast, and author of over 75 publications including the 2015 Routledge text, *Suicide in Schools: A Practitioner's Guide to Multi-level Prevention, Assessment, Intervention, and Postvention*. He lives in Evanston, IL with his wife and three children and can be found on Twitter as @socworkpodcast.

Ngoh Tiong Tan is Professor and former Dean at Singapore University of Social Sciences and Chair of the Global Institute of Social Work. Dr Tan is Treasurer, International Association of Schools of Social Work, President of ConneXions International, and former Vice President of International Federation of Social Workers. He has authored and edited a number of books including: *Transforming Society, Asian Tsunami and Social Work Practice, Challenge of Social Care in Asia, Extending Frontiers, Human Rights Perspective, Social Work Around the World Volumes I, II and III*, and *Preparing for Marriage and Parenting Today*.

Carol Tosone, PhD, LCSW, is Professor at New York University Silver School of Social Work, recipient of the NYU Distinguished Teaching Award, Editor-in-Chief of the *Clinical Social Work* Journal, and a Distinguished Scholar in Social Work in the National Academies of Practice. Dr Tosone is editor of 5 books, as well as author of numerous professional articles, book chapters, and mental health training media. She is conducting a national study on the impact of COVID-19 on clinical practice, and has studied Manhattan clinicians post 9/11, New Orleans clinicians post Hurricane Katrina, and social workers in Northern Ireland during the Troubles.

JaLisa Williams, MSW, LCSW, is a fierce curator of intentional spaces and conversations regarding diversity, mindfulness, and liberation in the classroom, the community, and individually. Currently residing in Denver, JaLisa is a lecturer for Smith College School for Social Work focusing on community healing, social accountability, and radical social work practices. As a Black feminist scholar, she has intersected yoga with her calling for community healing in her small private practice Yemaya Innergy Therapeutics specializing in working with Black, Indigienous, Brown, and other folks of color. JaLisa imagines Black folks putting intention and action together to create magic.

Foreword

I had just finished my first supervision of the morning. My colleague, Sandra, was leaving the office as the phone rang. I waved goodbye to her and picked up the phone to hear the frantic voice of my brother, Peter.

"Are you alright?"
"Yes, I'm fine."

"Is Susan alright?"

"She's probably still at home, so, I'm sure she's fine. What are you going on about?"
"Didn't you see, a plane flew into the WTC."

I reassured him that I was fine and took the stairs up to the unit. I was the Unit Chief of a 44-bed drug and alcohol detox and rehab. The patients were in the lecture hall watching the news. Apparently, Nursing had given permission to continue watching the breaking news until the morning lecture began. Several nurses and therapists were standing in the rear of the hall. I nodded hello to the heads that turned to me. I arrived in time to see the second plane crashing into the tower. A collective groan arose. The shock and disbelief at what we were seeing was shared by everyone in the room, regardless of status—patient or staff. In that second awful moment on that sun-drenched morning, status and role fell away. We were one.

This was the start of my day on September 11, 2001. My job description was suddenly changed, in the way that war-time commanders know, from overseeing the delivery of treatment and program development to the care, safety, and morale of my patients and treatment team—nurses, doctors, therapists, and support staff. For all we knew, the nation was at war and the loss of the towers was only the beginning. In those hours and early days after the attack, the feeling of unity on the unit floor, in the subways and throughout the land was palpable.

Then on March 13, 2020 the world was suddenly facing a fatal and unrelenting virus, COVID-19, in a manner unimaginable except in science fiction or dystopian novels.

At this time, I was no longer in agency work but in private practice. My first response to the "shelter in place" was to continue to see my patients in person. As the death toll climbed in the world and particularly in New York City, the lack of sense to my policy grew clearer. My home is ten blocks from Colombia Presbyterian Hospital. The shrill sound of ambulances traveling to the ER was constant and unsettling, offsetting the growing silence of a city under siege. I finally decided that the heroics of seeing patients was untenable. However, I continued to see the most unstable and high-risk patients for another three weeks until the reality— that these were the very people most unlikely to mask, social distance, or take precautions—became unavoidable. By May, my practice was exclusively remote.

Thus began the life that continues to this day. I was startled that the quality of therapeutic relationship was not diminished or hindered by the move from treatment in Room to Zoom. In fact I found that the small screen allowed and forced me to focus even more closely on the spoken words, tone, and facial expressions / cues of my patients. Twenty-four months before, I would have argued that a quality of rapport would have been impossible. The fact that a third of my cases are new since the Time of Corona speaks to the utter viability of telemedicine to allow for the formation of intimate connection and alliance (something that I had scoffed at pre-COVID).

What was even more unexpected was the shift in what was being treated. It was as if the bulk of my patients had woken up, freed of the neurosis and discomforts that had driven them to my office. Instead the pressing issue was how to live in a world that had changed overnight and offered little hope of ever changing back.

In times like this, when social workers and patients are sharing the same global community trauma, *Shared Mass Trauma in Social Work: Implications and Strategies for Resilient Practice* goes to the heart of this experience and offers a way of understanding, responding to and intervening with the Other and Self in a world where the map of clinical response is outdated and insufficient. It offers ways to comprehend the experience of both Patient and Provider in the age of community disaster and also how to address, intervene and help both our patients and ourselves. This book will be great tool for understanding the unfolding of trauma as community disaster, with shared trauma distinguished from our previous understandings of vicarious trauma, burn-out, compassion fatigue, or secondary victimization.

If therapy is the provision of a safe and stable container in which to process change, then the process in the times of community disaster, war, pandemic, environmental crisis, is akin to having the container in the midst of a maelstrom, where the therapist is at risk from the same forces that imperil the patient. Both are simultaneously threatened, suffer disrupted routines, blurred boundaries, growth of fear and inhibition of self-care and efficacy.

To my colleagues in any of the helping professions, buy this book and read it carefully!

Shared Mass Trauma in Social Work offers insight and action plans for the client and therapist as they face mutual exposure to collective traumatic events and the simultaneous experience of powerlessness over safety, dysregulation, hyperarousal, and the death of hope. In a world where the underpinnings of normalcy and stability are eroding, this text provides more than words. It offers methods to find grounding and balance for the individuals on both sides of the desk. My testimony on the value of this book is based on the experience of being a provider in these times, who would have been well served by attending more closely to my needs, fears, and care. May the reader save and support themselves while continuing to treat and serve others.

Heraclitus "All is in flux"

Kevin Barry Heaney, LCSW, Psychotherapist in Private Practice
Former positions: Clinical Director, Safe Foundation.
Inpatient Rehab Unit Chief, Smithers/Addiction Institute of NY; and
Directer, Beth Israel, Stuyvesant Square, Intensive Outpatient

Introduction

Shared Mass Trauma in Social Work: Implications and Strategies for Resilient Practice is a labor of love inspired by the current COVID-19 pandemic and the variety of ways we responded to it as social workers. As you will see in this book and may have experienced yourself, our unique way of working with person in the environment systems is instrumental during times of shared trauma. The contributors to *Shared Mass Trauma in Social Work* demonstrate this as they share the creative ways we social workers work with and help clients during times, like COVID-19, of widespread crisis and trauma, often also helping ourselves in the process.

The concept of mass traumatic experiences being shared by practitioners and their clients is a relatively new one that has only been studied since the 1990s. We are still learning about its outcomes, which are becoming more frequent due to war, political and religious strife, terrorist attacks, mass shootings, police brutality, natural disasters compounded by climate change, pandemic, mass poverty and starvation, famine, drought, discrimination, genocide, and more. This book is a stepping stone toward understanding implications of mass trauma and developing strategies for resilient practice; and as such is crucial for continued social work practice in these times of frequent crises.

The aim of *Shared Mass Trauma in Social Work* is to arm social workers and other practitioners with the knowledge and tools with which to understand and work with shared trauma. Despite the potential impact of mass trauma, its effect is not always easy to delineate. We know it occurs when widespread trauma simultaneously affects both practitioners and their clients, confounding their joint processes. However, as Dr. Tosone and Mr. Cohen-Serrins describe in their chapter on research, this phenomena "represents a unique and profound experience with a plethora of potential outcomes."

This book, which is meant to provide social workers with clarity on what shared trauma is and how to work with it, is organized, for use both as a text and resource guide, in three parts which represent ways of looking at shared trauma, and includes features such as: practical tips for practice, a glossary of terms, and a sample shared trauma course syllabus with practice exercises and questions that make it a natural for educators.

Its first part, "Getting Started: Shared Trauma Perspectives," sets the stage with an in-depth look at the background and concepts that underlie and illustrate shared trauma, as well as an exploration of the research done to date. Fundamental to understanding shared trauma and its impact is conceptualizing the process as Drs. Tosone and Bloomberg undertake in the first chapter of the book—"Shared Trauma: An Essential Construct for Challenging Times." They begin by introducing and eluci-dating the history, definitions, theories, and contexts that surround shared trauma. Auspiciously, good news is also discussed—that opportunities for personal and professional growth as well as development of resilience exist within shared trauma. You will see that this thread of hope entwines the book. Do not be misled by the thread of hope, however. Despite its good news, trauma is traumatizing and can be difficult to read about and com-prehend. Take good care of yourself as you read and do so in manageable doses that do not overwhelm. The material can be unsettling even as it inspires hope.

The second chapter of Part I of the book, "An Investigation of Research on Shared Trauma," reviews research on shared trauma, iden-tifying key findings and suggesting avenues for further study. Dr. Tosone and Mr. Cohen-Serrins show the universality and scope of shared trauma, citing studies done in the US, Israel, and Northern Ireland on terrorism, mass shootings, war, political/religious strife, and natural dis-aster. They state that, "shared trauma infiltrates traditional boundaries between personal and professional life, and supplants a new reality where clinicians must grapple with novel symptomology in their clients, and within themselves," supporting the need for this book and at this time.

The second part of the book, "Battlegrounds of Shared Trauma: Trau-matic Events," looks at shared trauma through the lens of these distressing occurrences—pandemic, police brutality and racism, natural disaster, and war and terrorism, illustrating the myriad similarities and differences between how shared trauma is manifested in diverse circumstances. The first chapter of this section, "Frontline Devotion in a Shared Trauma: Partners of Doctors and Nurses Combatting COVID-19," is unique in that Drs. Siegel and Dekel explore trauma shared between frontline health care workers and their significant others. As was expected, it is clear from the chapter that the shared trauma experience trickled down from front-line doctors and nurses to their partners. Showing the power of resilience, their research also demonstrated that the support of the partners for the doctors and nurses they cohabitated with bolstered those frontliners and must also have influenced their interactions and shared trauma experiences with COVID-19 patients.

One of the more difficult chapters of the book, "Trauma, Policing, and United States Social Work Practice," comes next. Ms. Jette and Dr. Sacks struggle with the idea of shared trauma since white practitioners have not directly experienced slavery, racism, and racist police brutality. They may have compassion for those who have, but it is not their trauma so they do not share the experience of it with their Black clients. Moreover, social workers have a history of complicity with the police, which adds another layer of complexity to the issue. The way Jette and Sacks grapple with these issues demonstrates something akin to shared trauma and drama-tizes the need for work in this area. This chapter is a must-read for social workers.

In the chapter "Social Resilience and Natural Disasters: Effective Social and Community Response to Shared Trauma," Dr. Ngoh Tiong Tan looks at shared trauma through societal, communal, and individual lenses and points out how our interventions can help create resilience at all levels and also for the social workers involved. As he states in the chapter abstract,

> Drawing on the shared experiences of the worker and client to build social inclusion and social resilience responsibly is a powerful way to deal with trauma. Thus, 'meeting in the middle' highlights shared ownership of the process of recovery, and promotes effectively coping with trauma brought about by natural disaster.

You will see how he brings this alive in his chapter with case examples from the Asian Tsunami and Sichuan Earthquake.

Part II wraps up with "Shared Reality as a Result of War and Terror," where Dr. Nuttman-Shwartz explains that

> in order to know how to create a therapeutic relationship, either in the acute or chronic phase of a war/terror event, social workers must be aware of both their own and their clients' direct exposure responses. They must have an understanding of the 'shared concerns' concept, which is based on the very real physical danger posed by the concrete traumatic threat..."

Her case example of balloons and kites exploding along the Gaza/Israel border is gripping in that it shows how something as innocent as a kite or balloon can cause terror and confusion, creating a shared traumatic reality that affects both therapist and client. Read the chapter to see how they contend with this and in so doing progress toward personal and profes-sional growth.

The third part of the book, "Battlegrounds of Shared Trauma: Social Work Modalities," focuses on how we work, stressing that shared trauma can occur regardless of the type of social work we practice. It explores three—psychotherapy, group work, and community organizing—which depict why disseminating knowledge of shared trauma and ways to work with it are essential. This underlines the importance of this book for social workers and again reminds us that no matter what we do as helping professionals, we are affected by shared communal trauma.

The first chapter in this part, "Finding Our Way Together: Relational Therapy during a Global Pandemic," focuses on work done online with clients during COVID-19. Drs. Barry and Singer present case examples of psychotherapy done virtually during the pandemic with trauma survivors who were re-triggered by COVID-19. They suggest utilizing a relational therapeutic model to help these clients find meaning and heal. They also demonstrate how much more important the therapeutic relationship became during this time, so that in one case "success was redefined as moments where both Lily and Johanna [the client and the therapist] emerged feeling metaphorically held and comforted" and that the work done in psychotherapy sessions needed to be sensitive to this redefinition of success so that the focuses and goals of therapy could flexibly change, with the therapist dancing with the client to the beat of the COVID-19 times.

"Shared Trauma in a Group Context" also focuses on work done during COVID-19. Drs. Knight and Gitterman "...identify social work practice skills that lessen the risk [during groups] that shared trauma (ST) will surface in the first place and assist the worker in managing its manifestations when they appear." They note that this "management" of shared trauma manifestations is more complicated with groups than with individuals and that, despite this, most of the work done on ST to date has been related to work with individuals, leading to a dearth of guidance for social workers leading groups during times like COVID-19. Therefore, inclusion of group work is such an important benefit for social workers navigating shared trauma in the field. Read this chapter for concrete tips on how to approach groups during times of mass trauma, while riding the tide of crisis and balancing the principles of both mutual aid and trauma-informed care.

"Shared Trauma and Community Organizing" explores another arena of social work which has been under-represented in discussions on shared trauma. What Dr. Ngoh Tiong Tan demonstrated in his chapter on natural disasters—that shared trauma can be addressed in communities as well as with individuals—is amplified by Mss. Aloziem and Williams' chapter on community organizing. Their work focuses on the "ugly and traumatic history [that] has bled into a strange present that includes two pandemics that disproportionately plague Black people—the COVID-19 pandemic and the ever-present pandemic that is systemic state-sanctioned racism and racial inequity." To them, the term shared trauma

acknowledges that we—as Black women, social workers and community organizers—have reactions to the trauma histories of communities
we serve, COVID-19 discussions and racial injustice in community
organizing spaces, and we also have to contend with our own independent reactions to the intersection of these two pandemics.

This chapter adds to the knowledge base on shared trauma, informing
community organizers, social workers, other practitioners and educators
alike—as it exposes and magnifies the ever present, corrosive reality of
systemic oppression.

The final chapter, "In Conclusion: Lessons Learned Going Forward," fin-
ishes up by summarizing the lessons learned, tips and tricks, and opportunities for growth presented in each chapter, while also outlining the ways in
which shared trauma remains an evolving concept that has grown over the
years, becoming more well-known and understood, and guiding numerous
practitioners. It is my hope that *Shared Mass Trauma in Social Work* will
contribute to this process in ways that will 1) inspire research and evidence-
based practice, and 2) help social workers cope with dangerous and difficult
circumstances confronting communities all over the world, building social
resilience as they work with their clients and progress together along the way.

Part I

Getting Started: Shared Trauma Perspectives

Chapter 1

Shared Trauma

An Essential Construct for Challenging Times

Carol Tosone and Shari Bloomberg

In the therapeutic relationship, social workers provide a holding container for clients to process their challenges. Despite their best attempts to maintain neutrality, therapists may be personally triggered by the nature of a client's situations or something they say. Such experiences are often labeled as countertransference or secondary traumatic responses; these reactions are unidirectional, solely impacting therapists. The terms transference, in general, and traumatic transference, in particular, are reserved for clients' responses in relation to their interactions with clinicians. However, when clients and therapists are exposed to the same external catastrophe, be it a natural disaster, war, terrorism, or global pandemic, it is termed shared trauma. This chapter will examine the development of the construct of shared trauma, providing an understanding of the history, the dual impact on the clinician, as well as a consideration of shared trauma in the practice context, and the growth that can occur through shared trauma, both in the personal and professional realms.

Freud, Shared Trauma, and War

Initially, trauma symptoms started with a label of hysteria, more often attributed to women. In Freud's 1893 paper, "On the Psychical Mechanism of Hysterical Phenomena," he observed that hysterics repressed memories of intense, painful experiences, accompanied by the isolation of feelings associated with those experiences which were preserved in a "strangulated state." Repression, according to Freud, comes into play when the feelings associated with the experience are too intense, and may be expressed as a hysterical symptom, symbolic of the repressed memory. The cure involved the catharsis of memories of and affects related to the original event which were brought into consciousness. *Studies on Hysteria*, co-authored with Joseph Breuer in 1895, was the culmination of his seduction theory, but was abandoned shortly afterwards (1897) and replaced by infantile sexuality. Observing the ubiquity of childhood trauma in his patients, Freud asserted that the

DOI: 10.4324/9781003176947-2

unconscious mind of the child was unable to distinguish fact from fiction. Hence, infantile sexuality was a universal experience.

Freud did acknowledge adult onset trauma in the soldiers returning from World War I, observing that they were suffering from "shell shock." The symptoms they exhibited—nightmares, traumatic memories, chronic anxiety—provided the foundation for our understanding of trauma today. In traumatic and war neuroses, Freud (1919) asserted that the ego is defending itself against an objective danger from without, whereas in the transference neuroses of peace, the ego is defending itself from the libido. In a subsequent paper, Freud (1920) returned to the subject of war neuroses treatment in a memorandum presented to the Austrian War Ministry. He maintained that psychoanalysis could best treat shell shock and related trauma responses, as these experiences resonated with childhood traumatic experiences. With its roots in childhood trauma, psychoanalysis could help to explain why some men experienced shell shock while others did not.

Significantly, shared trauma has a history based in war. At the time of World War I, Freud was too old to be drafted into the army, but his three sons served on the battlefront. One of his three sons, Martin, spent time as a prisoner of war. While many psychoanalysts were drafted into the army, Freud treated soldiers and veterans at home; his work with the individual transformed into a study of community and the collective unconscious. Over time, Freud endured senseless wars, escalating anti-Semitism, and the threat of Nazi domination. The calamities that directly impacted him and his family were all interpreted by Freud in terms of his model of psychological conflict (Schorer & Ellinger, 2010). Schmideberg, a psychoanalyst living through the London Blitz of World War II, wrote an article (1942) about civilian life at that time and briefly mentioned the same traumatic experience impacting both 1) her as a person and a professional, and 2) her patients. Schmideberg (1942) observed that while some residents left during the raids, the majority remained, adjusting to the new traumatic reality of threats to safety. Baum (2010), in citing Schmideberg's work, notes that the phenomenon was not named until the 1991 Gulf War. At that time, the terms *shared traumatic reality* and *shared reality* were introduced to describe the interaction of the clinician's experience in response to their clients' work in the context of a communal disaster. Dekel and Baum (2009), studying the ongoing threat of terrorist attacks in countries such as Israel, posit that the terms shared reality or shared traumatic reality better capture the "chronic nature" of a traumatogenic environment rather than a single terrorist event, such as 9/11.

The scope and breadth of shared traumatic experience go well beyond the parameters of war, terrorist attacks, or violent sectarian and political conflict. Natural disasters, such as hurricanes, tornadoes, or wildfires, result in social workers living and practicing in a surreal catastrophic environment, along with their clients. During natural disasters, clinicians are called upon to provide a holding environment for their clients, while possibly facing the same destruction of their homes and offices, and injuries to loved ones that their clients experience (Faust et al., 2008). In March of 2020, COVID-19 was recognized as a global pandemic, bringing the world to an abrupt stop. Many clinicians pivoted to working from home, using telehealth to maintain client connections while managing their own personal stressors. Still, other providers worked on the front lines, caring for their patients while addressing their health concerns privately. Currently, many areas of the world are facing a resurgence with a new variant, Delta, and the uncertainty of the last 18 months continues.

Impact of Working with Trauma on the Clinician: Existing Constructs

Despite the hope or the goal that social workers will be able to work with clients—whether virtually, in private practice, or in an agency setting—and manage the impact of their trauma experiences, there are often residual effects. Numerous terms describe these reactions, including traumatic countertransference, enactment, secondary traumatic stress, vicarious trauma, compassion fatigue, and burnout. These can be overlapping concepts, often used interchangeably and imprecisely. Differentiating between them is essential in understanding the clinician's experiences and how to address their needs best.

Let us first consider the constructs of enactment and traumatic countertransference. Theodore Jacobs initially conceptualized an *enactment* as the involvement of transference and countertransference between patient and therapist, often through nonverbal means. An enactment occurs when both the therapist and patient unconsciously "play out" psychic conflicts that must be worked out therapeutically (Severo et al., 2018). Herman (2015) noted that countertransference reactions may not always be traumatic, but if so, she referred to them as *traumatic countertransference*. She further proposed an example wherein a therapist dealing with an overwhelming traumatic client presentation might bend their therapeutic framework. Under the intense pressures of the patient's corresponding traumatic transference, the therapist may respond by advocating for the client, extending the length of the therapy session, or connecting with the patient at night or when away from the office. The therapist thereby takes on a rescuer role, disempowering the patient and sidestepping the reflection that needs to take place for both parties.

Secondary traumatic stress, vicarious trauma, compassion fatigue, and burnout are all potential conditions that the therapist may experience when working with traumatized clients. Figley (1995) described secondary traumatic stress as a secondary trauma that results from indirect exposure to trauma, such as hearing a client recount the specific traumatic event(s). He first wrote about a type of burnout or "secondary victimization" in the early 1980s when studying a phenomenon where therapists were exhibiting similar symptoms to the traumatized clients they were treating (Figley, 1983). Subsequently, it has been observed that secondary traumatic stress can occur suddenly, bringing about post-traumatic stress disorder (PTSD)-like symptoms, including anxiety, depression, avoidance, and hyperarousal, which a clinician may experience when listening to a client share a traumatic experience. Secondary trauma risk factors include neophyte clinicians with limited experience or clinicians with a personal trauma history (Creamer & Liddle, 2005).

Compassion fatigue has been described as the "cost of caring" for others in emotional pain (Figley, 2015). The use of the word compassion, Figley (2015) explained, refers to a feeling of deep sympathy and sorrow for another stricken by suffering or misfortune with a strong desire to alleviate the pain. The term had already been used for frontline workers, including nurses and emergency personnel, to describe the type of burnout experienced in the line of duty. It occurs when the caregiver does not take the time to recharge and engage in self-care. Compassion fatigue affects therapists on three levels; cognitively, they may struggle with concentration, negativity, and harmful thoughts; emotionally, with feelings of powerlessness, guilt, or rage; and behaviorally with nightmares, hypervigilance, and expressions of frustration and impatience (Figley, 2015). Therapists suffering from compassion fatigue may blame the victim (client) or avoid the work, overwhelmed by the suffering, discomfort, and hardship. Sometimes practitioners blame themselves for not being "enough," damaging their self-esteem and self-image. Compassion fatigue can also cause somatic distress, including headaches, stomachaches, difficulties with sleep, and physical and emotional exhaustion (Berzoff & Kita, 2010). As with secondary traumatic stress, those with insecure attachments or a history of traumatic life events are more susceptible to compassion fatigue (Racanelli, 2005; Creamer & Liddle, 2005). Examples of compassion fatigue are evident in frontline workers, and were especially so during the early days of the COVID-19 pandemic; exhausted hospital staff, with limited personal protective equipment, worked around the clock caring for the sickest patients. Those who believe that the world is unsafe and feel helpless to make a change may also suffer from vicarious trauma.

Vicarious trauma is defined as the "permanent transformation in the inner experience of the therapist that comes about as a result of empathic engagement with clients' trauma material" (Pearlman & Saakvitne, 1995, p. 31). This occurs when clinicians absorb clients' traumatic and difficult images and emotions, and slowly include them within their own memory recollection (McCann & Pearlman, 1990). This transformation alters or shifts the way the therapist views the world, impacting five key areas: trust, safety, control, esteem, and intimacy. Vicarious trauma is cumulative, building over time as the therapist develops an empathetic engagement with clients as they process traumatic experiences. Yet, the onset of symptoms can be sudden and abrupt with the clinician's beliefs about the world profoundly changed by being repeatedly exposed to layers of traumatic material. Social workers experiencing vicarious trauma react to ongoing client traumatic experiences, as well as the traumatized history of a traumatized population (Trippany et al., 2004).

Burnout is a defensive response to prolonged occupational and/or work-related interpersonal situations, resulting in psychological pain (Jenkins & Baird, 2002). It was first coined in the mid-1970s by Herbert Freudenberger, an American psychologist, after observing the volunteer staff at a free clinic for those with drug addictions. He noted the volunteers presented as exhausted and depressed, with notable physical symptoms (Freudenberger, 1974). Leiter and Maslach (1988) outline a gradual, pathological process whereby symptoms of emotional exhaustion can develop due to the psychological strain of working with multiple stressors. They included cynicism, boredom, loss of compassion, erosion of idealism, and a reduced sense of professional accomplishment and commitment as core features of burnout. Today we understand burnout as the physical and emotional deterioration that workers encounter through low job satisfaction, often leaving them feeling overwhelmed and powerless at work. Unlike the other terms, burnout does not suggest that our worldview has been harmed or that we cannot maintain compassion for others. Burnout is often cited as a reason for one leaving mental health and health care professions. The immediate antidote to burnout can often be a change in the workplace.

Understanding Shared Trauma

Shared trauma differs from the constructs above in describing the collective experience of the social worker and the client living and/or working in the same community. Unlike secondary traumatic phenomena, the practitioner and client face exposure to the same externally traumatic and threatening experiences (Nuttman-Shwartz, 2016; Tosone, 2012, 2021). This speaks to the dual nature of the trauma, in both the clinician's personal and professional lives. The term *shared traumatic reality* refers to this primary and secondary exposure to trauma. Sometimes it is of a chronic nature; that is, the environment is traumatological, as in regions where terrorism is frequent and ongoing. A notable example includes Northern Ireland practitioners exposed to the Troubles, a 30-year period of sectarian violence. (Baum, 2013; Dekel & Baum, 2009; Dekel et al., 2016; Tosone et al., 2012). Like vicarious trauma, shared trauma can cause permanent alterations in the clinician's existing mental schema and worldview. Therefore, these therapists are potentially more susceptible to post-traumatic stress, blurred professional and personal boundaries, and increased self-disclosure.

Whether it be a violent conflict, natural disaster, or a worldwide pandemic, both the social worker and the client face the same challenges and insecurities, including concern for loved ones, possible loss of home or office, and potential health issues. A comprehensive experience, shared trauma is the affective behavioral, cognitive, spiritual, and multimodal responses of practitioners exposed to the same collective trauma as their clients. However, it is essential to note that shared trauma does not imply that the clinician's response will be identical to the client's. Clinicians and clients can be variably impacted by the same simultaneous events (Tosone, 2012).

Shared traumatic experiences often blur boundaries and upend routines, changing the physical parameters for therapeutic work. The shift in the established pattern allows the social worker and client to have a common experience. The more recent shared trauma of COVID-19 necessitated shifting to a telehealth platform. Clinicians in areas with hurricanes or other natural disasters often cannot see clients in their office space due to transportation constraints or damage to the physical locations. Boulanger (2013) described clinical office space as "the physical container, a treatment, the familiar place where patients find sanctuary... free from the constraints of reality" (p. 35). Bloomberg (2021) noted that as a therapist using telehealth from home, "the clients saw the inside of my home as I saw the inside of theirs. The doorbell would ring, a child or pet would join the session, or the next-door neighbor would loudly be mowing their lawn" (p. 73). Thus the new normal limited the ability to maintain a safe, controlled therapy environment.

In times of trauma, not only are physical boundaries blurred, but people loosen their physical appearance standards. During the recent pandemic, clients who usually dressed professionally or always wore makeup no longer did so, taking a more casual stance. Clients would have their therapy sessions while sitting on their beds, hiding in their bathrooms, or sitting in the car for privacy (Bloomberg, 2021). This loosening of personal boundaries encouraged clients to become more familiar with the clinician. Clients would often inquire as to the well-being of the therapist and the therapist's family. In this manner, the shared trauma created a new therapeutic intimacy. As Tosone (2011) stated, "I found myself engaging on a deeper level and revealing more than usual" (p. 26). Self-disclosure and mutual discussion of the traumatic event were more likely and acceptable in these unique situations (Bauwens & Tosone, 2010). While such a stance can be positive, it is also critical that the motivation for sharing remains focused on the client's best interest rather than the clinician's personal need (Tosone et al., 2012).

The shared trauma that clinicians experience has additional effects. Social workers may find they are immersing themselves in their work as a means of coping with the collective trauma, such as clinicians who volunteered to do crisis counseling post-9/11. Workday boundaries may also become pervious. During the COVID-19 pandemic, for instance, clinicians working from home reported challenges setting limits on their workdays, often scheduling clients at their convenience. This flexibility inhibited the clinician's ability for self-care. Other therapists reported being preoccupied with their struggles in home-schooling children or worrying about the health of loved ones. Post-9/11, Tosone et al. (2003) found that with some clinicians, the high degree of emotion and preoccupation with their own feelings made it challenging to assist others. She further noted that these feelings resulted in desensitization toward patients, causing a lack of empathy, less tolerance, and even anger at patients' expressions of rage and anxiety, leading them to question their future in the profession.

Shared Trauma in Context

Shared trauma can occur in a variety of practice settings and configurations. Those in private practice may have a different experience than those working within an agency context. Social workers who also supervise staff or students may have a different experience than those who do not serve as supervisors. Even within the same organizational structure, clinicians working on the front line of the COVID-19 pandemic will likely have a different experience from those providing administrative support or supervision off-site, the latter workers not needing to interact directly with COVID patients or their families.

For private practitioners, there can be a sense of isolation as they navigate the traumatic experience with patients, but perhaps without the benefit of debriefing with nearby colleagues. Faust et al. (2008) reflected vividly on their experience of returning home to New Orleans post-Hurricane Katrina and finding destroyed homes, closed practice locations, and displaced patients. Others returned to "wade through the rubble of their ravished communities and only the disrepair of their homes and offices" (Bauwens & Tosone, 2014, p. 209). During the most recent pandemic, those in private practice were left to suddenly pivot to a new normal, and determine how to support their clients while moving to a virtual platform.

While clinicians working in agencies benefit from shared responsibility, they also have the pressure of meeting the needs of the agency funders and those that the agency serves. In times of crisis, the demand for mental health services rises, straining the existing services and personnel. As clinicians address their own experiences in the trauma, they might not be available to meet the growing demand, nor have the agency support to pursue necessary self-care practices. During Hurricane Sandy and the recent COVID pandemic, New Jersey and New York mental health agencies have anecdotally reported large waiting lists as people seek services. Additionally, agencies are hierarchical structures. If a supervisor is facing a challenging personal experience, they may not be available to provide the required supervision for their supervisee. If a supervisor and a supervisee had a strenuous relationship pre-pandemic, the additional traumatic stress of the crisis will put undue pressure on the fragile relationship. Additionally, supervisors have the added responsibility of looking out for their own clients and staff, and the clients of those they supervise. Agencies must also ensure that their funders are content with their crisis response and fulfill the needs outlined in the grants awarded.

Although the challenges described above sound daunting, positive realizations can come out of the shared trauma experience; processing the trauma with the client can help social workers achieve a sense of universality of experience, leading to increased self-disclosure and enhanced intimacy in the therapeutic relationship. Maintaining a work schedule can also give structure and routine in a time of chaos. Graduate social work students reported that working for an agency and attending their field placement provided optimism, fostered determination, and even offered relief in a time of shared trauma (Tosone et al., 2003).

Holding Environments: Personal and Professional

Supervisors, agency-based administrators, colleagues, and professional organizations all play an essential role in providing professional holding environments to help clinicians feel less isolated and provide reinforcement. During a time of shared trauma, it is critical that agencies and social work clinical programs demonstrate flexibility in managing work assignments and caseloads, providing material supplies as needed (e.g., masks, glove cleaning products), and allowing workers to have the time necessary to address their personal situations. Clinicians reported disappointment with agencies and supervisory personnel for not attending to the mental health needs of their staff during the COVID-19 pandemic. Professional organizations were also found to be lacking in their responses to the pandemic, in terms of providing adequate trauma training and mental health resources for their members (Tosone & Cohen-Serrins, 2021). As was found with New Orleans social workers practicing in a post-Hurricane Katrina environment, additional training, trauma education, and other forms of support are critical during a shared traumatic experience (Tosone et al., 2014).

Reactions to a traumatic experience are highly personal. As stated by Ursano et al. (1994), "The psychological responses of individuals to trauma vary greatly. The meaning of any traumatic event is a complex interaction of the event itself and the individual's past, present, and expected future, as well as biological givens and social context" (p. 45). Moreover, clinicians react uniquely to a shared traumatic experience based on their personal connections to the event. Clinicians living and working in New York City will have had a different experience with 9/11 than those in other parts of the country. Proximity to the collective disaster was positively correlated with compassion fatigue and secondary traumatic stress among New York City social workers (Boscrino et al., 2004). Interestingly, unlike other collective traumatic events, the COVID pandemic was not limited to any particular region or group, and could be characterized as a global shared trauma.

While no one was immune to the impact of COVID-19, many individuals in Black and Brown communities faced the additional trauma of not having access to resources. This reality is not unique to the trauma of COVID as it has appeared throughout traumatic historical events such as Hurricane Katrina. Together with the ongoing racial tensions between marginalized communities and law enforcement, the disparity has created a separate shared trauma that clinicians who identify as part of these communities also must contend with and address (Audate, 2021; Edwards, 2021; Franco, 2021; James, 2021; Morgan-Mullane, 2021). We support the entire mental health community by looking at the individual and their specific experiences and needs. The following case example illustrates the overlapping secondary traumatic stress constructs, and contrasts them with the unique aspects of shared trauma.

The Constructs in Context: A Case Illustration

Penny has been working in the field as a licensed clinical social worker for the past five years. She reports struggling with one client in particular, an 82-year-old Jewish cisgender woman living alone in New York City. The client, Rachael, has recounted a history filled with multiple traumatic events, both personal and collective. During the Holocaust, Rachael was a child in hiding. She struggled throughout her childhood to bond with her mother, who remained cold, aloof, and deeply scarred by her Holocaust experience. Rachael later found herself in a physically abusive and loveless marriage, which ended with the death of her husband 15 years prior. The marriage bore two daughters, both of whom Rachael has been estranged from since her husband's death.

Penny is aware the client, Rachael, is lonely, isolated, and rarely leaves her apartment since the onset of the COVID-19 pandemic. While working via telehealth, Rachael has been commenting on Penny's home environment, and inquiring about Penny's marital status and if she has children. Penny knows she struggles with a preoccupation with the client's situation, challenges in boundary setting, and an overall sense of increased anxiety for herself and her family as a result of the pandemic. Penny finds it difficult to listen to her client's anxiety about contracting COVID, and tends to "space out" when that is the focus of their discussion. Penny admits that she feels sorry for the client, and due to the flexible nature of telehealth, she has more leeway in terms of setting and maintaining boundaries with her client. Penny has excused her client, who has slept through their morning appointments several times and allowed Rachael to reschedule rather than holding her financially accountable for the missed session. These actions, the result of Penny's countertransference, impact the therapeutic work.

Penny also questions if she is experiencing secondary traumatic stress. As she hears the client's recitation of her traumatic experiences, Penny notes feelings of increasing anxiety and hyperarousal, and finds herself recounting Rachael's graphic descriptions of her physical abuse at the hands of her husband. Penny finds herself grateful when Rachael forgets a session, as she often wants to avoid their sessions. Processing her experience with a supervisor and colleagues, Penny has a better understanding of secondary traumatic stress, and feels supported to continue her work with Rachael.

Since the start of the pandemic, Penny has found herself working more hours and having an increased, more difficult caseload. Rachael is just one example of her many difficult cases. Penny reports feeling overwhelmed, unable to keep up with paperwork, and with diminished time for family. Penny has been less mindful of boundaries, often finding herself speaking to clients in the evenings or on weekends as the lines between work and personal time have blurred due to working from home.

Penny has had changes to her self-care routines as well. No longer able to attend the gym, she has found a sharp decrease in her level of physical activity. Due to the pandemic, she has spent less time with friends and no time on relaxing activities. Losing her avenues for self-care while extending herself professionally has left her feeling exhausted, irritable, and struggling to find a balance between work and her personal life. Although her supervisor has been sympathetic to Penny's situation, the supervisor also reports similar work issues and is helpless to reduce the number of assigned cases. The supervisor comments that they are both struggling with compassion fatigue, but yet remain committed to the work.

Penny shares with her supervisor that she feels "worn down" by Rachael's hopeless and futile worldview, now exacerbated by her forced isolation and loneliness due to COVID. In return, Penny, who specializes in domestic violence, has noticed her own feelings of mistrust of others and a lack of control over life occurrences. Penny is questioning her view of the world as a safe place. She finds herself unable to stop thinking about the artwork and writings the client has shared, and thinks about the images long after the session has concluded. Penny is finding that Rachael's insights about the world and relationships resonate with her own experience. From this perspective, Penny's experience could be described as vicarious traumatization.

However, it is not just her experiences with the client or the pandemic impacting Penny, as she has been feeling dissatisfaction with her workplace. The onboarding of a new executive director, together with a change in the administration, has left many in the agency feeling unsupported and unappreciated. Seeking support from her immediate supervisor regarding the issues of secondary trauma and vicarious trauma presents its own challenges as described above. Penny's supervisor has a parallel experience in terms of feeling "under water" without adequate support or resources from administration. These feelings of mistrust have caused an agency-wide low level of morale, a reduced commitment to the work and the agency, and an overall sense of dissatisfaction. To address the burnout Penny is experiencing, she is looking for a different position where she feels supported and professionally nurtured.

In working with Rachael, Penny operated as part of an agency. The agency provided strict rules and boundaries about the therapeutic relationship. Guidance about charging for missed sessions and not communicating via email or text was part of the enforced agency policies. Had Penny worked in private practice, especially within the realm of the shared trauma of COVID-19, she would have had more flexibility about where and when to enforce the boundaries. Seeking professional guidance and supervision among her peers or in private supervision would aid Penny in navigating the difficult terrain.

How does the shared trauma experience between Penny and her client shape the therapeutic relationship? The lockdown due to the COVID-19 pandemic impacted both Penny and her client in similar ways. They shared the same sense of uncertainty or anticipatory anxiety regarding the future and the concerns about contracting COVID-19, and Penny found herself triggered by her client's articulation of her fears. Since moving to telehealth, there was a loosening of the boundaries regarding appointment times and self-disclosure. Responding to the client's concerns, Penny has been forthright in disclosing her health status and how COVID-19 has impacted her and her family.

Penny and her client have an additional layer of shared trauma. As Penny strongly identifies with her Jewish faith, the client's experience during the Holocaust resonates with Penny as she grew up in the shadow of the genocide. This type of collective trauma, much like other forms of large-scale devastating events, impacts a community or society of people. Still, unlike those experiencing the trauma simultaneously, this type of collective trauma experience also has historical, cultural, and transgenerational components (Hirschberger, 2018).

Beyond Trauma: Professional Post-Traumatic Growth and Shared Resilience

Penny's case demonstrates the complexities of working in a shared traumatic reality, underscoring the need for social workers to gain both awareness of this phenomenon and tools that enable working effectively within its framework. The good news is that in addition to the negative aspects of trauma work described in Penny's work with her client, there are opportunities for positive growth from a personal or collective trauma.

Post-traumatic growth is defined as a "positive psychological change experienced from the struggle with highly challenging circumstances" (Tedeschi & Calhoun, 2004, p. 1). Tedeschi and Calhoun (1996) identified five areas that result in growth after a trauma: 1) new possibilities, 2) relating to others, 3) personal strength, 4) appreciation for life, and 5) spiritual change. Clinicians working with trauma survivors reported positive consequences such as increased self-confidence, independence, resilience, emotional expressiveness, sensitivity, compassion, and deepened spirituality (Nuttman-Shwartz, 2014). Bauwens and Tosone (2010), in their study of Manhattan clinicians post-9/11, found that participants attributed the trauma of 9/11 as the impetus for enhancing self-care and connection, changing clinical modalities, forging new skills, and enhancing compassion and connection in the therapeutic relationship. They define these positive changes as *professional post-traumatic growth*. One experienced trauma-focused clinician shared anecdotally that working remotely through the COVID pandemic challenged her to use different skills and strengths. The experience also gave her the perspective to realize that working in person was unnecessary, and she was happier working remotely. She chose to leave and pursue a different position allowing her to work on a full-time telehealth platform. Preliminary results from the COVID-19 quality of professional practice survey are consistent with anecdotal accounts of professional post-traumatic growth. Respondents largely reported satisfaction with a telehealth delivery of service, and some changed from agency-based work to private practice to enhance their autonomy over client care (Tosone & Cohen-Serrins, 2021).

Shared trauma also needs to be understood in the context of shared resilience. In shared resilience, clinicians derive positive experiences from exposure to traumatic events both directly and through their work with clients: the term suggests that a reciprocal mutual aid can occur between client and clinician. Shared resilience in traumatic reality allows the therapist to have increased bonding, empathy, and compassion due to the shared experience of "being in the same boat" (Nuttman-Shwartz, 2014). In their study of clinicians post-9/11, Tosone et al. (2011) noted that respondents had a more robust ability and urgency to care for themselves in the work setting, and a renewed appreciation for the profession.

How is shared resilience accomplished? Mechanisms meant to create a work/life balance are a necessity. The clinician must engage in forms of self-care to ensure they are allowing themselves time to process and renew. Social and professional support can also make a significant contribution. Professional and educational organizations, colleagues, and personal help from family and friends can influence work quality and post-traumatic experience (Tosone et al., 2012).

The goal of this chapter was to explore the trauma that clinicians can experience due to their work, and the shared trauma that occurs due to exposure to collective disasters. The trauma that a client brings into a room can impact the clinician in many ways, either negatively, positively, or a combination. Social workers must be familiar with these concepts and have the self-awareness to recognize the challenges they create. Only through addressing these difficulties and seeking the appropriate support can we provide our clients with the best treatment possible.

References

Audate, T. (2021). The pandemic within the pandemic of 2020: A spiritual perspective. In C. Tosone (Ed.), *Shared trauma, shared resilience during a pandemic: Social work in the time of COVID-19* (pp. 271–280). Springer Nature.

Baum, N. (2010). Shared traumatic reality in communal disasters: Toward a conceptualization. *Psychotherapy: Theory, Research, Practice, Training*, 47(2), 249–259. https://doi.org/10.1037/a0019784.

Baum, N. (2013). Professionals' double exposure in the shared traumatic reality of wartime: Contributions to professional growth and stress. *British Journal of Social Work*, 44(8), 2113–2134. https://doi.org/10.1093/bjsw/bct085.

Bauwens, J., & Tosone, C. (2010). Professional posttraumatic growth after a shared traumatic experience: Manhattan clinicians' perspectives on post-9/11 practice. *Journal of Loss and Trauma*, 15(6), 498–517. https://doi.org/10.1080/15325024.2010.519267.

Bauwens, J., & Tosone, C. (2014). Post-traumatic growth following Hurricane Katrina: The influence of clinicians' trauma histories and primary and secondary traumatic stress. *Traumatology*, 20(3), 209–218. https://doi.org/10.1037/h0099851.

Berzoff, J., & Kita, E. (2010). Compassion fatigue and countertransference: Two different concepts. *Clinical Social Work Journal*, 38(3), 341–349. https://doi.org/10.1007/s10615-010-0271-8.

Bloomberg, S. (2021). Reflections on Covid-19, shared trauma and domestic violence. In C. Tosone (Ed.), *Shared trauma, shared resilience during a pandemic: Social work in the time of COVID-19* (pp. 69–78). Springer Nature.

Boscrino, J. A., Figley, C. R., & Adams, R. E. (2004). Compassion fatigue following the September 11 terrorist attacks: A study of secondary trauma among New York City social workers. *International Journal of Emergency Mental Health*, 62, 57–66.

Boulanger, G. (2013). Fearful symmetry: Shared trauma in New Orleans after Hurricane Katrina. *Psychoanalytic Dialogues*, 23(1), 31–44. https://doi.org/10.1080/10481885.2013.752700.

Breuer, J., & Freud, S. (1956). On the psychical mechanism of hysterical phenomena (1893). *The International Journal of Psychoanalysis*, 37, 8–13.

Calderon-Abbo, J. (2008). The long road home: Rebuilding public inpatient psychiatric services in post-Katrina New Orleans. *Psychiatric Services*, 59(3), 304–309. https://doi.org/10.1176/ps.2008.59.3.304.

Creamer, T. L., & Liddle, B. J. (2005). Secondary traumatic stress among disaster mental health workers responding to the September 11 attacks. *Journal of Traumatic Stress*, 18(1), 89–96. https://doi.org/10.1002/jts.20008.

Dekel, R., & Baum, N. (2009). Intervention in a shared traumatic reality: A new challenge for social workers. *British Journal of Social Work*, 40(6), 1927–1944. https://doi.org/10.1093/bjsw/bcp137.

Dekel, R., Nuttman-Shwartz, O., & Lavi, T. (2016). Shared traumatic reality and boundary theory: How mental health professionals cope with the home/work conflict during continuous security threats. *Journal of Couple & Relationship Therapy*, 15(2), 121–134. https://doi.org/10.1080/15332691.2015.1068251.

Dekel, S., Hankin, I. T., Pratt, J. A., Hackler, D. R., & Lanman, O. N. (2015). Post-traumatic growth in trauma recollections of 9/11 survivors: A narrative approach. *Journal of Loss and Trauma*, 21(4), 315–324. https://doi.org/10.1080/15325024.2015.1108791.

Edwards, R. (2021). An intimate portrait of shared trauma amid COVID-19 and racial unrest between a Black cisgender femme sex worker and her Black cisgender femme therapist. In C. Tosone (Ed.), *Shared trauma, shared resilience during a pandemic: Social work in the time of COVID-19* (pp. 303–312). Springer Nature.

Faust, D. S., Black, F. W., Abrahams, J. P., Warner, M. S., & Bellando, B. J. (2008). After the storm: Katrina's impact on psychological practice in New Orleans. *Professional Psychology: Research and Practice*, 39(1), 1–6. https://doi.org/10.1037/0735-7028.39.1.1.

Figley, C. R. (1983). Catastrophe: An overview of family reactions. In C. R. Figley & H. I. McCubbin (Eds.), *Stress and the family*: Vol. 2. *Coping with catastrophe* (pp. 3–20). Brunner/Mazel.

Figley, C. R. (Ed.). (1995). *Compassion fatigue: Coping with secondary traumatic stress disorder in those who treat the traumatized*. Brunner/Mazel.

Figley, C. R. (2015). *Treating compassion fatigue*. Routledge.

Franco, D. (2021). COVID-19 as post-migration stress: Exploring the impact of a pandemic on Latinx transgender individuals in immigration detention. In C. Tosone (Ed.), *Shared trauma, shared resilience during a pandemic: Social work in the time of COVID-19* (pp. 313–321). Springer Nature.

Freud, S. (1919). *Introduction to Psycho-Analysis & the War Neuroses*. The Standard Edition of the Complete Psychological Works of Sigmund Freud, 17: 205–216.

Freud, S. (1920). *Addendum to Introduction to Psycho-Analysis & the War Neuroses*. The Standard Edition of the Complete Psychological Works of Sigmund Freud, 17: 277–286.

Freud, S. (1971). On the psychical mechanism of hysterical phenomena: A lecture (1893). PsycEXTRA Dataset. https://doi.org/10.1037/e417472005-086.

Freud, S., & Breuer, J. (1971). Studies on hysteria (1893–1895). Chapter I. On the psychical mechanism of hysterical phenomena: Preliminary communication (1893) (Breuer and Freud). PsycEXTRA Dataset. https://doi.org/10.1037/e417472005-070.

Freudenberger, H. J. (1974). Staff burn-out. *Journal of Social Issues*, 30(1), 159–165. https://doi.org/10.1111/j.1540-4560.1974.tb00706.x.

Herman, J. L. (2015). *Trauma and recovery: The aftermath of violence, from domestic abuse to political terror*. Basic Books.

Hirschberger, G. (2018). Collective trauma and the social construction of meaning. *Frontiers in Psychology*, 9. https://doi.org/10.3389/fpsyg.2018.01441.

Jacobs, T. J. (1986). On countertransference enactments. *Journal of the American Psychoanalytic Association*, 34(2): 289–307.

James, K. J. (2021). Black lives, mass incarceration, and the perpetuity of trauma in the era of COVID-19: The road to abolition social work. In C. Tosone (Ed.), *Shared trauma, shared resilience during a pandemic: Social work in the time of COVID-19* (pp. 281–290). Springer Nature.

Jenkins, S. R., & Baird, S. (2002). Secondary traumatic stress and vicarious trauma: A validational study. *Journal of Traumatic Stress*, 15(5), 423–432. https://doi.org/10.1023/a:1020193526843.

Leiter, M. P., & Maslach, C. (1988). The impact of interpersonal environment on burnout and organizational commitment. *Journal of Organizational Behavior*, 9, 297–308.

McCann, I. L., & Pearlman, L. A. (1990). Vicarious traumatization: A framework for understanding the psychological effects of working with victims. *Journal of Traumatic Stress*, 3(1), 131–149.

Morgan-Mullane, A. (2021). COVID-19 and the injustice system: Reshaping clinical practice for children and families impacted by hyper-incarceration. In C. Tosone (Ed.), *Shared trauma, shared resilience during a pandemic: Social work in the time of COVID-19* (pp. 291–302). Springer Nature.

Nuttman-Shwartz, O. (2014). Shared resilience in a traumatic reality. *Trauma, Violence, & Abuse*, 16(4), 466–475. https://doi.org/10.1177/1524838014557287.

Nuttman-Shwartz, O. (2016). Research in a shared traumatic reality: Researchers in a disaster context. *Journal of Loss and Trauma*, 21(3), 179–191. https://doi.org/10.1080/15325024.2015.1084856.

Pearlman, L. A., & Saakvitne, K. W. (1995). *Trauma and the therapist: Countertransference and vicarious traumatization in psychotherapy with incest survivors*. Norton.

Racanelli, C. (2005). Attachment and compassion fatigue among American and Israeli mental health clinicians working with traumatized victims of terrorism. *International Journal of Emergency Mental Health*, 7(2), 115–124.

Schmideberg, M. (1942). Some observations on individual reactions to air raids. *International Journal of Psychoanalysis*, 23, 146–176.

Schorer, J., & Ellinger, C. (2010, July 23). *Sigmund Freud: Conflict & Culture From the Individual to Society*. Library of Congress. www.loc.gov/exhibits/freud/freud03a.html.

Severo, C. T., Laskoski, P. B., Teche, S. P., Bassols, A. M., Saldanha, R. F., Wellausen, R. S., Rodrigues Wageck, A. A., Costa, C. P., Rebouças, D. B., Padoan, C. S., Barros, A. J., Nunes, M. L., & Eizirik, C. L. (2018). Conceptual and technical aspects of psychoanalytic enactment: A systematic review. *British Journal of Psychotherapy*, 34(4), 643–666. https://doi.org/10.1111/bjp.12386.

Tedeschi, R. G., & Calhoun, L. G. (1996). The posttraumatic growth inventory: Measuring the positive legacy of trauma. *Journal of Traumatic Stress*, 9(3), 455–472. https://doi.org/10.1002/jts.2490090305.

Tedeschi, R. G., & Calhoun, L. G. (2004). Post-traumatic growth: Conceptual foundations and empirical evidence. *Psychological Inquiry*, 15(1), 1–18. https://doi.org/10.1207/s15327965pli1501_01.

Tosone, C. (2006). Therapeutic intimacy: A post-9/11 perspective. *Smith College Studies in Social Work*, 76(4), 89–98.

Tosone, C. (2011). The legacy of September 11: Shared trauma, therapeutic intimacy, and professional post-traumatic growth. *Traumatology*, 17(3), 25–29. doi:10.1177/1534765611421963.

Tosone, C. (2012). Shared trauma. In C. Figley (Ed.), *Encyclopedia of Trauma*. Sage Publishers.

Tosone, C. (2021). Introduction. In C. Tosone (Ed.), *Shared trauma, shared resilience during a pandemic: Social work in the time of COVID-19* (pp. 1–14). Springer Nature.

Tosone, C., & Cohen-Serrins, J. (2021). *COVID-19 quality of professional practice survey*. Unpublished research findings.

Tosone, C., Lee, M., Bialkin, L., Martinez, A., Campbell, M., Martinez, M. M., Charters, M., Milich, J., Gieri, K., Riofrio, A., Gross, S., Rosenblatt, L., Grounds, C., Sandler, J., Johnson, K., Scali, M., Kitson, D., Spiro, M., Lanzo, S., & Stefan, A. (2003). Shared trauma. *Psychoanalytic Social Work*, 10(1), 57–77. https://doi.org/10.1300/j032v10n01_06.

Tosone, C., Nuttman-Shwartz, O., & Stephens, T. (2012). Shared trauma: When the professional is personal. *Clinical Social Work Journal*, 40(2), 231–239. https://doi.org/10.1007/s10615-012-0395-0.

Tosone, C., McTighe, J. P., & Bauwens, J. (2014). Shared traumatic stress among social workers in the aftermath of Hurricane Katrina. *British Journal of Social Work*, 45(4), 1313–1329. https://doi.org/10.1093/bjsw/bct194.

Trippany, R. L., Kress, V. E., & Wilcoxon, S. A. (2004). Preventing vicarious trauma: What counselors should know when working with trauma survivors. *Journal of Counseling & Development*, 82(1), 31–37. https://doi.org/10.1002/j.1556-6678.2004.tb00283.x.

Ursano, R. J., McCaughey, B. G., & Fullerton, C. S. (Eds.). (1994). *Individual and community responses to trauma and disaster: The structure of human chaos*. Cambridge University Press. https://doi.org/10.1017/CBO9780511570162.

An Investigation of Research on Shared Trauma

Carol Tosone and Julian Cohen-Serrins

Trauma occupies an enormous space within the human service sector, and especially among those in healthcare and social service occupations. Traumatic experiences can take on physical and psychosocial forms, can be deeply subjective (Boals, 2018) and collectively felt across generations (Lev-Wiesel, 2007). However, what is consistent about trauma is that it can be destructive if left unaddressed and is nuanced enough that it requires specified approaches to remedy (van der Ham et al., 2021; Karatzias et al., 2019). This chapter will focus on a type of trauma specific to clinicians and others providing direct services. Often referred to as shared trauma or shared traumatic reality, this genre of trauma can be understood as the mutual exposure to a collective traumatic event by both a clinician and client (Tosone, 2011).

Typically, shared trauma takes the form of large-scale events that affect entire geographic areas, such as natural disasters, human-made disasters, terrorist attacks, or wars. Global exposure to COVID-19 suggests that shared trauma is experienced by social workers and other helping professionals working with various client populations. Shared trauma captures a unique dynamic and scenario that often runs counter to the traditional distinctions of both trauma and its role in clinical work. This may explain why shared trauma was formulated and operationalized so much later than other types of traumas, and although there is room to infer its existence in the DSM-5 (APA, 2013), it is not explicitly named or defined. However, addressing this type of trauma has the potential to alleviate some of the suffering that clinicians face throughout these events.

Shared trauma differs from vicarious or secondary trauma, which is defined as when the communication of a client's traumatic experience has a traumatic effect on the clinician (Tosone et al., 2012; Tosone, 2011). The critical elements of this distinction lie in the nature and timing in which a traumatic event affects the client and clinician. When conceptualizing secondary or vicarious trauma, the client has already experienced a traumatic event, and is relaying their lived experience to the clinician. This type of trauma is dependent upon the clinician not having directly

DOI: 10.4324/9781003176947-3

experienced what their client is relaying to them, but still having a subjective traumatic reaction within themselves. Shared trauma, on the other hand, relies on the same collective traumatic event being experienced by both the client and clinician. The traumatic event has a dual effect on the clinician by impacting both their professional and personal lives. This creates a complex situation where the clinician must remain professionally capable of supporting their traumatized client, while also coping with their own, personal experience of that trauma.

Even with the nuances that define shared trauma, it is a phenomenon that has the potential to occur in any location and during any large-scale traumatic event in the modern era. While the true frequency of shared trauma is nearly impossible to accurately measure, identical terms for shared trauma have been developed and studied in scholarly research. This suggests that even if defined by another term, shared trauma frequently occurs in large-scale traumatic events around the world. A survey of scholarly literature suggests that the term shared trauma was introduced and adopted in the United States following 9/11 (Saakvitne, 2002; Altman & Davies, 2002; Tosone et al., 2003), and later used in research pertaining to Hurricane Katrina (Boulanger, 2013; Tosone et al., 2015) and the Troubles in Northern Ireland (Campbell et al., 2021; Duffy et al., 2019). However, in Israel, an area that has been in perpetual conflict since its inception, shared trauma has been called double exposure, shared traumatic reality, and shared reality (Baum, 2010; Baum, 2012; Baum, 2014). Each of these terms is synonymous with shared trauma, and each demonstrates that shared trauma infiltrates traditional boundaries between personal and professional life, and supplants a new reality where clinicians must grapple with novel symptomology in their clients, and within themselves. These alternate terms also emphasize that shared trauma is a frequent enough occurrence to warrant further study, and to review the circumstances in which this phenomenon has been researched thus far.

Finally, through an informed and careful review of the literature, there is evidence to suggest that because the term shared trauma is not yet fully established among scholars and practitioners, research on shared trauma has been undertaken by existing terms such as compassion fatigue (Boscarino et al., 2004; Tosone et al., 2010) or vicarious trauma (Eidelson et al., 2003). For example, because vicarious trauma has a bit more notoriety, and is also an occupationally based type of trauma (McCann & Pearlman, 1990), if researchers were to only examine the transfer of a client's trauma to a clinician and not identify the causal traumatic event as either personal or collective, then it would be easy to miss that the researchers are discussing shared trauma. Additionally, it would be beneficial for a meta-analysis to be conducted to formulate how many articles under the name of other types of trauma actually fall under the rubric of shared trauma.

A prime example of shared trauma remaining erroneously unidentified in research can be shown in a study conducted in former Yugoslavia, where during a violent and multifactional civil war, researchers examined the role of music therapy for therapists who provided clinical services during the war (Harris, 2016). Shared trauma was not named in the study and therefore including it among the literature on the topic would be improper. However, when examined in the context of shared trauma, this study was exploring the ways therapists coped with a shared traumatic event and focused on how the duality of that event affected both their professional and personal lives simultaneously. This is the definition of shared trauma and has been common in every study on the topic. It is therefore valid to consider that, if this study had been conducted by researchers familiar with shared trauma, it may have been denoted as such and directly explored in the study.

With the onset of the global COVID-19 pandemic, a deeper exploration of shared trauma has never been more warranted. Likely every active clinician has been affected in some way by this pandemic, and due to its longevity, lethality, and destruction the impacts of shared trauma will need to be adequately measured and addressed. This chapter aims to speak to these needs by examining where shared trauma has been studied in the past, what methodologies were employed, and among which types of providers. The chapter will conclude with a discussion of the implications of shared trauma if left unaddressed, protective factors against shared trauma, and future directions to ensure that we can continue to examine this vital topic and support providers in their essential work.

Research on Shared Trauma: Locations, Methodologies, Populations

Locations of Research

United States

Shared Trauma in the United States has been explored across different types of large-scale traumatic events such as natural disasters, mass shootings, and acts of terrorism. The first exploration of the topic occurred around the September 11th terrorist attacks (Tosone et al., 2003), where social work clinicians in New York City navigated how the attack would affect their clients' sense of safety as well as their own (Tosone, 2011). Student clinicians specifically reported feeling powerless over their own sense of safety, dysregulated, and hyperaroused (Tosone et al., 2003). This represented not only a new level and type of trauma in their lives, but also a distinct reversal of how these clinicians saw themselves, chiefly as individuals grounded with a strong grasp of what was needed to sustain their psychosocial wellbeing (Tosone et al., 2003). The shared traumatic research around the September 11th terrorist attacks also found that student clinicians were experiencing a reactivation of past traumas (Tosone et al., 2003). This meant that not only did the shared traumatic event erode their ability to feel safe and grounded, but it was acute enough to elicit the impacts of any past experiences. After time had passed, many, but not all, reported feeling a sense of connection, and strength in realizing that they were not alone in their experiences and feelings. Some of these individuals described a new sense of motivation and resilience akin to what is often referred to as post-traumatic growth (Tosone et al., 2003).

The Post 9/11 Quality of Professional Practice Survey (PQPPS) explored the long-term impact of 9/11 on 481 Manhattan social work clinicians living and working in the area at the time of the traumatic event (Tosone et al., 2011). Examining the risk and protective factors associated with both primary and secondary/vicarious trauma, the PQPPS included established measures on compassion satisfaction, resiliency, and attachment styles, as well as questions specific to 9/11 personal experiences and professional practice, supervision, and training. Shared traumatic stress was operationalized by the mean scores of the Posttraumatic Checklist-Civilian Version for PTSD (PCL-C) (Weathers et al., 1994) and the secondary trauma/compassion fatigue subscale of the Professional Quality of Life (ProQOL) (Stamm, 2005), rescaled to give equal weight to both constructs. Findings included that insecure attachment, and greater exposure to traumatic life events in general, and 9/11 in particular, were predictive of higher levels of shared traumatic stress. Resilience served as a mediator for the relationships between attachment, traumatic life events, and shared traumatic stress, potentially lessening their impact.

A thematic analysis of the PQPPS open-ended responses from 201 participants who were invited to "add any additional comments you choose related to your personal and professional September 11 experiences" revealed the following themes: 1) greater ability and urgency to care for themselves; 2) renewed appreciation for the profession; 3) greater recognition of the limits of the professional relationship; 4) past traumas served to prepare for or complicate recovery from 9/11; and 5) the collective nature of the trauma brought about blurred therapeutic roles and increased self-disclosure (Bauwens & Tosone, 2014). Being the first such terrorist attack in the United States, this particular shared traumatic event also elucidated that those existing concepts such as burnout, secondary or vicarious trauma, or even direct trauma were inadequate to explain the experience of clinicians during this event (McTighe & Tosone, 2015).

Shared trauma was next examined after Hurricane Katrina with 244 New Orleans clinicians. A significant finding was that the combination of physical devastation, along with the breakdown of social structures and basic needs, caused social work clinicians substantial strain to both survive and professionally function well enough to meet the acute needs of their displaced and underserved clients (Tosone et al., 2015). Indeed, many of the findings were similar in that clinicians had difficulty feeling safe and grounded in both their personal and professional lives, and many of those who had experienced past traumas re-experienced their effects (Tosone et al., 2015). There was also further evidence that those with more secure attachments were more resistant to the acute effects of the trauma (Tosone et al., 2015). While this cannot be controlled among clinicians, it does suggest that increased attention to clinician trauma history is a necessity in ensuring that this workforce is able to provide urgently needed care.

However, there were some divergences from the study on those working in New York City during the September 11th terrorist attacks. Particularly, during the study on Hurricane Katrina there was no relationship found between resilience and a history of traumatic experiences (Tosone et al., 2015). While this does not disprove the potential for post-traumatic growth, nor its importance in the study of shared trauma, it does demonstrate how it can be specific and variable to a given traumatic event. Finally, one of the more unique findings suggests that resource deficiencies caused by the hurricane left clinicians without the means to improve their conditions, and instead they were forced to rely on internal, professional, or communal supports to foster resiliency and continue to work (Tosone et al., 2015; Bauwens & Tosone, 2014).

Shortly after Hurricane Katrina, shared trauma was explored on what has now become a far too frequent event, mass shootings, notably in the wake of the Virginia Tech shootings which killed over 30 people and wounded many others (Day et al., 2017). Although this was not the first mass shooting in a school setting, at the time it was one of the few, and media exposure was intense in the United States. Research on this type of shared traumatic experience focused both on how the event was a surprise to clinicians, and on how it would change their professional behaviors and habits (Day et al., 2017).

The study on the Virginia Tech shooting was qualitatively structured, and therefore focused on how this specific event caused detrimental effects. However, the findings from this study aligned with previous research findings on shared trauma such as not feeling comfortable alone or feeling unsafe in the workplace, and positive effects such as feeling substantially more attuned to their clients' symptoms surrounding the event (Day et al., 2017). Finally, the first explorations of shared trauma after a mass shooting reiterated the critical importance of having organizational structures, resources, and policies in place prior to a shared traumatic event. Yet, clinicians in the Virginia Tech study stated that their workplace was caught off guard by the event and had little resources to respond in a timely manner, which ultimately led to increased burnout and clinician turnover (Day et al., 2017).

Currently, shared trauma is being explored in reference to the COVID-19 pandemic (COVID-19 Quality of Professional Practice Survey; CQPPS). Although this research is ongoing, some literature has explored how the pandemic has altered the physical spaces where clinical interactions take place, difficulties in creating safety and grounding while working, and what types of self-care strategies are feasible during the conditions of the pandemic (Tosone, 2021). COVID-19 represents what may be the most extensive and well-defined example of shared trauma in the last century. In fact, it is improbable for any working healthcare provider to not have experienced this shared traumatic event or be affected by it. Due to the rare combination of pervasiveness, lethality, and invisibility, this pandemic exemplifies the manifold nature of shared trauma. Furthermore, what has been made clear by research on this topic thus far is that the shared traumatic effects of the COVID-19 pandemic will be felt by clinicians of all types, and unless further research and resources are allocated to address this shared traumatic event, its effects will be devastating to some of the largest and most essential sectors of the global economy.

Israel

In Israel, shared trauma may have been defined under differing terms, but it has largely been explored in relation to the same circumstance or ongoing traumatic event. Specifically, Israel has been in a state of conflict for much of its existence (Fraser, 2015), and although there are some episodic differences within the greater conflict, they have been mostly related to Israel's territory and sovereignty (Fraser, 2015). Indeed, Israel has been the second largest producer of research on shared trauma and continues to fund research on this topic (Tosone et al., 2012).

Because of the frequency and duration of conflicts in Israel, research on shared trauma has identified that while the shared traumatic effects are felt among clinicians, there was also evidence to suggest a type of tolerance or acclimation to these events over time (Tosone et al., 2012). Specifically, it was noted that over time, clinicians begin to build resilience to future shared traumas (Tosone et al., 2012). This should not be interpreted to mean that inaction toward shared traumatic events is a viable option, but rather it speaks to the capacity of individuals and communities, especially those in health and social service occupations, to experience post-traumatic growth and resilience during large-scale traumatic events. In fact, Tosone et al. (2012) suggest that both destigmatizing and self-disclosure related to shared trauma can be empowering and healing for clinicians.

Other studies on shared trauma from Israel have included the effects of traumatic events in Israel on social workers and nurses, as well as potential solutions for mitigating the traumatic effects of such events. For example, Baum (2014) and Somer et al. (2004), qualitatively address how practice during frequent or ongoing shared traumatic events numbs clinicians, causing a lapse in empathy towards their clients, as well as a spiraling effect as such a lapse causes clinicians to doubt their professional capabilities (Baum, 2014; Somer et al., 2004).

Cohen et al. (2006) examined the same issues from a quantitative standpoint by providing 53 clinicians working in a hospital during several concurrent terrorist attacks in Israel with a battery of scales for secondary trauma, PTSD, and burnout (Cohen et al., 2006). Cohen and colleagues confirmed earlier findings by Baum and Somer et al. but added that repeated exposure to a shared traumatic event within a close time period does not affect the degree of secondary trauma (Cohen et al., 2006).

Comparative studies in Israel, such as Lev-Wiesel et al.'s (2009) study, examined shared traumatic effects between nurses and social workers practicing during the Second Lebanese War through a survey of scales measuring personal resources, dissociation, post-traumatic stress, post-traumatic growth and vicarious trauma (Lev-Wiesel et al., 2009). The study contained 76 nurses and 128 social workers working in the area around Haifa, which is close to the Lebanese border (Lev-Wiesel et al., 2009). The results from this study suggested that nurses have a significantly higher degree of post-traumatic growth while the other measures were not significantly different, leading to a call for more research into resiliency and post-traumatic growth in different healthcare professionals (Lev-Wiesel et al., 2009).

Lastly, there have been studies done in Israel about how to best respond to shared traumatic events, meaning methods or interventions to mitigate their effects. Two such studies are Dekel and Baum's (2010) commentary and Shamai and Ron's (2009) qualitative study. Dekel and Baum's commentary, a conglomeration of similarities in how shared trauma has manifested across the globe, points to specific commonalities that have led to protection from the effects of shared trauma (Dekel & Baum, 2010). They pointed to the need for a close network of support, outlets for expression, and organizational mechanisms such as improved supervision and creating more teamwork opportunities (Dekel & Baum, 2010).

Shamai and Ron's qualitative study was comprised of a grounded theory type of interview with 29 social workers within three types of agencies, all of which were providing current care to those who had been affected by a recent terrorist attack (Shamai & Ron, 2009). The study's goal was to explore when, and for how long, to target interventions for clinicians experiencing a shared trauma. Their findings suggested that similar to the principles of crisis counseling, the effects were most severe in the immediate aftermath of the shared traumatic event, and what was most disrupted was the clinician's sense of feeling grounded in their role, routine, and resources (Shamai & Ron, 2009). Overall, due to the frequency of shared traumatic events in Israel, there have been several groundbreaking studies of shared trauma, as well as a large enough quantity of studies for the scientific process to begin to identify commonalities and variances. This makes the body of research on shared trauma from Israel an invaluable contribution to the field.

Northern Ireland

The conflict in Northern Ireland, known as the Troubles, was ongoing for years (Cohen, 1994). Since the introduction of social services in the region, the opportunities for shared traumatic experiences have been abundant. The Troubles represent an extraordinary grouping of ethnic, religious, national, and geographic conflict. Duffy et al. (2019), conducting a mixed method study, recruited 102 practitioners who had practiced during the Troubles for an online survey, as well as 28 practitioners for a semi-structured interview. The area of focus for this study centered on if and how practitioners adjust to the dislocation and dysregulation caused by working in a shared traumatic environment (Duffy et al., 2019). This study suggests the importance of training and resources for practitioners working during a shared traumatic event, as well as the power of peer support systems in bolstering resilience (Duffy et al., 2019).

Campbell et al. (2021) reported the results of those 28 semi-structured interviews of a diverse range of social service workers who had practiced during the Troubles. Notably, the study was mostly comprised of Catholic social workers who worked in child and family service settings (Campbell et al., 2021). The results of this study demonstrated that clinicians in the region had to frequently negotiate their ability to safely provide care for clients, carefully balancing personal connections and relationships with both combatants and clients (Campbell et al., 2021). The familiarity of clinicians in the region with knowledge of several elements of the conflict compounded the duality of shared trauma, demonstrating how difficult and complex clinical work can be during such a prolonged and violent event.

Campbell et al.'s (2021) study also showed the potency of trying to seek stability, even if that means just a different mindset, in mitigating the effects of shared trauma. Particularly, in Northern Ireland this meant attempting to take a strongly objective stance in their work and trying to remove their work from the political conflicts (Campbell et al., 2021). This coping mechanism with shared trauma is unique to the Troubles and may have been developed due to a lack of organizational support and clinical supervision. While this would be difficult to definitively prove, any lack of structural and organizationally based support would be severely detrimental while practicing in a shared traumatic environment.

Research Methodologies

Qualitative Methods

Qualitative research is likely the most commonly employed type of methodology for investigating shared trauma. Although there is a wide range of qualitative methodologies that may fit well for exploring shared trauma (Gooberman-Hill et al., 2011), according to a review done by the authors, the qualitative methods most used have been structured and semi-structured interviews. Typically, interviews are coded by researchers and developed into themes or textual analyses, and then interpreted in accordance with specified research questions (Padgett, 2016).

In the case of shared trauma, interviews seek to explore themes (or divergences) about the effects of the shared traumatic event on clinicians' personal and professional lives. In past research this has meant developing questionnaires that target complexities caused by the specific traumatic event that would not be otherwise apparent, personal accounts of how those events affected clinicians, and what resources or factors helped them endure. One specific example is Seeley's (2008) research, which focused on the clinician's capacity for empathy with clients around issues of trauma. Using rigorous qualitative methods, Seeley's study displayed both the positive empathic side of shared trauma, while also finding that shared trauma can have a cyclical dynamic where clients and clinicians can project their anxieties onto each other (Seeley, 2008).

The use of qualitative methods is particularly well suited to exploring shared trauma for several reasons. First, qualitative methods allow researchers to generate original questions that can lead to nuanced understandings, and do not require the burden of psychometrics and validation. Questions can be tailored to a specific traumatic event, highlight both the uniqueness of that event, and inversely potentially showcase commonalities across shared traumatic events. Furthermore, qualitative methods allow for the researchers to gauge the participant's body language, tone of voice, and engagement with the questions. These aspects of the research process provide investigators access to highly subjective and otherwise immeasurable aspects of the research.

Although qualitative methods have been favored by past researchers, and have garnered many valuable insights, qualitative methods do carry some issues and risks when studying shared trauma. First, researchers must be mindful of the potential for doing harm to participants, namely by either re-traumatizing participants or creating unintended adverse effects during the interview process. The former concern must be at the forefront of the researcher's attention as shared traumatic events are felt across so many of the aspects of a participant's life that duress can be easily triggered unintentionally. Second, because these qualitative methods require tailored questions, it is possible that a researcher who has not adequately prepared could ask questions that are in some way insensitive, erroneous, or offensive. There is the potential for this to be a particularly sensitive area for researchers exposed to the same shared trauma being studied—their ability to negotiate nuanced communication with participants may be affected by their own trauma response. Avoiding these issues should be a matter of adequate preparation (pilot testing, member checking, etc.); however, these mistakes could derail a study and cause harm.

Finally, qualitative methods require direct interaction between the researcher and participants. This means that researchers need to garner trust and rapport with participants to gain useful and insightful information. While this is an issue for any qualitative researcher (Padgett, 2016), when discussing workplace issues, researchers must be aware of hesitancy from participants, especially those who share experiences of when their workplace may not have provided adequate support or when the participant may not have been optimally performing their duties. Therefore, qualitative research on shared trauma implores researchers to be as thorough and rigorous as possible in keeping their sample anonymous and maintaining credibility with participants.

Quantitative Methods

Quantitative research on shared trauma is less frequent than qualitative research and has emerged more recently. Previously discussed studies in Israel have come from Dekel et al. (2016), Pruginin et al. (2017), Freedman et al. (2018), and Baum (2014), while in the United States they have come mostly from Tosone et al. (2016). The objective for using quantitative methods in relation to shared trauma would be to operationalize shared trauma, validate existing scales, and produce generalizable results for quantitative analyses. The use of hypothesis testing is particularly valuable for research on shared trauma as it allows for researchers to build an increasingly specified and accurate knowledge base about shared trauma.

Currently, there are two validated scales that measure shared trauma, the first developed in the United States by Tosone et al. (2016) and the second in Israel by Baum (2014). Tosone et al.'s shared trauma scale utilizes a 14-question five-point Likert scale called the Shared Trauma/Professional Posttraumatic Growth Inventory (STPPG) that can be adapted to a specific traumatic event (Tosone et al., 2016). This validated scale, developed for use with mental health professionals, generally asks participants about both personal and professional perceptions about participants' status, reactions, and behaviors (Tosone et al., 2016).

The STPPG contains three subscales related to how the shared trauma has impacted their therapeutic techniques, personal lives, and professional post-traumatic growth. The subscale questions related to therapeutic technique specifically ask about self-disclosure, professional boundaries (between personal and professional life), and grieving. The subscale related to growth includes questions about the following: 1) appreciation for their profession; 2) seeking more practice knowledge; 3) the perimeters of what their profession can achieve; 4) their ability to empathize with clients' experiences of the shared traumatic event and trauma in general; 5) if the shared traumatic experience alters their practice orientation and allows them to make their workload more manageable; 6) if they are triggered by their clients' experiences of the shared traumatic event, or by their trauma in general; and 7) if they find themselves hoping to avoid approaching the shared traumatic event (Tosone et al., 2016).

Baum's 40-question scale is organized into five domains: intrusive anxiety, reduced empathy, inappropriate or exorbitant preoccupation with work, overly expanding one's professional role, and inappropriate alterations of the location and time of work (Baum, 2014). Baum's scale also uses a five-point Likert scale. The domains on intrusive anxiety and decreased empathy each contain ten questions; the domain on inappropriate alterations in the location and time of work contains seven questions; the domain on inappropriate or exorbitant preoccupation with work contains four questions; and the domain on overly expanding one's professional role contains nine questions (Baum, 2014). The scale has been adapted to several different shared traumatic events in Israel (Baum, 2014), however the United States has a wider array of shared traumatic events than Israel.

The generalizability of quantitative research on shared trauma allows researchers to perform a variety of comparisons and techniques to assess a scale's adaptability across different shared traumatic events. By allowing quantitative comparisons of scores among different clinicians we can begin to predict how, and to what extent, a certain type of shared traumatic event will impact certain clinicians. Quantitative analyses such as multiple regression, which relies on the reduction of a complex phenomenon like shared trauma, also allow for different types of comparative analyses with other phenomena such as post-traumatic stress, burnout, or secondary trauma. Therefore, quantitative research on shared trauma has a unique ability to further refine and differentiate shared trauma, and thereby further establish it as an imperative area of research.

However, imbedded along with the benefits of quantitatively focused research on shared trauma are potential pitfalls and limitations that must be acknowledged. First, quantitative data alone cannot display the full effect of shared trauma in the way qualitative data can. Because quantitative data is by its definition depersonalized and reduced into numerical form, it fails to adequately explain the depth of suffering that shared trauma can entail. Missing this emphasis can reduce the impact of the research and in turn the impetus to address it. Second, quantitative data is rigid as the adjustment of a question's wording or altering answer choices from a scale can compromise its generalizability, reliability, and validity. Qualitative data, by contrast, thrives in its ability to be tailored to the specific circumstances of a study. Therefore, quantitative data has the potential to become outdated as new shared traumatic events occur in new conditions.

Mixed Methods

Mixed methods research has become increasingly more common and is often hailed as the most comprehensive methodological choice for social science research (Dattilio et al., 2017). When considering mixed methods studies on shared trauma, it is important to first understand explicitly what this type of research entails. Mixed methods studies imply the complementarity of both quantitative and qualitative methods towards research questions (Creswell & Clark, 2017).

If both methods do not align and provide pertinent information, then it is not a true mixed methods study. For example, if one of the methods is redundant or the methods only answer tangential questions related to the study, then it is not a properly performed mixed methods study, and should not be considered as such. Furthermore, the results of a mixed methods study must integrate the findings from both qualitative and quantitative methods in such a way that it avoids the appearance of being two separate studies (Creswell & Clark, 2017). Such integration is often shown in what is called a joint display, or a graphical representation, like a table or image, that depicts the integration of both methods (Creswell & Clark, 2017).

Mixed methods studies related to shared trauma, such as Duffy et al.'s (2019) study in Northern Ireland or Dekel et al.'s (2016) study in Israel, are limited but growing in number. Having both elements in a single study is ideal for investigations of shared trauma because purely quantitative methods can lose its humanistic appeal and impact and purely qualitative studies can be overly subjective and lack comparative ability.

A properly executed mixed methods study addresses both previously mentioned concerns, without the need to compare dissimilar results from separate studies where study conditions and the passage of time compromise the ability to glean actionable information. Additionally, mixed methods research on shared trauma heightens its specificity by allowing researchers to address many components of a research question more effectively. For example, if a researcher wanted to explore the degree to which a shared traumatic event affected clinicians' ability to feel safe at work, a mixed method study would be ideal.

Mixed methods research is clearly an optimal approach for exploring shared trauma, as it is for many social science studies. However, it too has a notable drawback. Mixed methods studies need to be carefully designed so both methods complement each other, and neither method can be abridged or lack rigor; doing so degrades the quality of the research and the standing of mixed methods research in the scientific community (Creswell & Clark, 2017). These considerations mean that mixed methods studies often take more time to plan and implement as well as requiring researchers to have adequate expertise in both methodologies.

Narratives and Commentaries

One of the more common types of professional literature found on shared trauma is first-person narratives and commentaries. This type of literature does not seek to produce qualitative or quantitative data, nor does it even claim to be scientific. Instead, these reports seek to provide direct experiences, reflections, and recommendations for practice during shared traumatic experiences. An obvious critique of this literature is its indifference to any kind of methodology or rigor. There is no ability or intent for narratives and commentaries to be validated, or even checked for accuracy. While it should be noted that this kind of literature does not claim to be scientific, it can be featured in scholarly periodicals, and therefore is easily subjected to critique from the scientific community.

Despite being non-scientific, this type of literature can be insightful and inclusive of perspectives from individuals who may not have the resources to produce scientific writing. Their insights, perhaps even more vividly than in qualitative research, demonstrate some of the most urgent and current issues facing clinicians during shared traumatic events. In fact, this type of literature is the most responsive to the onset of a shared traumatic event, and can voice a collection of perceptions in a timely enough manner to rapidly effect conditions and resources for clinicians experiencing that trauma.

Some of the most prominent and impactful shared traumatic events have been written about from scholars and practitioners in the field in the form of commentaries. Indeed, commentaries on shared trauma have been ubiquitous and while a full listing would be arduous, a sample of some of the most prominent have been: Saakvitne's and Tosone et al.'s commentaries on therapists' experiences of September 11th terror attacks (Saakvitne, 2002; Tosone, 2002), Altman and Davies' psychoanalytic interpretations of September 11th terror attacks (Altman & Davies, 2002), Rao and Mehra's refection of working during Hurricane Sandy in New York City (Rao & Mehra, 2015), reflections of counselors who worked on campus during the Virginia Tech shootings (Day et al., 2017), or Faust et al.'s and Boulanger's accounts of the mass destruction caused by Hurricane Katrina in New Orleans (Faust et al., 2008; Boulanger, 2013). Each of these commentaries shows both the depth of impact that the shared traumatic event caused, as well as an account of how the event manifested in occupational settings.

Research Populations and Locations

The research on shared trauma has taken place among a select group of clinicians and study locations. A majority has been performed on social workers. While this is reasonable, as social workers are often performing clinical work, they are still overrepresented in the research on shared trauma. Outside of social workers, shared trauma research tends to be focused on a conglomeration of mental health professionals such as licensed mental health counselors, licensed professional counselors, and what some of the literature simply refers to as "therapists" (Baird et al., 2016). While the term is unacceptably vague, it demonstrates how much of the research on shared trauma is focused on mental health providers.

However, there is mention of non-mental health professionals in the literature, namely nurses in studies that do not utilize the terminology of shared trauma, but de facto involve it (Kleis & Kellogg, 2020; Niiyama et al., 2009). This represents an understudied but perfectly valid area for future research. In fact, thus far we have yet to see a study about shared trauma that identifies physicians, nurse-aids, first responders (who are not social workers), or any member of what is referred to as the "allied health" professions (McPherson et al., 2006). While non-mental health providers may not be engaging in psychotherapy with clients, they still do encounter mental health issues and would be vulnerable to a shared traumatic experience.

The location of shared trauma research is somewhat more varied than the types of professionals being researched. Currently, research has been performed in hospital settings (Kleis & Kellogg, 2020), community mental health centers (Bauwens & Tosone, 2014), and among private practitioners (Tosone et al., 2003; Tosone, 2021). More recently, during the COVID-19 pandemic, shared trauma has been explored in a plethora of professional settings. An edited book on shared trauma (Tosone, 2021) among social workers practicing during the COVID-19 pandemic revealed that it has been recorded in relation to: identifying moral distress in acute care settings (Cerone, 2021), maintaining robust boundaries in domestic violence centers (Bloomberg, 2021), maintaining the importance of empathy while remotely training new social workers (Sapiro, 2021), understanding the effects of disruption on school-based clinicians (Sedillo-Hamann et al., 2021), highlighting the futility of the current criminal justice system (James, 2021), and recognizing the risks that child welfare workers take on a daily basis (Williams, 2021).

Each of these settings has notably different structures, resources, and dynamics. Such variations may alter how a shared traumatic event is experienced, and what factors will be necessary to foster post-traumatic growth. Because of their divergences, we can establish that shared trauma can be felt in any of these settings and likely within any setting that is providing healthcare or social services. Forthcoming research will require a multitude of methodologies and substantial sample sizes to properly demonstrate the full effects of shared trauma due to the COVID-19 pandemic.

Effects of Shared Trauma and Protective Factors

The effects of shared trauma, at a cursory level, mirror many common aspects of the sequelae of trauma (Walton et al., 2017), namely hyperarousal, flooding, social withdrawal, anxiety, and professional boundary issues (Tosone, 2019; Tosone et al., 2012; Day et al., 2017). However, because of the unique elements that define shared trauma, it is an especially complex type of trauma and likewise has some distinctive effects. It is important to keep in mind that shared trauma is primarily viewed as a workplace issue, even though it impacts clinicians' personal lives as well. Consequently, this chapter now focuses on the unique effects of shared trauma as it relates to the work environment.

A helpful way to distinguish these effects is to consider, in two related domains, how shared trauma affects individual psychosocial functioning with clients and how it affects the clinician's relationship to the organization. First, it can obscure appropriate workplace boundaries between clients and clinicians (Cohen-Serrins, 2021). Due to the dysregulation and distress caused by the traumatic event, a clinician may deviate from what are typical or appropriate workplace boundaries such as by overly identifying and disclosing their personal concerns with clients, or conversely, being overly restrictive and protective of boundaries with clients, causing the clinician to appear disconnected or isolated from their professional responsibilities.

Another way this can become evident would be through notably increased countertransference, or when a clinician reacts, behaviorally, emotionally, or cognitively towards their client in conscious or subconscious ways (Tosone, 2019). For example, if during a shared traumatic event a client reminds a clinician of their parent, and consequently the clinician starts to interact with that client in a similar way to how they would with that parent, the clinician is experiencing countertransference. While countertransference is a common, and even expected, aspect of clinical work, during a shared traumatic event, a new type of countertransference may appear and at a new intensity. This may be noticeable to the client and may even be inappropriate in a professional clinical space. Therefore, as a shared traumatic event unfolds, it is essential to provide heightened attention and supervision toward countertransference.

The other domain centers on to how the individual clinician may relate to their work environment during and after a shared traumatic event. This primarily refers to feelings of physical and psychological safety in the workplace. Research in this area has defined psychological safety as the perception that the work environment will not be overly punitive and that employees' psychosocial needs such as protection from discrimination and support for some assemblage of work/life balance will be met (Frazier et al., 2017).

During a shared traumatic event physical and psychological safety can be compromised and its effects can be displayed in several ways such as a clinician being more withdrawn from interactions with co-workers and supervisors or becoming more easily agitated with clients and co-workers. At the core of such reactions is a disruption in feeling grounded or secure in the work environment. Because we spend so much time in the work-place, and as it can have a profound role in our identity (Vallas & Christin, 2018), when the workplace becomes more dangerous or threatening, the notion of typical behavior seems disjointed or impossible.

While routine and learning allow clinicians to hone their skills and capabilities to take on stress, a shared traumatic experience produces the inverse conditions, causing one to potentially regress or at least experience fear and anxiety. However, what must be kept in mind is that the shared trauma is not only occurring in the workplace. The clinician's life, material possessions, and loved ones are also threatened by this event, and yet the clinician is still being asked to function professionally, namely, to support others for the duration of the traumatic event. Past research has indicated that the level of dysregulation, danger, and countertransference caused by a shared traumatic experience can force clinicians to leave their place of work, known as turnover (Willard-Grace et al., 2019), or remain in their positions and suffer the psychosocial consequences of shared trauma (Tosone, 2021). Either of these outcomes is detrimental to clinicians, their clients, and the organizations employing them.

Future Directions and Considerations for Research on Shared Trauma

Populations and Events

As new shared traumatic events occur, research will be needed to deter-mine potential commonalties and divergences. After examining the litera-ture, there is a clear lack of representation among shared traumas. For example, there have been wars outside of the United States and Israel which have occurred since the advent of healthcare and social services. Wars such as those in the Congo, the Middle East, and East Asia all have the potential to cause shared traumatic events, and because of their taking place in countries not yet researched in relation to shared trauma, new and potentially vital information is not being collected.

As new shared traumatic events must be explored, so too must the range of professionals being studied increase. Mental health professionals and nurses do not nearly represent the full range of health and social service providers. For example, psychiatrists and psychologists have not had any notable focus in the shared trauma literature, and yet provide substantial clinical work for a variety of patient populations. Another area for further exploration would be to examine shared trauma in specific subsections of employees. For example, it may be necessary to determine how employees at certain levels within an organization are each affected by a shared trauma, or if employees of various demographic identities experience these events differently. The more nuanced our knowledge is about how different populations and events interact with shared trauma, the more acceptable and effective future approaches can be.

Methodological Improvements and Considerations

Future methodological considerations require more granular approaches to probe deeper into shared trauma and more accurately into its effects. From a quantitative standpoint, this means that existing shared trauma scales need to be further validated and refined. If the current scales tend to lose reliability and validity over time, then the existing scales will need to be refined. However, this can only be determined if they are employed in new locations and among new populations. The development of new scales, although enticing, is likely unnecessary as the two existing scales have thus far been both psychometrically sound and adaptable (Tosone et al., 2016; Baum, 2014).

Regarding qualitative methodologies, future research would benefit from going beyond structured or semi-structured interviews. Qualitative methods align well with creative forms of communication such as photovoice, mapping techniques, and observational methods like ethnographies or observational studies (Padgett, 2016). These techniques do not require participants to verbalize their perceptions and impacts of shared trauma, and are effective methods for communicating about such experiences (Perryman et al., 2019).

Further Exploring Protective Factors

The final section of this chapter relates to what future researchers should consider when developing interventions and resources to support those experiencing shared trauma. At the individual level, further research into attachment style and shared trauma could be insightful for determining how an individual clinician's relationship to their work and their workplace may facilitate reactions to a shared traumatic event. Attachment style is one of the most important psychosocial aspects of one's development (Meyer & Pilkonis, 2001). It may relate to how one is able to remain resilient in the face of shared trauma or how acute a negative reaction is to it.

Further research is necessary on the intrinsic factors that may foster or inhibit resilience during a shared traumatic event. For example, spirituality has been used during numerous large-scale traumatic events to bring alleviation of suffering and increase fortitude to those most affected (Walker & Aten, 2012). Spirituality relates to one's beliefs about what non-material or supernatural forces determine or influence the events in our lives. An operationalization of how different levels and types of spirituality moderate one's reaction to shared traumatic events could both elucidate spirituality-based interventions and provide insight into how effective intrinsic sources of resilience can be to mitigate the effects of shared trauma.

When considering organizationally rooted approaches to shared trauma, it is currently unknown to what extent a positive organizational culture promotes clinician wellbeing during a traumatic event and, inversely, if a toxic organizational culture has a significantly detrimental effect. Future research exploring organizational dynamics and cultures in relation to shared trauma could both add to the existing literature about their importance in healthcare and social service workplaces, as well as provide a catalyst for creating preventative interventions and systems to address shared trauma. While we cannot control the severity or frequency of these events, if future research can develop highly effective means to mitigate their effects, we could potentially limit the damages shared traumatic events cause to clinicians themselves, the organizations they work for, and the communities that they serve.

References

Altman, N., & Davies, J. M. (2002). Out of the blue: Reflections on a shared trauma. *Psychoanalytic Dialogues*, 12(3), 359–360.

American Psychiatric Association. (2013). *Diagnostic and statistical manual* (5th edn). American Psychiatric Association.

Baird, K., & Kracen, A. C. (2016). Vicarious traumatization and secondary traumatic stress: A research synthesis. *Counselling Psychology Quarterly*, 19(2), 181–188.

Baum, N. (2012). Trap of conflicting needs: Helping professionals in the wake of a shared traumatic reality. *Clinical Social Work Journal*, 40(1), 37–45.

Baum, N. (2014). Professionals' double exposure in the shared traumatic reality of wartime: Contributions to professional growth and stress. *The British Journal of Social Work*, 44(8), 2113–2134.

Bauwens, J., & Tosone, C. (2014). Posttraumatic growth following Hurricane Katrina: The influence of clinicians' trauma histories and primary and secondary traumatic stress. *Traumatology*, 20(3), 209.

Bloomberg, S. (2021). Reflections on COVID-19, domestic violence, and shared trauma. In C. Tosone (Ed.), *Shared trauma, shared resilience during a pandemic* (pp. 69–77). Springer.

Boals, A. (2018). Trauma in the eye of the beholder: Objective and subjective definitions of trauma. *Journal of Psychotherapy Integration*, 28(1), 77.

Boscarino, J. A., Figley, C. R., & Adams, R. E. (2004). Compassion fatigue following the September 11 terrorist attacks: A study of secondary trauma among New York City social workers. *International Journal of Emergency Mental Health*, 6, 57–66.

Boulanger, G. (2013). Fearful symmetry: Shared trauma in New Orleans after Hurricane Katrina. *Psychoanalytic Dialogues*, 23(1), 31–44.

Bradley, M., & Chahar, P. (2020). Burnout of healthcare providers during COVID-19. *Cleveland Clinic Journal of Medicine*. doi:10.3949/ccjm.87a.ccc051.

Campbell, J., Duffy, J., Tosone, C., & Falls, D. (2021). 'Just get on with it': A qualitative study of social workers' experiences during the political conflict in Northern Ireland. *The British Journal of Social Work*, 51(4), 1314–1331.

Cerone, V. L. (2021). COVID-19 and moral distress/moral anguish: Therapeutic support for healthcare workers in acute care. In C. Tosone (Ed.), *Shared trauma, shared resilience during a pandemic: Social work in the time of COVID-19* (pp. 21–31). Springer.

Cohen, M. (1994). Religion and social inequality in Ireland. *The Journal of Interdisciplinary History*, 25(1), 1–21.

Cohen, M., Gagin, R., & Peled-Avram, M. (2006). Multiple terrorist attacks: Compassion fatigue in Israeli social workers. *Traumatology*, 12(4), 293–301.

Cohen-Serrins, J. (2021). How COVID-19 exposed an inadequate approach to burnout: Moving beyond self-care. In C. Tosone (Ed.), *Shared trauma, shared resilience during a pandemic: Social work in the time of COVID-19* (pp. 259–268). Springer.

Creswell, J. W., & Clark, V. L. P. (2017). *Designing and conducting mixed methods research*. Sage Publications.

Dattilio, F. M., Edwards, D. J., Messer, S. B., & Fishman, D. B. (2017). Mixed methods research offers a more powerful gold standard for evaluating psychological treatments. *The Behavior Therapist*, 40(4), 151–154.

Day, K. W., Lawson, G., & Burge, P. (2017). Clinicians' experiences of shared trauma after the shootings at Virginia Tech. *Journal of Counseling & Development*, 95(3), 269–278.

Dekel, R., & Baum, N. (2010). Intervention in a shared traumatic reality: A new challenge for social workers. *British Journal of Social Work*, 40(6), 1927–1944.

Dekel, R., Nuttman-Shwartz, O., & Lavi, T. (2016). Shared traumatic reality and boundary theory: How mental health professionals cope with the home/work conflict during continuous security threats. *Journal of Couple & Relationship Therapy*, 15(2), 121–134.

Duffy, J., Campbell, J., & Tosone, C. (2019). The Northern Irish study: Voices of social work through the Troubles. In J. Duffy, J. Campbell, & C. Tosone (Eds.), *International Perspectives on Social Work and Political Conflict* (pp. 38–49). Routledge.

Eidelson, R. J., D'Alessio, G. R., & Eidelson, J. I. (2003). The impact of September 11 on psychologists. *Professional Psychology: Research and Practice*, 34(2), 144–150.

Faust, D. S., Black, F. W., Abrahams, J. P., Warner, M. S., & Bellando, B. J. (2008). After the storm: Katrina's impact on psychological practice in New Orleans. *Professional Psychology: Research and Practice*, 39(1), 1.

Fowler, K. L., Kling, N. D., & Larson, M. D. (2007). Organizational preparedness for coping with a major crisis or disaster. *Business & Society*, 46(1), 88–103.

Fraser, T. G. (2015). *The Arab-Israeli conflict*. Macmillan International Higher Education.

Frazier, M. L., Fainshmidt, S., Klinger, R. L., Pezeshkan, A., & Vracheva, V. (2017). Psychological safety: A meta-analytic review and extension. *Personnel Psychology*, 70(1), 113–165.

Freedman, S. A., & Tuval Mashiach, R. (2018). Shared trauma reality in war: Mental health therapists' experience. *PloS one*, 13(2), e0191949.

Gooberman-Hill, R., Fox, R., & Chesser, T. J. S. (2011). What can qualitative approaches bring to trauma outcome research? *Injury*, 42(4), 321–323.

Harris, B. T. (2016). Trauma and creative healing: Reflections on providing music therapy in post-war Bosnia and Herzegovina. *Journal of Applied Arts & Health*, 7(2), 253–261.

James, K. J. (2021). Black lives, mass incarceration, and the perpetuity of trauma in the era of COVID-19: The road to abolition social work. In C. Tosone (Ed.), *Shared trauma, shared resilience during a pandemic: Social work in the time of COVID-19* (pp. 281–290). Springer.

Karatzias, T., Murphy, P., Cloitre, M., Bisson, J., Roberts, N., Shevlin, M., & Hutton, P. (2019). Psychological interventions for ICD-11 complex PTSD symptoms: Systematic review and meta-analysis. *Psychological Medicine*, 49(11), 1761–1775.

Kleis, A. E., & Kellogg, M. B. (2020). Recalling stress and trauma in the workplace: A qualitative study of pediatric nurses. *Pediatric Nursing*, 46(1), 5–10.

Lev-Wiesel, R. (2007). Intergenerational transmission of trauma across three generations: A preliminary study. *Qualitative Social Work*, 6(1), 75–94.

Lev-Wiesel, R., Goldblatt, H., Eisikovits, Z., & Admi, H. (2009). Growth in the shadow of war: The case of social workers and nurses working in a shared war reality. *British Journal of Social Work*, 39(6), 1154–1174.

Lichner, V., & Lovaš, L. (2016). Model of the self-care strategies among Slovak helping professionals–qualitative analysis of performed self-care activities. *Humanities and Social Sciences*, 5(1), 107–112.

McCann, I. L., & Pearlman, L. A. (1990). Vicarious traumatization: A framework for understanding the psychological effects of working with victims. *Journal of Traumatic Stress*, 3(1), 131–149.

McPherson, K., Kersten, P., George, S., Lattimer, V., Breton, A., Ellis, B., & Frampton, G. (2006). A systematic review of evidence about extended roles for allied health professionals. *Journal of Health Services Research & Policy*, 11(4), 240–247.

McTighe, J. P., & Tosone, C. (2015). Narrative and meaning-making among Manhattan social workers in the wake of September 11, 2001. *Social Work in Mental Health*, 13(4), 299–317.

Meyer, B., & Pilkonis, P. A. (2001). Attachment style. *Psychotherapy: Theory, Research, Practice, Training*, 38(4), 466.

Mitchell, J. T., & Everly, G. S. (1997). *Critical incident stress debriefing (CISD): An operations manual for the prevention of traumatic stress among emergency service and disaster workers* (2nd edn, revised). Chevron Publishing Corporation.

Niiyama, E., Okamura, H., Kohama, A., Taniguchi, T., Sounohara, M., & Nagao, M. (2009). A survey of nurses who experienced trauma in the workplace: Influence of coping strategies on traumatic stress. *Stress and Health: Journal of the International Society for the Investigation of Stress*, 25(1), 3–9.

Padgett, D. K. (2016). *Qualitative methods in social work research*, Vol. 36. Sage Publications.

Panagioti, M., Panagopoulou, E., Bower, P., Lewith, G., Kontopantelis, E., Chew-Graham, C., & Esmail, A. (2017). Controlled interventions to reduce burnout in physicians: A systematic review and meta-analysis. *JAMA Internal Medicine*, 177(2), 195–205.

Perryman, K., Blisard, P., & Moss, R. (2019). Using creative arts in trauma therapy: The neuroscience of healing. *Journal of Mental Health Counseling*, 41(1), 80–94.

Pruginin, I., Findley, P., Isralowitz, R., & Reznik, A. (2017). Adaptation and resilience among clinicians under missile attack: Shared traumatic reality. *International Journal of Mental Health and Addiction*, 15(3), 684–700.

Rao, N., & Mehra, A. (2015). Hurricane Sandy: Shared trauma and therapist self-disclosure. *Psychiatry*, 78(1), 65–74.

Saakvitne, K. W. (2002). Shared trauma: The therapist's increased vulnerability. *Psychoanalytic Dialogues*, 12(3), 443–449.

Sapiro, B. (2021). Teaching social work practice in the shared trauma of a global pandemic. In C. Tosone (Ed.), *Shared trauma, shared resilience during a pandemic: Social work in the time of COVID-19* (pp. 323–329). Springer.

Sedillo-Hamann, D., Chock-Goldman, J., & Badillo, M. A. (2021). School social workers responding to the COVID-19 pandemic: Experiences in traditional, charter, and agency-based community school agency settings. In C. Tosone (Ed.), *Shared trauma, shared resilience during a pandemic: Social work in the time of COVID-19* (pp. 135–144). Springer.

Seeley, K. M. (2008). *Therapy after terror: 9/11, psychotherapists, and mental health*. Cambridge University Press.

Shamai, M., & Ron, P. (2009). Helping direct and indirect victims of national terror: Experiences of Israeli social workers. *Qualitative Health Research*, 19(1), 42–54.

Somer, E., Buchbinder, E., Peled-Avram, M., & Ben-Yizhack, Y. (2004). The stress and coping of Israeli emergency room social workers following terrorist attacks. *Qualitative Health Research*, 14(8), 1077–1093.

Stamm, B. H. (2005). *The Proqol manual: The professional quality of life scale: Compassion satisfaction, burnout & compassion fatigue/ secondary trauma scales*. Sidran Press.

Tedeschi, R. G., & Calhoun, L. G. (1996). The posttraumatic growth inventory: Measuring the positive legacy of trauma. *Journal of Traumatic Stress*, 9, 451–471.

Tosone, C. (2002). On the eve of 9/11: Reflections from a New York colleague. *Newsletter of the National Membership Committee on Psychoanalysis in Clinical Social Work*, Fall.

Tosone, C. (2006). Therapeutic intimacy: A post-9/11 perspective. *Smith College Studies in Social Work*, 76(4), 89–98.

Tosone, C. (2011). The legacy of September 11: Shared trauma, therapeutic intimacy, and professional posttraumatic growth. *Traumatology*, 17(3), 25–29.

Tosone, C. (2019). Shared trauma and social work practice in communal disasters. In J. Duffy, J. Campbell, & C. Tosone (Eds.), *International perspectives on social work and political conflict* (pp. 50–64). Routledge.

Tosone, C. (Ed.). (2021). *Shared trauma, shared resilience during a pandemic: Social work in the time of COVID-19*. Springer.

Tosone, C., Bialkin, L., Lee, M., Martinez, A., Campbell, M., Martinez, M., Charters, M.et al. (2003). Shared trauma: Group reflections on the September 11th disaster. *Psychoanalytic Social Work*, 10(1): 57–77.

Tosone, C., Minami, T., Bettmann, J. E., & Jasperson, R. A. (2010). New York City social workers after 9/11: Their attachment, resiliency, and compassion fatigue. *International Journal of Emergency Mental Health*, 12(2), 103–116.

Tosone, C., McTighe, J., Bauwens, J., & Naturale, A. (2011). Shared traumatic stress and the long-term impact of September 11th on Manhattan clinicians. *Journal of Traumatic Stress*, 24 (5), 546–552.

Tosone, C., Nuttman-Shwartz, O., & Stephens, T. (2012). Shared trauma: When the professional is personal. *Clinical Social Work Journal*, 40(2), 231–239.

Tosone, C., McTighe, J. P., & Bauwens, J. (2015). Shared traumatic stress among social workers in the aftermath of Hurricane Katrina. *British Journal of Social Work*, 45(4), 1313–1329.

Tosone, C., Bauwens, J., & Glassman, M. (2016). The shared traumatic and professional posttraumatic growth inventory. *Research on Social Work Practice*, 26 (3), 286–294.

Vallas, S. P., & Christin, A. (2018). Work and identity in an era of precarious employment: How workers respond to "personal branding" discourse. *Work and Occupations*, 45(1), 3–37.

van der Ham, A. J., van der Aa, H. P., Verstraten, P., van Rens, G. H., & van Nispen, R. M. (2021). Experiences with traumatic events, consequences and care among people with visual impairment and post-traumatic stress disorder: A qualitative study from the Netherlands. *BMJ Open*, 11(2), e041469.

Walker, D. F., & Aten, J. D. (2012). Future directions for the study and application of religion, spirituality, and trauma research. *Journal of Psychology and Theology*, 40(4), 349–353.

Walton, J. L., Cuccurullo, L. A. J., Raines, A. M., Vidaurri, D. N., Allan, N. P., Maieritsch, K. P., & Franklin, C. L. (2017). Sometimes less is more: Establishing the core symptoms of PTSD. *Journal of Traumatic Stress*, 30(3), 254–258.

Weathers, F. W., Litz, B. T., Huska, J. A., & Keane, T. M. (1994). *PTSD checklist—civilian version*. National Center.

Willard-Grace, R., Knox, M., Huang, B., Hammer, H., Kivlahan, C., & Grumbach, K. (2019). Burnout and health care workforce turnover. *The Annals of Family Medicine*, 17(1), 36–41.

Williams, D. S. (2021). Shared traumatic stress and the impact of COVID-19 on public child welfare workers. In C. Tosone (Ed.), *Shared trauma, shared resilience during a pandemic: Social work in the time of COVID-19* (pp. 249–257). Springer.

Part II

Battlegrounds of Shared Trauma: Traumatic Events

Chapter 3

Frontline Devotion in a Shared Trauma

Partners of Doctors and Nurses Combatting COVID-19

Alana Siegel and Rachel Dekel

A highly contagious coronavirus—soon called COVID-19—broke out in Wuhan, China, in December 2019, and was declared a global pandemic by March 11, 2020 (WHO, 2020). COVID-19 is a highly contagious disease that targets the respiratory system, and can lead to fever, difficulty breathing, aches, loss of taste and smell, and result in a host of complications (WHO, 2021). COVID-19 has taken a staggering toll on global public health; as of the start of April 2021—15 months into the outbreak—there were over 131.1 million ill and more than 2.85 million deaths worldwide.[1] The global ramifications of the pandemic have been devastating: crippling economies (The World Bank, 2020), overwhelming healthcare systems and leading to healthcare crises (Blumenthal et al., 2020), mandating lockdowns and closures of businesses, schools, and universities (Kaplan et al., 2020), and unleashing hardships of food, housing, and employment (Center on Budget and Policy Priorities, 2021).

Within weeks of the outbreak, the doctors and nurses working on the hospitals' frontlines were overwhelmed (Schwirtz, 2020). While "frontline worker" can be defined as "employees within essential industries who must physically show up to their jobs" (Tomer & Kane, 2020), here we will focus on the doctors and nurses working in the frontlines of hospitals as they battled COVID. Indeed, these frontliners were suddenly and unexpectedly faced with a virus with an unclear etiology and pathology, high numbers of sick and dying patients with no known cure, and having to make life-saving decisions for hundreds of critically ill patients, all while afraid of falling ill themselves (Kisner, 2020). Doctors and nurses working in the frontlines of hospitals have been at especially high risk for catching the virus. Indeed, in a study examining the prevalence of COVID-19 in frontline workers in the United States and the United Kingdom, it was found that they were at a significantly higher risk of contracting the virus, as there were 2,747 cases per 100,000 frontline healthcare workers compared to 242 cases per 100,000 people in the general community (Nguyen et al., 2020). This was evident in additional countries: a study which gathered data from 37 countries found that nearly 300,000 healthcare

DOI: 10.4324/9781003176947-5

workers had been infected and over 2,500 healthcare workers had died from the coronavirus as of August 15, 2020 (Erdem & Lucey, 2020).

Doctors and nurses felt especially at risk due to not having sufficient protective gear such as N95 masks, face shields, and plastic gloves—some even wore garbage bags for protection—(Bowden et al., 2020), and there were an insufficient number of ventilators for patients (Schwirtz, 2020). Frontline workers were also overburdened by the number of patients who would take a sudden turn for the worse, leading to the deaths of dozens of patients each day (Brown & Borter, 2020). Due to the mandatory isolation of patients—as visiting family members were prohibited—doctors and nurses were also put in the unique position of arranging phone calls where patients could say goodbye to loved ones before they passed away. Many frontliners described the personal toll this devastating experience took on them (Goldstein & Weiser, 2020). Due to these multiple stressors, many frontline workers reported burnout (Chen et al., 2021), PTSD (Gavin et al., 2020), anxiety, depression (The Physicians Foundation, 2020), hopelessness, and fatigue (Li et al., 2020) as a result of their work.

In addition to the struggles at the hospital, frontline workers were confronted by another fear: to not spread the virus to their families upon returning home from work (Wu et al., 2020). A study of the families of healthcare workers found that their household members were twice as likely as the general public to fall ill with COVID as a result of their exposure to the virus at work (Shah et al., 2020). Indeed, while some frontliners found alternative options for housing (i.e., hotels, apartments), this was not an option for many healthcare workers for a variety of reasons (i.e., lack of availability or finances, desire to remain with loved ones, responsibility for young children, etc.) thereby increasing risk of exposure to loved ones (Vielkind, 2020).

The families of frontliners were also under stress, with one study finding high levels of anxiety (33.7%) and depression (29.35%) symptoms in family members (Ying et al., 2020). Additionally, many partners were devastated by the sudden loss of their frontliners to COVID-19 (Gold, 2020). Many of the healthcare workers who died left behind children and spouses who were stunned and overwhelmed by their loved one's quick demise; oftentimes the frontliner went from healthy and able to deceased within days or weeks (Sacks, 2021).

The current study focuses on the spouses and romantic partners of frontline doctors and nurses working in hospitals in the New York City (NYC) area during the outbreak of COVID. We choose this population for several reasons. First, while there are many studies that are focused on the doctors and nurses themselves, we wanted to broaden the perspective and to look at their spouses coping with stress and trauma both through a general social work system lens as well as a family-systems lens, focusing on individuals in the context of their family units (Papero, 2017; Sutphin et al., 2013). Moreover, as this book focuses on shared trauma, and while many studies examine the effects of this situation on therapists and their clinical work, we wanted to focus on the effects of this situation on the significant others. As there is a strong bidirectional connection between both partners' functioning, we believe this will facilitate better understanding of both the frontliners' and their partners' experience in an acute crisis. In order to do this, we aimed to learn about the onset of the crisis from the perspective of their partners. Finally, we also reflect on our experience interviewing the participants as we together navigated a shared trauma, and how this affected our research process.

Shared Trauma

As frontliners were navigating this crisis, there simultaneously unfolded a shared trauma, which occurs when professionals both live and work in the same community as the people whom they serve so that they are exposed to and threatened by the very same disaster or collective trauma as their clients (Lavi et al., 2015). Most studies on shared trauma have been focused on mental health professionals and highlight that therapists are exposed to this collective trauma both as private citizens, members of a family, as well as professionals who are aiming to treat their patients in the aftermath of the event (Saakvitne, 2002). The professionals may experience conflicts of loyalty in choosing between their professional obligations to clients and their needs or wishes to remain beside family members and loved ones during an emergency (Dekel et al., 2016). Mental health professionals were found to be at risk for emotional distress both during and in the immediate aftermath of the traumatic event, including burnout, insecurity about their professional abilities, and guilt due to a shared trauma overload (Tosone et al., 2012). At the same time, professionals may feel in better contact with their clients' emotions and even experience a renewed commitment to the profession and to their patients in the aftermath of a shared trauma both have experienced (Lavi et al., 2015).

Despite the "sharedness" aspects of the phenomena, most studies have focused on mental health professionals, while few studies have focused on the patients or on the significant others of the professionals within the shared traumatic reality (Dekel & Nuttman-Shwartz, 2014, p. 224). In this chapter we are seeking to extend the theory of shared trauma as we apply it to professional doctors and nurses in frontline positions and their spouses and partners. Similarly to their patients, the frontliners are also navigating their fears of infection, loss of income, job uncertainty, and balancing of work/family (Madani, 2020). Just like the patients they were treating, the shocking and sudden onset of the pandemic was a major stressor for both the doctors and nurses, as well as for their partners and families (Arnetz et al., 2020). Although they were at higher risk than the general population, the frontliners were also afraid for their family's stress and potential contagion of the virus (Wu et al., 2020). In our study, the professionals, partners, and the patients they cared for in the hospital all lived in the same geographic area as the hospitals in which they worked.

In widening the scope of shared trauma, we aim to focus on the intimate relations of those working on the frontlines, not what happens to these professionals in treatment settings as is typically studied (Lavi et al., 2015; Tosone et al., 2015). Given the second author's previous research on professionals in southern Israel (Nuttmann-Shwartz & Dekel, 2009) as well as on spouses (Dekel et al., 2005; Schelleles & Dekel, 2001; Dekel et al., 2015; Dekel et al., 2017), we were especially interested in the effects of acute crisis on the relations of those working on the frontlines of the COVID crisis in the outbreak of an early epicenter. Indeed, previous research on shared trauma found that "the family domain was the vulnerable space for the participants. Workers found it difficult to function in their professional roles as long as they are not sure that their own family members are safe" (Dekel & Nuttman-Shwartz, 2014, p. 235). Therefore, we focused on the shared trauma of the New York outbreak from the perspective of the spouses of those on the frontlines, how they were affected, and how they coped with a shared intensive life-threatening event.

Our study aimed to learn about:

1   How was the partner impacted by the frontliner's duties in this shared traumatic reality?
2   What was the partners' experience during the pandemic, especially during the period of time (approximately 12 weeks) that their loved one was on the frontlines?
3   How were self-care and coping strategies used in times of acute stress?
4   What were the partner's perceptions of the support of both hospital and governmental systems while navigating the crisis?

Participants

This qualitative study was conducted with 29 spouses or romantic partners of doctors and nurses who had been working on the frontlines with COVID patients in NYC hospitals during its outbreak from February 29–June 1, 2020. The city was one of the earliest epicenters of the coronavirus in the United States (Thompson et al., 2020). A citywide lockdown was declared in NYC on March 22, 2020 (Ramachandran et al., 2020). There were 203,000 cases reported within the first three months of the NYC outbreak, and one-third of patients who were hospitalized during this time passed away from COVID (Thompson et al., 2020). Of the frontline workers interviewed, 22 were doctors, and 7 were nurses. The frontliners worked in medical units which included the Emergency Room, Obstetrics,

Nephrology, Pulmonology, Rheumatology, Gastroenterology, Internal Medicine, and Rehabilitation Medicine. Several of the frontliners were placed by their hospital administration from Pediatric or Surgery departments, and had little experience working with adults or respiratory issues.

While both 25 married spouses and 4 cohabiting partners were interviewed, for the sake of simplicity they will often be described here in the text as a "partner." Of the partners interviewed, 12 were female and 17 were male. They ranged from age 29–71 years (M = 38.8). The couples had been together between 3 and 45 years (M = 13.5). Twenty couples had children together, averaging 1–2 children per family. Twenty-seven couples were of heterosexual sexual orientation, and two couples were of gay male sexual orientation. Racially, 22 partners identified as Caucasian or Jewish, 3 of the partners identified as Asian, and 2 as Latina. None of the partners were frontline workers; their professions included (but were not limited to) mental health, dentistry, education, law, technology, childcare, and entertainment. Four of the spouses were sick with COVID early in the pandemic, two of whom believe they contracted the virus as a result of their partner's work. One spouse was widowed after losing her husband to COVID at the start of the pandemic, which he contracted at work.

Ethical considerations

All participants agreed to voluntarily participate in the study, and signed consent forms. The partners were given a brief explanation of the study's aims. All names and identifying information about the partner, the frontliners, and places of employment have been omitted. At the end of the informed consent, partners were provided with the contact information of mental health professionals, should they need support for emotional distress in the aftermath of the interview. This study was approved by the Bar-Ilan University Institutional Review Board.

Procedure

Participants were recruited via snowball sampling. In order to be eligible for the study the partner needed to be at least 25 years old, fluent in English, have a spouse or partner who is a doctor or nurse treating COVID patients in New York hospitals, and to not be a frontliner treating COVID patients in a New York hospital. Data was then gathered via semi-structured interviews that were conducted over Zoom or telephone, and recorded. All interviews were conducted in English by the first author and lasted between 30 and 50 minutes. The interviews were then transcribed by the first author or one of four university students. All participants were asked the same ten questions. These questions included, but were not limited to, inquiring about levels of stress, coping strategies, how the pandemic impacted daily life, and what challenges have been faced. Partners were also asked about their relationships and pandemic experiences: *What has been your experience during the COVID pandemic? In what way, if any, has your partner's job impacted your daily life since the pandemic began? What challenges have you faced throughout this pandemic? What coping strategies have you used to navigate the pandemic?*

Collecting data from the partner was a fascinating experience, as they shared a yet unheard-of experience and had an intimate-yet-still-outsider view of the pandemic. The partners' risk of infection was far greater than that of the general population, coupled with the knowledge that their partner could potentially fall ill or die as a result of their work. All of the partners had frontliners who were working intensive and long hours, and for that reason had to balance their own careers, household tasks, and often childcare largely solo. It was an honor to speak with them. Some of the interviews were exceptionally and unexpectedly emotional and difficult. In one interview, I [the first author] was unaware that I was going to be speaking to the widow of a nurse who had recently died from coronavirus which he contracted at work. After decades together, she was suddenly and shockingly without him. She wept throughout the interview, and it was devastating to hear about her painful loss. This was a very emotional interview to complete, as her suffering and grief were evident. I felt myself at a loss for words, and was overcome by a strong desire to assist her and lessen her enormous pain. I felt acutely aware of the differences in our pandemic experiences: I did not have a family member on the frontlines, whereas due to the bravery of her husband, she was now faced with a life without her beloved partner.

Findings

Data analysis resulted in the following four main themes:

Theme 1: The Partner as an Emotional Container for an Overwhelmed and Fearful Frontliner

The doctors and nurses shared their frightening experience of being on the frontlines in conversations with their partners.

One spouse shared:

> "He was the most anxious, nervous, overwhelmed I have ever seen him. He's the prototypical surgeon, where he's very cool, calm and collected, not a super emotional person, very cool under pressure, and this was like, he had unbelievable anxiety. When I say anxiety, he was anxious, nervous, thinking about this constantly."

Another wife observed:

> "*I have never seen him so disheartened. And we've been married for 45 years. I have never seen him so despondent and so helpless. He would often come home and had a really despondent feeling. I think he felt that there was little being done. People were so sick. There was nothing predictable about this. It was just a horrible thing.*"

Many partners reported that the frontliners were not properly trained or equipped to deal with a lot of the things they were facing, and that they were uncertain how to manage this new and overwhelming virus. Indeed, within the hospital the frontliners witnessed scenes of chaos unfold. A husband described his wife's experience of watching patients die of suffocation:

> "*She had these patients that she had to put on oxygen, but they weren't on wall oxygen, they were on tanks and the tanks would run out pretty quickly without any good way of keeping track. You have to put somebody on a tank and then you have to go deal with the next ten people. And in the meantime, the people who you put on the tank at the start of the shift are dead. And so, for me, my biggest memory of her talking about this is this image that she painted of people in the waiting room, and nobody knows when they died because their tanks ran out and they suffocated. And she's stepping over them, trying to figure out what to do.*"

This husband painted a particularly graphic and detailed description of what his wife experienced, and I [the first author] felt haunted by the image of rooms of people who had suffocated to death inside of a hospital.

Frontliners also shared with their spouses the experience of watching many patients code at the same time:

> "*A few of the days she was code leader. This was the scariest responsibility that she had. In the hospital, if someone has an acute emergency event, like if someone had a heart attack or stroke—in the case of COVID it was mostly a heart attack—they would call a code. The code team has to drop everything and run to the room where code is being called and do CPR and try to resuscitate the patient. Or to insert the breathing tube. That was scary, she was the leader of that team. She was witnessing the death firsthand. In COVID almost no one survived these codes. That was frightening in terms of her health, and also emotionally she witnessed a lot of people die.*"

Not only were frontliners witnessing mass patient deaths, but they were also devastated by the loss or illness of their bosses and colleagues at the hospital to COVID, "*My husband told me that like, there were I think 400 staff members out, they had tested positive, and they were out in quarantine, like they were all getting sick, all of the doctors, so staffing became very difficult.*" Shared another partner, "*He ended up losing the chairman at his hospital... They did everything for him and he passed away... I mean that was horrible. That was definitely the worst of it for him.*"

It appears that the frontliners were confronted with stress, trauma, and death in proportions that many had never before experienced. As such, they came home to their partners feeling fatigued, pained, and over-whelmed by what they had experienced at work.

Theme 2: The Partner's Increased Responsibilities in Support of the Frontliner

The stressed and overtaxed frontliners led to the partners taking on most—if not all—of the cleaning, cooking, errands, and (for some cou-ples) childcare responsibilities in order to decrease the pressure on the spouse after their hospital shift. Given the long hours and emotional and physical exhaustion that the frontliner was facing, partners regularly reported managing the household solo.

A husband shared, "*I was picking up a lot of slack, in terms of, like the days when she's at work, I'm operating like a single parent.*" Another partner shared her stress on many levels: "*Fear and anxiety, having to tolerate uncertainty about the future, physical separation of our family, having to balance work with personal challenges, having to manage some of the logistical challenges of living elsewhere, and arranging childcare.*"

Other partners made the choice—and had to rearrange their lives—to separate from their spouses for the safety of a pregnancy or a newborn and moved in with family members, "*I was seven months pregnant, so I moved out of our house. We separated for the period of time where the surge was happening in New York, and I moved in with my parents who also live in Manhattan across town, and I stopped seeing my husband in person for that time.*"

Additionally, many of the partners were balancing these responsibilities with their own careers, which were now taking place remotely at home. Many partners spoke about the challenges of balancing home responsi-bilities with their own careers:

> "*I think it's been pretty tough mostly because we have a two-year-old. And I've been mostly dealing, most of the burden was on me for the first two months. I just graduated from an MBA program. The first two months I was still a student, so I needed to still do all the exams and all the work and be with my baby basically 24/7. So that was pretty exhausting.*"

Because of the frontliner's exposure to COVID, many partners did not allow babysitters or family members to provide much needed support, out of fear of infecting others:

> *"It was literally 24/7 me with the kids. I had pretty much no interaction with other adults because with him, you know, I prioritize being able to see him* [her husband] *over being with other family because I wanted him to be with the kids and see them. I knew that was good for him, and it was good for me to be able to see him and have the help from him, but with his kind of continued exposure, I didn't feel safe going to my parents or going to my sisters or, you know, my in-laws... anyone... I really kind of cut everyone out from interaction during that time. It was incredibly isolating."*

Partners also reported feeling socially isolated or excluded as a result of the frontliner's job, as friends, neighbors, and family feared becoming infected with COVID should they interact with the frontliner's family, *"We have been treated differently by some of the people we know because of what my wife does for a living... the kids and the parents who would otherwise feel free to hang out with us have been a little more hesitant."* Other partners were scared of transmitting the virus to others due to their partner's job:

> *"I didn't want to be a vector* [i.e., one who transmits a disease]. *So, for me it was all of a sudden one day life changed and I started working from home and I very quickly stopped sending my son—we have a two-year-old who was going to daycare for ten hours a day—and I pulled him because I didn't want him infecting anybody in case he was infected or a vector."*

Multiple partners shared their feelings of being stigmatized or of feeling others distance themselves out of fear of contagion, as well as their own feelings of discomfort which kept them at a distance from others.

The partners were stressed and burdened across many dimensions—family, career, socially—as a result of the frontliners' job. However, partners shared their strong desire to *"be a support system for him and trying not to show him that I was really worried while he was here."* All partners also expressed their extreme pride for the sacrifices and dedication of their loved ones on the frontlines, and their desire to be as helpful as possible while the frontliners cared for coronavirus patients. Many partners shared the sentiment that *"to be the partner of somebody who is actually able to make a humongous difference in the face of the unfathomable definitely gave me a lot of pride."*

The partners were quickly faced with the responsibility of balancing many needs independently without the support of their friends or family.

Yet all did so and provided extensive support to their partner on the frontlines, despite the many stresses faced.

Theme 3: Self-Care: Differences in Partners' Responses

All partners were asked the following two questions in their interview: *What coping strategies have you used to navigate the pandemic? Are there any coping strategies from this pandemic that you plan to use moving forward; if so, what?* Partners listed techniques, and common strategies included strategies done by oneself, with one's partner, and also via supports external to their couple. Solo coping strategies included: exercise ("*I think the things that were most successful for me definitely were staying as active as possible. I noticed that when I was exercising regularly, each day, I was feeling less stressed or just less anxious*"); meditation and mindfulness ("*just trying to live in the moment with each other with the time that we had*"); creating structure in day-to-day life ("*a quarantine daily checklist. I was craving order*"); focusing on gratitude ("*I think gratitude is the biggest one; I've always really been big on appreciating what I have and how lucky I am and how privileged I am to have the things that I do*"); cooking ("*we've been cooking a lot more*"); spending time outside ("*I definitely have found that the more time I can spend outside, the more mentally healthy we've been*"); abstaining from media and social media ("*I stopped really reading the news*"); and establishing a routine ("*I also have a little bit of a routine and that helps me kind of cope*"). Some partners found communication with their frontliner to be helpful ("*we communicate a lot and we've always been really good about that*"). Others mentioned looking for external support: speaking with loved ones ("*staying in connection with friends and family*"); and speaking to a therapist ("*I have a regular therapist that I continue to see remotely during the pandemic, which was helpful*").

While many of the partners had coping strategies to share, several requested a definition of "a coping strategy" and then struggled to identify strategies they used. As one partner asked: "*What would be an example of a coping strategy?*" Shared another, "*I don't know. I've never really thought of coping strategies.*" Others did not understand how they could be useful, "*I don't see any changes. I don't need more coping than what I am doing now.*" Others did not make coping strategies a priority, "*I can't say that I've been good at the self-care side of things. I have not been good at making time for reading or anything that would let me unplug, it just, it has not been able to be a priority.*"

Multiple partners—interestingly, all male—mentioned the use of maladaptive strategies, such as substances or food: one partner shared how he made use of a collection of alcohol that had been given over the years by dinner guests: "*My liquor cabinet is gone.*" Shared another husband, "*I definitely drink more than I used to; it's just harder for me to resist as there is alcoholism in my family. And I've always done a pretty good job, I think, of keeping that at bay. But it is harder to keep that at arm's length when you're stuck at home stressed out for months."* Another partner turned to marijuana, *"I was using marijuana more than I usually do. Smoking and edibles one to three times a week, and normally it is zero to one time a week."* Another husband turned to food, *"One of my early coping mechanisms was that I ate anything I wanted to eat. Probably ate more ice cream than I should of, so I should probably stop that so I don't gain a ton of weight."*

Three of the 29 partners worked in the mental health profession—two as psychologists and one as a social worker. The therapists discussed their coping strategies as a continuation of what they had been doing in their lives prior to the pandemic, *"The same ones that I have always been using."* These professionals used strategies on themselves that they also used with patients. As one psychologist answered, *"I'm using my DBT (Dialectical Behavior Therapy) brain to categorize things differently."* The therapists detailed mindfulness and gratitude strategies, regular exercise, and focusing on the present, rather than the future unknowns. They also shared using yoga, breathwork, and positive reframing strategies to keep out negative thoughts. Having patients to focus upon was very helpful. As the social worker shared: *"My work saves me. There is a level of dissociation when I just have to focus on my patients."* The partners with a background in mental health were able to quickly mobilize and utilize the coping strategies that they spent years learning about and also hours reviewing with their patients. However, as seen with the partners, the use of coping strategies was not a given, nor did all partners understand how they could be used in times of stress.

Theme 4: The Trickle-Down Effect of a System-Wide Strain onto the Partners

The partners shared the lack of support and disappointment in various systems in which they had previously placed their trust, such as the hospital in which the frontliner worked, as well as in the local and state governments. The deficiencies of these systems trickled down onto the frontliners, which then affected their partners.

Partners reported a chaotic response from the hospital administration:

"A lot of it was just stressful for her, which came on to me too because they didn't know what procedures they should put into place, what they were they going into, nor did they have enough PPE... they really had to reinvent kind of how they work with patients and just so, there was there was all the, you know, and that created so many different stressors."

Not only was there not enough protective gear, but the plan of action was unclear as well:

> *"She would be listening to hear what was going to happen and what the plan was in terms of who is going to be deployed even, and the leadership either wasn't saying, or just didn't know, and then they would send people out to be deployed and they would tell them, initially, you're going to do this tour. You know, you're going to be deployed for two weeks and do three four days stints and then you'll be done. And they would just leave them out."*

In the beginning, one partner shared that the frontliner was even discouraged from wearing a mask:

> *"It was really interesting to see the dynamic between the hospital administration and the hospital staff. That it was a very different response. That there was even time where the hospital administration was saying, 'This is your own responsibility to take care of your health and not to wear masks because it scares the patient.' And any result in defying this rule of not wearing masks would end in the termination or sort of reprimand. So, it was really disheartening to see the divide and you know, it's always been there, but the administration was really concerned with money. They weren't concerned about their employees at all, until it became news.... You know, all of these brave souls putting their lives on the line and yet they were feeling like they were just disposable."*

Partners were resentful of the hospitals deploying the frontliner into COVID units, which was a virus that some of the doctors and nurses had little to no background in caring for (i.e., pediatricians, surgeons, etc. as opposed to pulmonologists or emergency room physicians). As one spouse explained:

> *"Being on the frontline was something she did not sign up for. It's beautiful to think that 'we are frontline workers, and we are going to run into the burning building. We are OB/GYNS, we didn't sign up to be an ER doctor, we didn't go into trauma.'"*

Echoed a second wife, *"He's not necessarily the profile of a doctor who would definitely be treating COVID, meaning he's not in the ER, he's not an emergency specialist and he's not a critical care specialist, you know, he's a surgeon."* Shared another partner, *"I think he [the frontliner] felt like he was not properly trained or equipped to deal with a lot of the things he was dealing with and it was hard and bad. I think it was a really difficult experience."* There was anger at the management of the hospital, lack of training and support, as well as fury and fear over the lack of sufficient personal protective equipment such as N95 masks and full-body gear.

The partners also shared their deep disappointment in the government:

> *"We are dismayed by the response of the New York State Government to the pandemic. I am very frustrated by it. The mayor mishandled it. Feel like I was planted on another planet. I never expected it. It was years in the making."*

The partners worried about their frontliners, as,

> *"it's pretty clear that there was no one* [governmentally] *in charge, and no one that is making decisions, no one that is guiding this ship and this ship is just aimlessly, kind of like sailing into the unknown, is definitely worrisome."*

Whereas the partners previously trusted in the government, now they shared they *"don't feel like the government is doing everything it can to protect you. That's what's really stressful about this."* Another partner was disappointed in the political culture, *"I think one of the biggest things is just here, in the US, is the political culture of COVID and the politicization of COVID has been really upsetting to her and frustrating."*

This system-wide failure not only fell on the frontline doctors and nurses, but it also impacted their families. As one partner stated, *"I knew how she was feeling, and it was just impossible to not kind of be stressed for her and I just knew that she was in a dangerous environment."* The partners feared for the safety, health, and even lives of their partners. One wife shared: *"I'd say this has been an extremely stressful situation.... I was constantly worried and preoccupied by his safety."* Almost all of the partners described the experience of having a partner on the frontlines as the most stressful experience of their lives.

Discussion

This study has provided insight into how the partners navigated the shared trauma with their frontliners. While a majority of partners reported the outbreak of the pandemic to be one of the most stressful times in their life, they also spoke of their immense pride in their frontliners' hard work and sacrifice. Not one single partner threatened to leave the frontliner during this acute crisis, but instead shouldered the burdens of their career, home-based tasks, and often childcare, all while offering support to their frontliners. Even when overwhelmed by systemic failures or their frontliner's fear or anxiety, partners focused on offering various means of support. In many ways, the partners navigated the same shared trauma as the frontliners and their patients in enduring the pandemic and its many stressors, such as the fear of their family and friends becoming ill, the unknown of what was to come, shortages of supplies, and the need to care for loved ones during a crisis.

In the first theme, the partner was found to provide exceptional emotional support for the frontliner, who felt overwhelmed, anxious, and fearful of what they were experiencing at work. The frontliners were confronted with a new virus that was resulting in the illness and death of never-before-experienced levels, and shared with their emotions, fatigue, and experiences with their partners. In the second theme, the partners took on high levels of practical support via taking on the majority of home-based tasks and childcare, in addition to their own careers. While 15 years of research on dyadic coping in close relationships has found that stress from outside the relationships—such as workplace stress—is negatively associated with relationships satisfaction and quality, and that it can be strongly predictive of divorce, poor communication, and the well-being of each partner (Bodenmann, 2000, 2005), this study found that acute stress led to high levels of support, teamwork, and loyalty. This may be due to the kind of stress the couple was experiencing and means of coping used: supportive coping—wherein one partner is confronted with a stressful event and is supported by the other—as well as common dyadic coping—when both partners are confronted with the same stress (Randall & Bodenmann, 2009) may have played a role in unifying the partners; in this case, both the partner and frontliner were utilizing the same common dyadic coping via the shared trauma of the virus.

Indeed, partners have also been found to have a protective role in the face of PTSD (Crevier et al., 2015), depression, and as a buffer against life stressors (Choi & Ha, 2011) via promoting shared resilience (Nuttman-Shwartz, 2014). In a meta-analysis of risk and protective factors for healthcare workers and military members in confronting outbreaks (such as HIV and SARS), it was found that those who were single or not living with family were at higher risk of acute distress, substance use, PTSD, depression, and anxiety (Vyas et al., 2016). It is possible that our findings point to how, in the face of an acute crisis, the partners were giving each other high to total levels of support as both the partner and the frontliner were confronted by a global pandemic during its outbreak in their neighborhoods. This could indicate resilience, possibly as a result of posttraumatic growth. Future studies should include a longitudinal design following these couples and their transactional of support, in order to better understand processes of support, as well as to examine other types of shared trauma.

Our results found differences in the use of self-care strategies. While some partners readily referenced techniques they use, others did not understand or make use of any kind of strategy, and some used maladaptive methods to manage their stress. The therapists interviewed here discussed their coping strategies as a continuation or extension of their professional training which they used regularly with their own patients and which is recognized in the self-care literature (Mills et al., 2020; Rokach & Boulazreg, 2020). In addition to the specific strategies discussed, the partners experienced the social support of their frontliners and oftentimes from their families as they navigated the pandemic; the social support of loved ones has found to be a key factor in navigating COVID-related stress (Babore et al., 2020; Saltzman et al., 2020). In line with other studies (Wardell et al., 2020), the partners here also used substances as a support strategy to deal with feelings of stress, depression, loss of social connectedness, or living alone (i.e., when separated from the frontliner) as they navigated the pandemic. Our results point to how there is a wide range of uses of self-care, and many of the partners found it to be helpful and adaptive in the face of enormous stress. At the same time, more education is needed as to what are useful strategies, and how to replace maladaptive techniques with adaptive methods, especially in the face of a crisis.

Our final theme found that the strains and failures of the hospitals and governments trickled down onto the partners. While the partners had previously trusted in these various systems, they found themselves disappointed, resentful, and angered by what the frontliner had experienced. Initial failures at the start of the pandemic included: 1) a lack of preparation; 2) no coordinated response in combatting the virus, restricting contact tracing of the virus, and shutting down the schools and city; 3) a lack of necessary PPE (especially masks) and also ventilators and supplies needed for patients (Kuchler & Edgecliffe-Johnson, 2020). The findings from our study reinforce the need for a system-wide perspective (Bronfenbrenner, 1974), and the vital importance of considering the experiences of the frontline workers, their families, and communities in the context of the trauma (Maercker & Hecker, 2016). The pandemic has reinforced the complex, nested, and interconnected systems in which both professionals and laypersons exist and operate, and to the extent these systems were stretched to their limits and experienced a cascade of failures and stresses during the outbreak (OECD, 2020). This is a phenomenon that is familiar to social workers who are taught to notice this interconnectedness as they work with clients.

Our findings can be conceptualized through the lens of this systems perspective (Bronfenbrenner, 1974; Payne, 2002)—a theory which examines the client holistically within the context of the various groups, dynamics, and environments in which he or she lives. Meaning, it is important for social workers who are interacting with or treating various groups of frontline workers, as well as professional and semi-professional workers, to give special attention to the partners' experience throughout the pandemic as well. In addition to their fears of their frontliners or themselves becoming sick or even dying, the partners also took on the majority of home and childcare responsibilities to decrease the pressure on the spouse after their hospital shift, all while balancing their own professional needs. They were living with partners who are greatly stressed by their jobs and were carrying their tension into the romantic relationship. While it is past the scope of this study, the shared trauma of the COVID outbreak may eventually result in secondary traumatic stress (STS) for the frontline partners. STS is "the natural consequent behaviors and emotions resulting from knowing about a traumatizing event experienced by a significant other—the stress resulting from helping or wanting to help a traumatized or suffering person" (Figley, 1993, 1995). It would be beneficial to continue to assess the partners for STS as they continue to navigate the pandemic. Furthermore, social workers may also want to give attention to potential posttraumatic growth (Tedeschi & Calhoun, 1996) that the couples have experienced as a result of this crisis. For example, the crisis may have led the partners to pull together, and to support one another in their coping.

It is also vital that social work renew its focus on practicing and teaching self-care techniques for the family as a whole. Without successful strategies in place, practitioners can face higher rates of burnout, compassion fatigue, vicarious trauma, secondary traumatic stress, or even posttraumatic stress disorder; however, using such strategies can enhance the ability to manage workload, professional development, and also to manage the stress of patients (Martin et al., 2019). Self-care can serve as an important buffer for those working in stressful environments between the professional and personal domains (Dugan & Barnes-Farrell, 2017). As seen in our study, those with training and practice in using self-care strategies were able to adapt to using these same techniques in times of acute stress. This suggests the importance of education of self-care, and how these strategies can potentially be effectively and quickly utilized in times of crisis.

Social workers may also wish to approach their work with frontliners, their spouses, and families from the perspective of trauma-informed care. This can include screening for trauma, minimizing distress and maximizing autonomy, and working with trauma-informed multidisciplinary teams and referrals (Reeves, 2015). Social workers may want to focus on increasing community, peer, and social support for the frontline families. Moreover, it is vital to increase hospital administrators' awareness of the need to support frontlines workers and their spouses (Smith et al., 2016).

In order to navigate the coming days of the shared trauma of the pandemic, it is important for social workers to seek both personal support and peer supervision. Social workers should reflect on how to identify their own stress and risks, and to reach out for support when needed. Further training on shared trauma, self-care, and navigating both acute and chronic crisis would be beneficial to social workers (Tosone et al., 2012). Additionally, having trauma-focused supervision is crucial. Supervisors and other social workers must learn how to identify staff and workers who are at higher risk while working in a trauma-focused setting (Menschner & Maul, 2016). The supervisors should consider how they distribute case-loads and assignments, especially during times of chronic stress (Tosone et al., 2015). Places of work may wish to put programs in place to support their employees, or safe spaces like "oasis rooms" or areas for staff to rest and recharge (Hecht, 2021). If the above supports are lacking, social workers are recommended to advocate for change at their places of work, schooling, and other professional associations (Tosone et al., 2012). Yet even in the face of shared trauma, social workers, their peers, and super-visors might also wish to consider the potential for enhancing their resi-lience and capacity for growth in the face of stress, otherwise known as "shared resilience," or the positive experiences that can be derived from a traumatic event—whether directly or in working with patients. For exam-ple, in navigating a crisis alongside a patient, the clinician may experience more growth and satisfaction from their work, as well as professional development. The clinician may also experience a deepened bond with their patient (Nuttman-Shwartz, 2014).

As with all studies, there were limitations to our research. It would be of interest to interview an even larger number of partners than the 29 inter-viewed here. Next, as our sample was largely Caucasian and heterosexual, further studies can interview partners from a more diverse range of racial, ethnic, and religious backgrounds. As our research took place in the aftermath of the crisis of the outbreak, it would be interesting to do a follow-up study in the months and years after the outbreak, to see how the partners have fared as the stresses of the pandemic became chronic. Research suggests that ongoing stressors are more detrimental to health and well-being than a short-term or occasional event (Lepore et al., 1997). This stress can have negative effects on an individual's health, emotions, immune, and nervous systems (Kemeny, 2003). While we examined the partners at the onset of the pandemic, coronavirus and its destructive effects continue, with no clear end date in sight.

As seen in our study, the partners of professionals working on the frontlines are a unique, stressed, and diverse population in need of further support and recognition. It would behoove social workers to recognize the spouses of frontliners as a diverse group in need of additional support in times of crisis (International Federation of Social Workers, 2021). Mental health professionals can provide support to these partners by acknowl-edging the unique stressors they have experienced in the pandemic. As the same time, frontline workers and their partners offered one another support as they together navigated an acute crisis, seemingly increasing couples' joint resilience. It is imperative to understand these frontline couples in the context of the systems in which they live and operate, and how their challenges and supports are due to, or reinforced by, these nested domains. As seen in the systems and hospital settings, there was not an equitable distribution of resources and wealth, and social workers can advocate on behalf of the frontline staff to receive the needed support, as well as to build networks of solidarity for the purpose of increased resilience and transformational change during a crisis such as the current pandemic (International Federation of Social Workers, 2021). Frontliners and their families continue to live and work in a shared trauma with the very people and communities which they are serving, and it is vital for social workers to provide care, support, and self-care strategies to this community as they battle the coronavirus pandemic in the days ahead.

Note

1 See Johns Hopkins University and Medicine Coronavirus Research Center: https://coronavirus.jhu.edu/.

References

Arnetz, J. E., Goetz, C. M., Arnetz, B. B., & Arble, E. (2020). Nurse reports of stressful situations during the COVID-19 pandemic: Qualitative analysis of survey responses. *International Journal of Environmental Research and Public Health*, 17(21), 1–12. https://doi.org/10.3390/ijerph17218126.

Babore, A., Lombardi, L., Viceconti, M. L., Pignataro, S., Marino, V., Crudele, M., Candelori, C., Bramanti, S. M.Trumello, C. (2020). Psychological effects of the COVID-2019 pandemic: Perceived stress and coping strategies among healthcare professionals. *Psychiatry Research*, 293. doi:10.1016/j.psychres.2020.113366.

Blumenthal, D., Fowler, E., Abrams, M., & Collins, S. (2020, October 8). COVID-19—Implications for the health care system. *The New England Journal of Medicine*. Retrieved from: www.nejm.org/doi/full/10.1056/nejmsb2021088.

Bodenmann, G. (2000). *Stress und Coping bei Paaren [Stress and coping in couples]*. Hogrefe.

Bodenmann, G. (2005). Dyadic coping and its significance for marital functioning. In T. Revenson, K. Kayser, & G. Bodenmann (Eds.), *Couples coping with stress: Emerging perspectives on dyadic coping* (pp. 33–50). American Psychological Association.

Bowden, E., Campanile, C., & Golding, B. (2020, March 25). Worker at NYC hospital where nurses wear trash bags as protection dies from coronavirus. *New York Post*. Retrieved from: https://nypost.com/2020/03/25/worker-at-nyc-hospital-where-nurses-wear-trash-bags-as-protection-dies-from-coronavirus/.

Bronfenbrenner, U. (1977). Toward an experimental ecology of human development, *American Psychologist*, 513–531.

Brown, N. & Borter, G. (2020, April 8). Speed of coronavirus deaths shock doctors as New York toll hits new high. *Reuters*. Retrieved from: www.reuters.com/a rticle/us-health-coronavirus-usa/speed-of-coronavirus-deaths-shock-doctors-as-new-york-toll-hits-new-high-idUSKBN21Q204.

Center on Budget and Policy Priorities. (2021, January 28). *Tracking the COVID-19 recession's effects on food, housing, and employment hardships*. Retrieved from: www.cbpp.org/research/poverty-and-inequality/tracking-th e-COVID-19-recessions-effects-on-food-housing-and.

Chen, R., Sun, C., Chen, J. J., Jen, H. J., Kang, X. L., Kao, C. C., & Chou, K. R. (2021). A large-scale survey on trauma, burnout, and posttraumatic growth among nurses during the COVID-19 pandemic. *International Journal of Mental Health Nursing*, 30(1), 102–116. https://doi.org/10.1111/inm.12796.

Choi, N. G., & Ha, J. H. (2011). Relationship between spouse/partner support and depressive symptoms in older adults: Gender difference. *Aging and Mental Health*, 15(3), 307–317. https://doi.org/10.1080/13607863.2010.513042.

Crevier, M. G., Marchand, A., Nachar, N., & Guay, S. (2015). Symptoms among partners, family, and friends of individuals with posttraumatic stress disorder: Associations with social support behaviors, gender, and relationship status. *Journal of Aggression, Maltreatment and Trauma*, 24(8), 876–896. https://doi.org/10.1080/10926771.2015.1069772.

Dekel, R., & Nuttman-Shwartz, O. (2014). Being a parent and a helping professional in the ongoing shared traumatic reality in southern Israel. In R. Pat-Horenczyk, D. Brom, & J. Vogel (Eds.), *Helping children cope with trauma: Individual, family and community perspectives* (pp. 224–240). Routledge.

Dekel, R., Goldblatt, H., Keidar, M., Solomon, Z., & Polliack, M. (2005). Being a wife of a veteran with posttraumatic stress disorder. *Family Relations*, 54, 24–36. http://dx.doi.org/10.1111/j.0197-6664.2005.00003.x.

Dekel, R., Levinstein, Y., Siegel, A., Fridkin, S., & Svetlitzky, V. (2015). Secondary traumatization of partners of war veterans: The role of boundary ambiguity. *Journal of Family*, 30(1), 63–71. https://doi.org/10.1037/fam0000163.

Dekel, R., Nuttman-Shwartz, O., & Lavi, T. (2016). Shared traumatic reality and boundary theory: How mental health professionals cope with the home/work conflict during continuous security threats. *Journal of Couple & Relationship Therapy*, 15(2), 121–134. https://doi.org/10.1080/15332691.2015.1068251.

Dekel, R., Siegel, A., Fridkin, S., & Svetlitzky, V. (2017). The double-edged sword: The role of empathy in military veterans' partners' distress. *Psychological Trauma: Theory, Research, Practice, and Policy*. https://doi.org/10.1037/tra0000265.

Dugan, A. G., & Barnes-Farrell, J. L. (2017). Time for self-care: Downtime recovery as a buffer of work and home/family time pressures. *Journal of Occupational and Environmental Medicine*, 59, e46–e56. doi:10.1097/JOM.0000000000000975.

Erdem, H., & Lucey, D. R. (2021). Healthcare worker infections and deaths due to COVID-19: A survey from 37 nations and a call for WHO to post national data on their website. *International Journal of Infectious Diseases*, 102, 239–241. https://doi.org/10.1016/j.ijid.2020.10.064.

Figley, C. R. (1993). Coping with stressors on the home front. *Journal of Social Issues*. https://doi.org/10.1111/j.1540-4560.1993.tb01181.x.

Figley, C. R. (Ed.). (1995). *Compassion fatigue: Coping with secondary traumatic stress disorder in those who treat the traumatized.* Brunner/Mazel Psychological Stress Series, No. 23. Brunner/Mazel.

Gavin, B., Hayden, J., Adamis, D., & McNicholas, F. (2020). Caring for the psychological well-being of healthcare professionals in the COVID-19 pandemic crisis. *Irish Medical Journal,* 113(4), 51.

Gold, J. (2020, December 22). We need to talk about the Covid-19 deaths of healthcare workers. *Forbes.* Retrieved from: www.forbes.com/sites/jessicagold/2020/12/22/we-need-to-talk-about-the-covid-19-deaths-of-healthcare-workers/?sh=75cc40103707.

Goldstein, J., & Weiser, B. (2020, April 14). "I cried multiple times": Now doctors are the ones saying goodbye. *The New York Times.* Retrieved from: www.nytimes.com/2020/04/13/nyregion/coronavirus-nyc-doctors.html.

Hecht, P. (2021). Repurposed, reassigned, and redeployed. In C. Tosone (Ed.), *Shared trauma, shared resilience during a pandemic: Social work in the time of COVID-19* (pp. 15–20). Springer.

International Federation of Social Workers. (2021). *Global social work statement of ethical principles.* Retrieved from www.ifsw.org/global-social-work-statement-of-ethical-principles/.

Kaplan, J., Frias, L., & McFall-Johnsen, M. (2020, September 23). Our ongoing list of how countries are reopening, and which ones remain under lockdown. *Business Insider.* Retrieved from: www.businessinsider.com/countries-on-lockdown-coronavirus-italy-2020-3.

Kemeny, M. E. (2003). The psychobiology of stress. *Current Directions in Psychological Science,* 12, 124–129.

Kisner, J. (2020, December 8). What the chaos in hospitals is doing to doctors. *The Atlantic.* Retrieved from: www.theatlantic.com/magazine/archive/2021/01/covid-ethics-committee/617261/.

Kuchler, H., & Edgecliffe-Johnson, A. (2020). How New York's missteps let Covid-19 overwhelm the US. *Financial Times.* Retrieved from: www.ft.com/content/a52198f6-0d20-4607-b12a-05110bc48723.

Lavi, T., Nuttman-Shwartz, O., & Dekel, R. (2015). Therapeutic intervention in a continuous shared traumatic reality: An example from the Israeli—Palestinian conflict. *British Journal of Social Work,* 1–17.

Lepore, S. J., Miles, H. J., & Levy, J. S. (1997). Relation of chronic and episodic stressors to psychological distress, reactivity, and health problems. *International Journal of Behavioral Medicine,* 4(1), 39–59. https://doi.org/10.1207/s15327558ijbm0401_3.

Li, W., Frank, E., Zhao, Z., Chen, L., Wang, Z., Burmeister, M., & Sen, S. (2020). Mental health of young physicians in China during the novel coronavirus disease 2019 outbreak. *JAMA Network Open,* 3(6). https://doi.org/10.1001/jamanetworkopen.2020.10705.

Madani, D. (2020, June 14). Therapists are under strain in COVID-19 era, counseling clients on trauma they're also experiencing themselves. *NBC News.* www.nbcnews.com/news/us-news/therapists-are-under-strain-COVID-era-counseling-clients-trauma-they-n1230956.

Maercker, A., & Hecker, T. (2016). Broadening perspectives on trauma and recovery: A socio-interpersonal view of PTSD. *European Journal of Psychotraumatology,* 7, 1–10. https://doi.org/10.3402/ejpt.v7.29303.

Martin, E. M., Myers, K., & Brickman, K. (2019). Self-preservation in the work-place: The importance of well-being for social work practitioners and field supervisors. *Social Work*, 65(1), 74–81.

Menschner, C., & Maul, A. (2016). *Key ingredients for successful trauma-informed care implementation.* Center for Health Care Strategies, Inc. Retrieved from: samhsa.gov/sites/default/files/programs_campaigns/childrens_mental_health/atc-whitepaper-040616.pdf

Mills, J., Ramachenderan, J., Chapman, M., Greenland, R., & Agar, M. (2020). Prioritising workforce wellbeing and resilience: What COVID-19 is reminding us about self-care and staff support. *Palliative Medicine*, 34(9), 1137–1139. https://doi.org/10.1177/0269216320947966.

Nguyen, L. H., Drew, D. A., Graham, M. S., Joshi, A. D., Guo, C. G., et al. (2020). Risk of COVID-19 among front-line health-care workers and the general community: A prospective cohort study. *The Lancet Public Health*, 5(9), e475–e483. https://doi.org/10.1016/S2468-2667(20)30164-X.

Nuttman-Shwartz, O. (2014). Shared resilience in a traumatic reality: A new concept for trauma workers exposed personally and professionally to collective disaster. *Trauma, Violence, and Abuse*, 466–475. https://doi.org/10.1177/1524838014557287.

Nuttmann-Shwartz, O., & Dekel, R. (2009). Challenges for students working in a shared traumatic reality. *The British Journal of Social Work*, 39, 522–538.

OECD. (2020, April 28). *A systemic resilience approach to dealing with Covid-19 and future shocks.* Retrieved from: www.oecd.org/coronavirus/policy-responses/a-systemic-resilience-approach-to-dealing-with-covid-19-and-future-shocks-36a5bdfb/.

Papero, D. (2017). Trauma and the family: A systems-oriented approach. *Australian & New Zealand Journal of Family Therapy.* https://doi.org/10.1002/anzf.1269.

Payne, M. (2002). The politics of systems theory within social work. *Journal of Social Work*, 2(3), 269–292.

Ramachandran, S., Kusisto, L., & Honan, K. (2020, June 11). How New York's coronavirus response made the pandemic worse. *The Wall Street Journal.* Retrieved from: www.wsj.com/articles/how-new-yorks-coronavirus-response-made-the-pandemic-worse-11591908426.

Randall, A. K., & Bodenmann, G. (2009). The role of stress on close relationships and marital satisfaction. *Clinical Psychology Review*, 29(2), 105–115. https://doi.org/10.1016/j.cpr.2008.10.004.

Reeves, E. (2015). A synthesis of the literature on trauma-informed care. *Issues in Mental Health Nursing*, 36(9), 698–709. doi:10.3109/01612840.2015.1025319.

Rokach, A., & Boulazreg, S. (2020). The COVID-19 era: How therapists can diminish burnout symptoms through self-care. *Current Psychology.* https://doi.org/10.1007/s12144-020-01149-6.

Saakvitne, K. (2002). Shared trauma: The therapist's increased vulnerability. *Psychoanalytic Dialogues: The International Journal of Relational Perspectives*, 12 (3), 443–449.

Sacks, E. (2021, January 1). A club nobody "wanted to join": How Covid widows are finding support through Facebook. *NBC News.* Retrieved from: www.nbcnews.com/news/us-news/club-nobody-wanted-join-how-covid-widows-are-finding-support-n1252478.

Saltzman, L. Y., Hansel, T. C., & Bordnick, P. S. (2020). Loneliness, isolation, and social support factors in post-COVID-19 mental health. *Psychological Trauma:*

Theory, Research, Practice, and Policy, 12, 55–57. https://doi.org/10.1037/tra 0000703.

Schelleles, S., & Dekel, R. (2001). Personality organization of post-traumatic stress disorders patients and their spouses. *Sichot*, XV, 208–218. (Hebrew.)

Schwirtz, M. (2020, March 30). Nurses die, doctors fall sick and panic rises on virus front lines. *The New York Times*. Retrieved from: www.nytimes.com/2020/03/30/nyregion/ny-coronavirus-doctors-sick.html.

Shah, K., Kamrai, D., Mekala, H., Mann, B., Desai, K., & Patel, R. S. (2020). Focus on mental health during the coronavirus (COVID-19) pandemic: Applying learnings from the past outbreaks. *Cureus*, 12: e7405. doi:10.7759/cureus.7405.

Smith, J. C., Hyman, S. M., Andres-Hyman, R. C., Ruiz, J. J., & Davidson, L. (2016). Applying recovery principles to the treatment of trauma. *Professional Psychology: Research and Practice*, 47(5), 347–355. https://doi.org/10.1037/pro0000105.

Sutphin, S. T., McDonough, S., & Schrenkel, A. (2013). The role of formal theory in social work research: Formalizing family systems theory. *Advances in Social Work*, 14(2), 501–517.

Tedeschi, R. G., & Calhoun, L. G. (1996). The posttraumatic growth inventory: Measuring the positive legacy of trauma. *Journal of Traumatic Stress*, 9(3), 455–472. https://doi.org/10.1002/jts.2490090305.

The Physicians Foundation. (2020, September 17). *Physician Survey: Part 2*. Retrieved from: https://physiciansfoundation.org/research-insights/the-physicians-foundation-2020-physician-survey-part-2/.

The World Bank. (2020, June 8). *COVID-19 to plunge global economy into worst recession since World War II*. Retrieved from: www.worldbank.org/en/news/press-release/2020/06/08/covid-19-to-plunge-global-economy-into-worst-recession-since-world-war-ii.

Thompson, C.N., Baumgartner, J., Pichardo, C., et al. (2020). COVID-19 outbreak—New York City, February 29–June 1, 2020. *Morbidity and Mortality Weekly Report*, 69: 1725–1729. http://dx.doi.org/10.15585/mmwr.mm6946a2external icon.

Tomer, A., & Kane, J. (2020, June 10). To protect frontline workers during and after COVID-19, we must define who they are. Brookings. Retrieved from: www.brookings.edu/research/to-protect-frontline-workers-during-and-after-covid-19-we-must-define-who-they-are/.

Tosone, C., Nuttman-Shwartz, O., & Stephens, T. (2012). Shared trauma: When the professional is personal. *Clinical Social Work Journal*, 40(2), 231–239. https://doi.org/10.1007/s10615-012-0395-0.

Tosone, C., McTighe, J. P., & Bauwens, J. (2015). Shared traumatic stress among social workers in the aftermath of hurricane Katrina. *British Journal of Social Work*, 45(4), 1313–1329. https://doi.org/10.1093/bjsw/bct194.

Vielkind, J. (2020, April 14). After fighting coronavirus, New York's health-care workers sleep away from home: Workers turn to hotel rooms, their cars and other arrangements to keep their families safe. *The Wall Street Journal*. Retrieved from: www.wsj.com/articles/after-fighting-coronavirus-new-yorks-health-care-workers-sleep-away-from-home-11586895678.

Vyas, K. J., Delaney, E. M., Webb-Murphy, J. A., & Johnston, S. L. (2016). Psychological impact of deploying in support of the US response to Ebola: A systematic review and meta-analysis of past outbreaks. *Military Medicine*, 181 (11), e1515–e1531. https://doi.org/10.7205/MILMED-D-15-00473.

Wardell, J. D., Kempe, T., Rapinda, K. K., Single, A., Bilevicius, E., Frohlich, J. R., Hendershot, C. S., & Keough, M. T. (2020). Drinking to cope during COVID-19 pandemic: The role of external and internal factors in coping motive pathways to alcohol use, solitary drinking, and alcohol problems. *Alcoholism: Clinical and Experimental Research*, 44(10), 2073–2083. https://doi.org/10.1111/acer.14425.

World Health Organization. (2020, April 27). WHO timeline—COVID-19. Retrieved from: www.who.int/news/item/27-04-2020-who-timeline—covid-19.

World Health Organization. (2021). *Coronavirus*. Retrieved from: www.who.int/health-topics/coronavirus#tab=tab_1.

Wu, Y., Wang, J., Luo, C., Hu, S., Lin, X., et al. (2020). A comparison of burnout frequency among oncology physicians and nurses working on the frontline and usual wards during the COVID-19 epidemic in Wuhan, China. *Journal of Pain and Symptom Management*, 60(1), e60–e65. https://doi.org/10.1016/j.jpainsymman.2020.04.008.

Ying, Y., Ruan, L., Kong, F., Zhu, B., Ji, Y., & Lou, Z. (2020). Mental health status among family members of health care workers in Ningbo, China, during the coronavirus disease 2019 (COVID-19) outbreak: A cross-sectional study. *BMC Psychiatry*, 20(1), 1–11. https://doi.org/10.1186/s12888-020-02784-w.

Chapter 4

Trauma, Policing, and United States Social Work Practice

Aimee Jette and Tina Sacks

The murder of George Floyd at the hands of a Minneapolis police officer in May 2020 (Hill et al., 2020) led to an unprecedented reckoning on policing, racial injustice, and trauma in the US and around the world. Many likened the cruelty of Mr. Floyd's killing to a modern-day lynching (Brown, 2020) harkening back to America's recent past in which Black people were terrorized to maintain a racial caste system (Carr, 2016). This system of terror undoubtedly leaves psychological, physical, and emotional scars as well as trauma, which is defined as exposure to an extraordinary experience that presents a physical or psychological threat to oneself or others and generates a reaction of helplessness and fear (American Psychiatric Association, 2013). Moreover, the disproportionate impact of police violence on racial and ethnic minorities may be described as a form of collective and historical trauma (Walters et al., 2011). These traumatic events (e.g., slavery, lynching, etc.) target specific communities and cause catastrophic upheaval, which has been posited to have pernicious effects that persist across generations through multiple mechanisms from the biological to the behavioral (Walters et al., 2011). As we will demonstrate throughout this chapter, despite violence being more visible recently due to increased video footage of police-civilian encounters, police violence toward Black people and other minoritized groups has a long history in the US.

To explore the implications of police violence on well-being, this chapter will 1) describe the history of policing as an instrument of racially targeted state control in the US, 2) describe the relationship between social work, policing and trauma, including shared trauma, 3) discuss how discrimination and violence by police specifically affects minorities as well as other groups, including women and LGBTQIA+ (lesbian, gay, bisexual, transgender, queer/questioning, intersex, asexual/agender) people, 4) describe the current challenges to implementing police reform, and 5) discuss how some social work practitioners (and other mental health providers) may experience (shared) trauma along with their clients, while others may struggle to understand the particularities of racial trauma and police violence. Throughout this chapter, we present case studies to facilitate analysis and discussion.

DOI: 10.4324/9781003176947-6

Brief History of US Policing

Like much of US history, the origins of American policing go back to the enslavement of African people. Specifically, modern policing emerged from slave patrols in which White slave owners controlled the movements of enslaved Black people through violence and fear. Although many scholars have traced this connection, the relationship between the history of slavery and contemporary policing is not well known among the lay public and social work scholars alike. Moreover, there is even less attention given to policing and its connection to another professional group, American social work. The profession of social work also has a long, complicated history that includes working on the front lines of the struggle for social justice as well as working as agents of social control (Abulhul, 2021; Piven & Cloward, 2012). Therefore, a discussion of policing and social work must begin with a thorough description of the origins and contemporary practices of both professions.

Policing in the US originates with settler colonialism and slavery. According to sociologist Evelyn Nakano Glenn (2015),

> The settler goal of seizing and establishing property rights over land and resources required the removal of indigenes, which was accomplished by various forms of direct and indirect violence, including militarized genocide. Settlers sought to control space, resources, and people not only by occupying land but also by establishing an exclusionary private property regime and coercive labor systems, including chattel slavery to work the land, extract resources, and build infrastructure.
>
> (p. 54)

Importantly, Nakano Glenn (2015) takes note of the fact that both the removal of Native peoples and the institution of chattel slavery served to establish property rights. Property rights play an important role in the American imagination, particularly with regard to using police officers to maintain control over property, space, and land. The enslavement and exploitation of African-descended people required the violent oversight of their physical bodies. The creation of Black bodies as property required someone to manage and control their movements through physical space and to prevent runaways from causing a loss of "property" and money to their owners.

In what Saadiya Hartman (1997) terms "the spatial organization of domination" (p. 68), slave owners created patrols to ensure that enslaved people could not move about freely. Hartman notes that one of the key characteristics of the US slave era was the maintenance of domination through controlling people's freedom of movement through physical space

(Hartman, 1997). Policing began as a system of racially targeted law enforcement that extended beyond slave patrols to include expert slave catchers, ordinary White citizens, overseers, constables, and local police. In fact, historian Sally Hadden notes that policing in the American South was fundamentally preoccupied with controlling the movement of enslaved people:

> The history of police work in the South grows out of this early fasci-
> nation, by white patrollers, with what African American slaves were
> doing. Most law enforcement was, by definition, white patrolmen
> watching, catching or beating enslaved persons.
>
> (Hadden, 2003, p. i)

Modern policing maintains many of these characteristics by patrolling where people are allowed to shop, walk, recreate, and simply exist.

The concept of race and the establishment of a hierarchy of racial differences were used to justify the degradation of enslaved and Indigenous peoples. Anthropologist Audrey Smedley notes:

> In the US, race ideology, as a body of beliefs and attitudes about
> human differences, evolved in the wake of the establishment of slavery
> only for Africans and their descendants. The invention of race was pri-
> marily a product of efforts to justify slavery and the continuing con-
> quest and exploitation of Native Americans on the basis of "natural"
> difference and inferiority. Race from its beginning was a mechanism
> denoting social ranking and inequality of human groups... When Chi-
> nese and Japanese immigrants began to arrive in North America in the
> 19th century, their physical features also became interpreted as evidence
> of an inferior race status.
>
> (Smedley, 2003)

The deployment of a racial hierarchy based on skin color and other physical characteristics differentiated policing in the US from its European antecedents (Hadden, 2003). Slave patrols emerged as appendages of slave owners, increasing the control over Blacks (Hadden, 2003). In the American context, race was the dominant and most important category upon which people were surveilled and controlled. Although poor White people and free Black people were subject to police authority, the regulation of the institution of slavery was the primary reason for police in the US during the slave era (Hadden, 2003).

Even after slavery was abolished in 1865, the logics of slavery, particularly the desire to control the movements of Blacks and other people of color through policing, remained. Under this system of rigid racial hierarchy, Black people and other people of color were often thought to be less than human and deserving of brutality and discrimination. In fact, many scholars have argued that pervasive anti-Blackness placed Black people outside of the human condition: "Black humanity is... 'a paradigmatic impossibility' because to be Black is to be 'the very antithesis of a Human subject'" (Wilderson, 2010, p. 9). Given this context, the murders of George Floyd, Ayanna Stanley, Eric Garner, and many other Black Americans may be understood as an extension of the logics of slavery and anti-Blackness that formed the foundation of American society and police practices.

Brief History of US Social Work: Social Control, Social Change, and Policing

Much like the profession of policing, the origins of social work are complex, particularly with regard to race and racism. Modern American social work emerged during the Progressive Era (1890–1920) to address rapid social changes associated with urbanization, industrialization, and immigration (Katz, 1996). Although a detailed history of social work is beyond the scope of this chapter, it is important to note that social workers have often aligned themselves with the state (Piven & Cloward, 2012). For example, social workers cooperated with the US government during the forced removal and incarceration of Japanese Americans during World War II (Park, 2020) and have been criticized for the disproportionate removal of Black, Indigenous, and Latinx children from families as a result of involvement in the child welfare system (Roberts, 2009).

Given the 2020 reckoning around structural racism and policing, social work has been called upon to reconsider its history of complicity and social control. Further, although the profession is bound by a code of ethics and a belief in social justice, social workers have long aligned themselves with policing and prisons. For example, even as recently as the summer of 2020, the National Association of Social Work championed social work's history of collaboration with the police (McClain, 2020). On the other hand, many social work scholars have suggested that the profession must come to terms with its origins as a mechanism of social control, particularly with respect to the carceral state. Carceral social work is defined as:

> a form of social work that relies on logics of social control and White supremacy and that uses coercive and punitive practices to manage BIPOC and poor communities. Carceral social work enacts these logics and practices in tandem with the penal arm of the state, condoning and in many cases collaborating or integrating with police, prosecutors, jails, prisons, juvenile and criminal courts.
>
> (Jacobs et al., 2021, p. 39)

As such, we must acknowledge social work's complicity with systems of coercive social control in order to consider how to fully address the trauma of state-sanctioned police violence. As social workers and healthcare providers, we must ask ourselves difficult questions, such as where do I fit in this system, what part do I play? Are there areas where I condone and collaborate with the police or carceral system? Is it possible that alignment with these systems reduces the amount of trauma I experience? Further, when a social worker or therapist works within the carceral system, is there a shared trauma between social worker and the persecuted? To answer this, we must consider different types of trauma and attempt to identify what, if any, shared trauma exists.

Is Police Violence a Shared Trauma?

Consider these examples: What if you follow the news and are impacted emotionally by coverage of police shootings and accounts of brutality? What if you have lost relationships with friends and peers after expressing your views? What if it happens in your community or to someone close to you? What if you work in a community that is repeatedly impacted by police brutality? What if you have a client who is struggling with a history of police brutality, and you are deeply moved by the explicit detail of their accounts? What if you are losing sleep, develop intrusive thoughts, or are constantly on edge after working with individuals directly impacted? Is police brutality a shared trauma?

We must first identify what shared trauma is, and what it is not. According to Tosone et al. (2012, p. 231), shared trauma "contains aspects of primary and secondary trauma, and more accurately describes the extraordinary experiences of clinicians exposed to the same community trauma as their clients." Boulanger (2013) suggests shared trauma arises when mental health practitioners and clients endure the same tragedy. Common environments where a shared trauma transpires are devastating natural disasters (hurricanes, tornadoes, floods), September 11th, or living and working in war zones—witnessing these events impacts clinicians and clients alike, profoundly altering how they look at the world. Shared traumatic reality describes a situation where social workers, therapists, and clients live in the same community impacted by disaster (Dekel et al., 2016).

Let's now consider several key elements of shared trauma. Primary trauma happens when someone witnesses or experiences a traumatic event. A victim of police brutality will experience primary trauma. Secondary trauma, vicarious trauma, and compassion fatigue (Zimering et al., 2003) may occur after hearing in-depth, vivid, recurrent accounts of human suffering. Akin to primary trauma, secondary trauma may cause PTSD-like symptoms such as hyperarousal or intrusive thoughts (such as recalling the client's story over and over). Secondary traumatic stress disorder may cause a "perceived threat to life or safety," just through witnessing accounts of the client's trauma (the clinician doesn't have to go through it firsthand) which results in physiological and emotional symptoms occurring through the empathetic connection to a client's account (Bell & Robinson, 2013). It is possible that a therapist or social worker will experience secondary trauma or even develop secondary traumatic stress disorder after listening to their clients' accounts of police brutality.

But what happens when a therapist or social worker lives in the same community impacted deeply by acts of police brutality, for example in Minneapolis, MN where George Floyd was murdered? Does this lay the groundwork for a shared trauma for therapists who are treating clients there? Yes and no. The history of slavery and its undeniable connection to policing impacts people in profoundly different ways and is based on the color of one's skin. If I am a White social worker who lives and works in Minneapolis and am exposed to secondary trauma from repeated eyewitness accounts of the murder of George Floyd, I do not directly experience anti-Blackness the way someone with a darker skin color would in the United States. Further, I do not have the generational lived experience of fearing for my life as Black and Brown individuals do. In many cases, it is likely I was raised with the belief that police are protectors, not agents of terror who violate human rights. George Floyd's murder will not impact me at the same level as Black and Brown social workers living in the same community who—in contrast to social workers like me who do not share the lived experience of police brutality—can be impacted by shared trauma as they work with their Black and Brown clients.

The authors suggest that this differentiation needs to be considered when reflecting on whether there is a shared trauma between clinician and client. According to Baum (2010), a shared trauma impacts everyone in the community simultaneously. Slavery and contemporary policing are inextricably linked and add to the degree of trauma that Black and Brown individuals are likely to experience in a community impacted by police brutality. It is incorrect to assume that all individuals in a given community are impacted the same way. The authors of this chapter posit that these exceptional experiences must consider whether individuals carry the embodied forces of the history of slavery, which conclusively depends on the color of one's skin and susceptibility to anti-Blackness in the United States.

Police Violence and Trauma

Although instances of police violence have become increasingly visible in the media and in the differences in political stances, social position, and lived experience, it is likely that Americans will have varying perspectives on police violence in particular and the criminal legal system in general. Moreover, as we will demonstrate throughout the remainder of the chapter, the impact of police violence affects ethno-racial minorities, women, and members of the LGBTQIA+ communities differently than members of majority communities. Given the pervasiveness of police violence including stop-and-frisk practices, deadly police-civilian encounters, and police harassment as we will see in the case studies of Khalon and Brian, social workers and other mental health practitioners must deepen their expertise and ability to treat trauma and shared trauma, particularly complex and post-traumatic stress syndrome.

Racial Disproportionality

Blackness has been purposely conflated with violence and criminality (Muhammad, 2019). As a result, there is a common misconception that police shootings mainly occur in the context of violent criminal behavior in low-income communities of color. There is a prevalent narrative that police officers need to protect themselves from (Black) men carrying weapons. Yet, when Ross (2015) analyzed police homicide data in the US Police-Shooting Database and the FBI's Supplemental Homicide Reports to explore the motivation for police shootings, he found that the risk of being shot by police is not a function of the crime rate. Rather, it is based on race/ethnicity. Strikingly, the probability of an unarmed Black man being shot in the US is almost 3.5 times higher than his unarmed White counterpart. Some counties in the US report that the ratio is as high as 20 to 1. The disparity in these numbers can be explained by factoring in differences in economic status, education level, and residential segregation between Blacks and Whites (Ross, 2015). For example, in urban communities where the socioeconomic divide is more significant and the number of Black community members is higher, the risk dramatically increases. Ross therefore concluded that police violence is correlated with race but not with the rate of violent crime in the area.

The police violence rate can also be predicted using a structural racism index. Structural racism includes residential segregation, disparities regarding education and incarceration, economic inequality, and employment incongruity (Mesic et al., 2018). Residential segregation is based on census data and considers the disparity between Black and White residents in a specific state. Education takes into account how many Black people have a college degree compared to White people. The incarceration rate includes how many Blacks and Whites are in jails and prisons. Economic inequality compares Blacks and Whites with respect to whether they live in poverty, their household income, and whether they rent or own their home. Employment incongruity evaluates the difference in unemployment between Blacks and Whites. Each state gets a rating between 1 and 100; the lower the number, the lower the likelihood of structural racism. The most notable indicators of the structural racism index were segregation, economic inequality, and employment incongruity. Interestingly, Mesic et al. (2018) found that the index could predict the difference in police shootings of unarmed Blacks and Whites. For example, the index ranged from a low of 25.9 in Montana to 74.9 in Wisconsin. For every ten-point rise in a state's index, the difference between police shootings of unarmed Blacks and Whites grew by 24%. The states with the highest index were Wisconsin (74.9), Minnesota (70), and New Jersey (68.5). These data therefore suggest a reconsideration of assumptions about police violence.

The following questions should be considered with respect to our own assumptions about police violence: What is the narrative that I grew up with around police violence and why it takes place? Are there specific images related to police violence that I hold in my mind? Are there conversations about police violence that I can recall with friends and family?

When a state ranks high on the structural racism index but shows an insignificant difference between police shootings of unarmed Blacks and Whites, racial profiling often manifests in other ways. Connecticut fits this profile since it has a structural racism index of 63.9 but a ratio of unarmed Black-to-White police shootings of 0. A common form of racial profiling is carried out during traffic stops. In a 2015 state report on traffic stop data, Connecticut minorities made up 46% of the driving population, yet accounted for 63% of traffic stops. In New Haven, CT, Black drivers were 2.9 times more likely to be pulled over than Whites, and the Latinx community 1.3 times more likely. In addition, it was found that Black and Latinx drivers were stopped and searched at a much higher rate than White drivers in Connecticut even though contraband was more likely to be found in a White driver's vehicle. Traffic stops also increased significantly during the day, when the color of one's skin is more obvious (Connecticut Racial Profiling Prohibition Project, 2015). Notably, in an analysis of 100 million stops across 21 state agencies between 2011 and 2018 that controlled for time of day, United States Black drivers were more likely to be stopped in daylight and less likely after sunset, suggesting that this kind of discrimination is happening nationwide. This is important to recognize because police violence and racial profiling—which often involve physical beatings, use of a weapon or taser, inappropriate sexual behavior, bullying, or threats—lead to physical, emotional, and psychological trauma and can have long-lasting negative effects on the victim (Pierson et al., 2020). According to the 2020 Police Violence Report (Mapping Police Violence, 2021),

> Some cities and states have begun to restrict or remove the police from traffic enforcement. In July 2020, the City of Berkeley passed legislation moving traffic enforcement duties from the police department to a new agency of unarmed civil servants. Other cities like Cambridge, MA, are considering similar measures. And in November 2020,

Virginia lawmakers passed HB 5058 which prohibits police from stopping cars for equipment violations like a broken light or tinted windows.

(n.p.)

Case Study: Khalon

Khalon is a 35-year-old African American cisgender male who resides in Hartford, Connecticut, US. He received an undergraduate degree in psychology from New York University and a master's degree in social work from Fordham University. He currently works as a social worker. He reported that he's had an excessive number of run-ins with the police. His earliest memory of police violence took place when he was 20 years old at Penn Station in New York City. Waiting for his next bus, Khalon sat down on a bench. Feeling safe enough to wait and rest, he pulled his baseball cap over his eyes. He awoke with a start as someone snatched the hat off his head. He reached out to grab his hat back when he realized a police officer was responsible. Suddenly, another police officer grabbed him, "and then they were on me. From there, it just escalated." The officers handcuffed him, grabbed him by all four limbs, and dragged him away, dropping him at one point and thereby causing him to fall on his face. "They put me in a cell; I was in the system for three days. I don't remember what the charges were." Finally, Khalon was released, with bruises on his wrists and a swollen face, unclear whether his injuries stemmed from being hit or dropped.

A couple of years later, when Khalon was walking down a crowded street with his buddy, "the officers rolled up on us, searched us, and didn't find anything." The White police officer who was in his early 40s said to Khalon, "Are you eyeballing me?" The context caught Khalon off guard, reminding him of something one would hear in the 1950s American South. Suddenly the police officer pulled out his gun and put it in Khalon's face. Khalon was unclear about what happened next. Later that year, he was in the city in the back of a cab when a police officer pulled the taxi driver over. The officer got Khalon out of the car, frisked him, searched the back of the cab, and then told the taxi driver that he'd received an anonymous tip that Khalon had weapons. Khalon remembers, "It just happened out of nowhere." When asked about traffic stops while driving his car, Khalon reports, "The stops for no reason... It happens too many times."

In recent years, Khalon spent time with friends in a town in Connecticut that was predominantly White (82%). As Khalon talked outside with his friend, a police officer pulled up and started asking him personal questions. Khalon remembers thinking, "I didn't do anything; you [the police officer] aren't offering any information about yourself." Eventually, the police officer left. A month later, he stood near his car in the same town after purchasing coffee at a local coffee shop. "I was on my phone with a [coffee]… in hand when a police officer drove up and started asking me what I was doing there." In another instance, at Khalon's place of employment where there was a mandated officer for a client he worked with, the officer told him that "Hispanics and Blacks in the city are better off dead because they are animals." Khalon realized that the officer might have had negative experiences in the past with the "certain minorities," but he was shocked at the officer's binary thinking.

When Khalon was asked what he feels is the most important thing a social worker / therapist should know when working with an individual who has been exposed to police violence, he replied that the social worker / therapist needs to understand the nuances of every situation and refrain from using blanket responses, "Having black-and-white thinking isn't helpful. You can have the opinion that it's awful. However, it's more helpful for me to go through the grey areas, look at it from all angles, and not judge what the police were thinking. Look at the whole thing honestly, openly discussing, without labeling."

When Khalon thinks about law enforcement now, he gets a visceral reaction: tightness in his shoulders, a lump in his throat, automatic thoughts come up such as, "why will they engage me?" While he recalls several encounters with police that were reasonable and thoughtful and didn't possess a blanket view that all Blacks are bad, he remains hypervigilant at navigating every encounter with a police officer by anticipating incorrect assumptions. He lives with an extra layer of anxiety and stress that his White counterpart Brian (who will be introduced in the next case study) does not.

Khalon suggests having a system in place for victims, an authentic advocate for follow-up. "When my face was swollen, I was alone in the jail cell for those days. Then I had to go back to school and explain my injuries; there was nobody to help me process it or offer empathy. It was just, that's what happens to Black people." It's therefore imperative not to normalize the experience of a victim of police violence. While Khalon received sympathy for his experiences, the underlying message was often, "this is just what Black males have to go through, this is how it is, and there's no way to fix it." Each experience should be explored without relegating it to an overarching theme of "this is just your experience because we see you as a Black male and a threat." Politicizing it and offering sympathy isn't the answer. "It just makes me feel like a victim. I can either be angry or helpless. I'd much rather be empowered."

Case Study: Brian

Brian is a 51-year-old White, cisgender male who resides in Guilford, Connecticut. He completed several undergraduate courses when he was in his late teens and decided to pursue a career in social service. He considers himself wealthy and reports that he has had 20–30 encounters with the police in the last 30 years. His earliest encounter took place at 20 years old when he received a charge of driving while intoxicated (DWI) in Rhode Island. "They treated me pretty decently, I was arrested, processed and jailed. In less than 24 hours, my friend posted the $500 bail." He wasn't asked to change his clothes, and he was alone in his cell. "They gave me coffee and a cigarette the next day, I thought it was a banquet." Brian has been pulled over for speeding about 15–20 times in his lifetime, both day and night, and his car has been searched by police officers several times. "One time I was doing 120 in a 55-mph [zone] driving a Ferrari 348." At more than twice the speed limit, he qualified for a $300 fine and up to 30 days imprisonment. The officer let him go with a $475 ticket and the advice, "You might want to slow down."

When Brian was arrested in Illinois on a drug charge, he remembers the experience as feeling traumatic due to the gravity of being incarcerated, but not necessarily due to his interaction with the police. "After they arrested me, the guy took my cuffs off and let me sit up front with him [in the police car]." He recalls being the minority race in the cell, sharing it with mostly Latino men. "I don't think it's something anyone really wants to experience, having your freedoms taken away." He was released the next day on a $5,000 bond posted by his family.

When asked if he ever felt victimized by police, Brian reported, "It was the opposite of that. Across the board, they were professional." When asked if he ever worried about getting pulled over: "I do feel intimidated by them, but mostly because I think they're just on an ego trip. They seem to get away with anything." He doesn't think through any potential inter-actions, however, and he doesn't have a visceral response, like Khalon. He doesn't wonder whether or not he will have to anticipate an incorrect assumption by an officer. "I don't like cops because they just want to bust my balls. To me, their function is nothing more than revenue makers. Now that I'm older, I know that I can just hire a lawyer."

When asked if the Black Lives Matter movement impacted his view of law enforcement, Brian answered: "It's shifted my view of police because it solidified what I already thought, in a more unfortunate way. They are worse now in my head because there is such an undeniable disparity between treatment. It's just wrong. I believe they do serve a function, absolutely. I wouldn't want to see an abolishment of the police. Part of keeping people in order is fear…"

Let's examine the cases of Khalon and Brian by looking at the central nervous system which consists of the sympathetic nervous system (freeze, flight, fight, fright, faint—emergency response) and parasympathetic ner-vous system (rest-and-digest). When one encounters acute stress, the sym-pathetic nervous system is engaged, resulting in an immediate release of the hormones epinephrine (adrenaline), norepinephrine, and cortisol. The heart rate increases, blood pressure rises, and the rate of breathing quickens. As blood rushes to the brain, pupils dilate, hands get cold and clammy, and the body may start trembling or shaking. Take a moment to recall the last time you experienced this in your body.

Consider Khalon and Brian starting their day out in parallel, moving through a morning routine, interacting with loved ones, getting a cup of coffee, and driving to work—an otherwise normal workday. On the way to work, a police officer pulls each man over. Brian's sympathetic nervous system causes his heart rate to increase; he can feel his adrenaline surge knowing he will be late for work. He's fairly confident he can navigate this with a mere conversation. After the incident, and because he has few traumatic memories connected to law enforcement, it takes about 45 minutes for his body to return to normal.

Khalon's lived experience, on the other hand, engages his sympathetic nervous system at a more profound level. When he sees the flashing lights, his heart starts racing, his hands get sweaty, and he becomes excessively focused on trying to figure out how to navigate all the different scenarios that could play out. His physical body is prepared for freeze, flight, fight, fright, faint, and he knows he must remain calm and clear-headed. His muscles tighten. After the incident, and because he has many traumatic memories connected to law enforcement, it takes about 24–48 hours for his body to return to a normal state. During this period, he operates in a state of hypervigilance, a component of post-traumatic stress disorder (PTSD) that increases the startle reflex. In the short term, it will take longer for his hormone levels, heart rate, and blood pressure to normalize. The increased stress will impact relationships at work and at home. In the long term, he has an increased risk for anxiety, depression, insomnia, heart attack, hypertension, and stroke. Take a moment to think about how your stress level impacts your relationships, both in and out of the home. How does stress impact your patience with and empathy for others? How do you imagine it will affect your client relationships or agency work? How can you use your lived experience with a triggered central nervous system and/or hypervigilance to connect with individuals you want to work with?

The Response of Police Officers to Sexual Violence

According to the Centers for Disease Control and Prevention (CDC), one in three women will experience sexual violence in their lifetime, and one third of female rape victims are sexually violated for the first time between the ages of 11 and 17, one in eight girls before age ten. One in four men will experience sexual violence in their lifetime. One-quarter of male rape victims experience their first victimization between the ages of 11 and 17 years old, and one quarter before age ten. As of 2019, the population of the US was reported to be 329 million (M) (Centers for Disease Control and Prevention, 2021). If one only considers those who are 18 and older (78% of the population, or 256.67M), 96M of those men and women will experience sexual violence in their lifetime. Of those 96M, 24M will have an initial experience between 11–17 years old and 12M under 10 years old. Yet, many victims do not report the violence, or the violence is not reported through proper channels by police. It is therefore likely that the number of victims of sexual violence in the US is underreported by the CDC.

Inappropriate reporting of sexual violence by police officers is a widespread problem that often arises due to their personal beliefs about the situation. That is, when officers respond to a domestic violence or sexual assault call while on duty, and the victim is female, officers tend to arrive with implicit biases. This extends to the nature of the crime and who was involved. As a result, decisions may be influenced by a victim who identifies as a cisgender female, a transgender woman, or a person of color and may therefore lead to aberrant reporting of the crime (Department of Justice, 2015). Consider the 2009 discovery of over 11,000 non-analyzed rape kits in storage at a police department in Detroit, Michigan by the Wayne County Prosecutor's Office. Analysis of the kits commenced six years later after a substantial award from the US Bureau of Justice Assistance. The cases were processed, and survivors were contacted. As of April 2021, all but 200 of the kits have been analyzed, with 2,616 DNA matches and the identification of 834 possible serial rapists (Department of Justice Office of Justice Programs, n.d.; End the Backlog, n.d.). To account for the oversight, some officers said that the adolescents were "lying to avoid getting in trouble," "got what was coming to them," or that it was "not really a rape" (Burns, 2019, n.p.). According to the Detroit Sexual Assault Kit Action Research Project Final Report, stakeholders were asked why so many kits were withheld from being sent for analysis. Almost all responded that gender was the main factor: "this is a crime that affects women, and in this city, that means Black women, poor Black women... there's a good chunk of the explanation right there" (Campbell et al., 2015). Indeed, when an officer discounts the violent act, it qualifies as a bias and is therefore considered unlawful discrimination under the Violence Against Women Act.

Targeted Police Violence against Women

Targeted violence against women by law enforcement is also a widespread problem in the US. Daniel Holtzclaw was a police officer who targeted Black women and girls while on duty between 2013 and 2014. He was found guilty in 2015 of 18 charges (rape / sexual battery of eight women) and subsequently sentenced to 263 years in prison in 2016 (Oklahoma City, 2020). This type of criminal activity by law enforcement is not uncommon. In a 2015 Associated Press investigation, 1,000 officers lost their licenses for sexual misconduct over a period of six years. Since most states don't have a way to identify, track or implement corrective action for sexual misconduct, this is likely an underestimation of the number of officers involved in sexual misconduct. Sarasota, Florida Police Chief Bernadette DiPino addressed the issue for the International Chiefs of Police and said, "It's so underreported and people are scared that if they call and complain about a police officer, they think every other police officer is going to be out to get them" (Sedensky & Merchant, 2015).

In addition to the fear of retaliation, certain childhood traumas can influence the likelihood of reporting violent acts against women by law enforcement. In the case of intimate partner violence (IPV), a child may be deeply impacted after witnessing her parent's interactions with the police. Consider the case illustration of a 33-year-old African American woman caught in a decade-long cycle of IPV (Brown et al., 2018). Her childhood memories include police forcibly removing her father from the house and an officer shaming her mother for staying in an abusive relationship after she dialed 911. She not only internalized the violence and inequities toward women, but was also hesitant to call for help when she found herself in a similar situation later in life.

Discrimination against LGBTQIA+ People

The history of policing LGBTQIA+ people originates in part from the criminalization of dressing in clothes of the opposite sex, which became popular in the mid-19th century. Just 50 years later, "gender inappropriateness" in the US was considered an illness carrying the weight of communal misconduct (Eskridge & Eskridge, 2009), potentially a criminal offense. The practice of "quality-of-life policing" encourages not only officers but whole communities to report behaviors such as disrupting the quiet in a public space. Since LGBTQIA+ youth who feel unsafe at home often spend time publicly congregating, law enforcement can exploit this as an opportunity to target them for loitering. Moreover, LGBTQIA+ people of color experience more arrests and police interventions than their White counterparts. In the West Village of New York City, the LGBTQIA+ community is largely White with less than 10% of residents who are African American or Latinx, yet approximately 77% of those stopped by police were African American or Latinx. One resident said, "I hate it, I hate it... It makes a lot of us stop coming out here... They don't treat straight people the way they treat gay people. They harass gay people" (Osborne, 2012).

Case Study: Z

Z is a 40-year-old queer individual who uses the pronouns they/them. They received an undergraduate degree in public administration and a master's degree in art therapy, which, like social work, has roots in activism. Z has a regular private practice in Westchester, New York. Z recalls their first encounter with the police when they appeared due to child neglect in Z's home. "When the police arrived, they told me I was the problem, that I was bad. And I didn't want to go to jail." Z was only 12 years old at the time. From that point forward, Z equated calling the police with making an unsafe choice. More recently, Z was walking in their neighborhood when they were accosted by a group of boys issuing slurs and violent threats. Z and their partner chose to call the police when they got home. "It was a double bind. I know the deal. I didn't feel comfortable sharing that I'm gay and transitioning. The officer just assumed I was hetero because my partner is a male and assured me that their behavior was normal, 'boys will be boys.'"

When Z was five years old, they were in the car with their mom on the way to a friend's house. An officer pulled Z's mom over for speeding. "My mom just shook and cried and needed my help getting stuff out of the glove box. I had no idea why she was so upset. After the encounter, we turned around and went home." They internalized the message that 911 was not to be called in an emergency, even if 911 was safe for others. The same scenario would play out three more times during Z's childhood. It wasn't until Z was in their 20s that they learned why.

When Z's mom was three years old, she witnessed her father being hit over the head with a gun and taken by men in trench coats in an unmarked car. He wouldn't return for weeks. "This was during the McCarthy period. My family was blacklisted. My mom couldn't even go to the grocery store because it would impact the owner in a bad way." Z refers to this period as six months of terrorism by law enforcement. Police surveilled the residence. The family forbade movies like *Dick Tracy* and the *Godfather* because the narratives were too close to the family's own situation. "My mom learned that people with power aren't safe. She learned that safety meant not getting involved in anything."

Z learned to channel their anxiety and generational trauma through creativity, theatre, and political activism. Z feels as though they have a coat of armor due to their work. "A client will hurl slurs at me during session. I've heard it all. Confrontation is part of what clients do." Z knows their protective factors are different from most of their clients. "I have power and privilege; I'm queer, White, lower-middle class. I live in a home that I paid for. That's a very different origin than many."

Work with homeless clients who identified as transgender shaped Z's early career in art therapy. Most engaged in sex work to survive. Almost all experienced sexual assault and had negative interactions with the police. "There's not a lot of trauma-processing around interactions with police at this level. It's mostly safety planning. Think Maslow's hierarchy of needs. They need food and shelter. Therapy is a luxury." For those who can begin to process their interactions with law enforcement, Z suggests narrative art therapy, which encourages clients to own all parts of their story, including the pain. "The last thing I want to do is call 911. I try to de-escalate a situation as much as possible, knowing that most clients do not see the police as a safe option." Z is committed to their work and has expanded their reach in political and social activism. They still regularly do creative work to process counter-transference and implicit biases that arise out of client-centered work. "This is a journey; we are all perfectly imperfect."

Mental Health Impact on Victims of Police Violence

There is a significant correlation between suicide attempts and police victimization. Those who have PTSD and have experienced sexual victimization are reported to be at high risk for suicidal ideation and attempted suicide (DeVylder et al., 2017). Similarly, people who are victimized by police, especially if the incident involves assault, will likely have related traumatic and psychological symptoms that increase the likelihood of attempted suicide.

These findings are especially important for social workers, whether in the clinical or administrative setting, who should take steps to assess client suicide risk. Consider including questions during an intake examination that probe for specific instances of trauma involving police victimization, such as 1) Has an officer ever hit, beaten, kicked, or dragged you? 2) Has a police officer ever used a gun, other weapon, or taser with you? 3) Has a police officer ever been sexually inappropriate with you? 4) Has a police officer ever bullied you, called you names, threatened you or employed racial/gender insults? 5) Has an officer ever responded inappropriately or in a delayed manner when you requested their help? (DeVylder et al., 2017).

Challenges for Police Reform

Hudson (2014), who served as a police officer for five years in Missouri, explains how broken the system is. Better training isn't the answer since racial sensitivity training and use-of-force reduction classes are attended regularly. If an officer receives disciplinary action, her friends and peers conduct the investigation, so there is no accountability. Hudson's peers referred to it as a "free vacation," and prosecutors, who generally share the same belief system as the courts, side with the police officer. There ultimately needs to be complete accountability for wrongdoing among the police officers in order to fix this failing system.

Case Study: Art Therapy with Police Officers

One of the authors of this chapter, Aimee Jette, participated in a response effort to gauge resilience in law enforcement agencies in the tri-state area (New York, Connecticut, and New Jersey) with the intention of offering self-care strategies. One officer shared about how his work has shifted: "Everyone's more on edge. I work the night shift so I can be home with my kids. My wife is a teacher. I'm more stressed on the job now. Then, I go home and my wife struggles with anxiety due to the COVID-19 pandemic. I don't know how to fix it. It's taking a toll on both of us." Officers have been worried about responding to calls, in light of restrictions on large gatherings. They expressed an overall lack of respect for the profession, which they are learning to grapple with. An exasperated officer reported, "We had to break up this huge party. Not only are you now exposed to everyone who's not wearing a mask, the kids actually taunt you. All the phones come out. They dare you to come in. How do you respond to that?"

On the topic of Black Lives Matter protests, "Yeah, we get stuff yelled at us a lot. But then you go into the local breakfast place and someone anonymously pays for your meal." A female officer replied, "I don't know how to respond, I have so many thoughts about all of it, but I can't say anything. You are damned if you do, damned if you don't. Holidays are the worst. Everyone takes their anger out on you. I'm just one person, I don't represent all cops."

To engender communication around their feelings and inner thoughts, they were asked to participate in an art therapy exercise. Using a paper mâché mask and markers, they used the outside of the mask to express how the world sees them. On the inside of the mask, they expressed how they really feel.

Sebastian

Outer mask: Sebastian drew three large blue storm clouds on the mask's forehead. "I have this constant battle about how I'm viewed and the impact I want to make." Next, he filled in the gaps with jagged yellow scribbles, which he reported as "lightning because it's so tumultuous." Next, he added sharp long brown eyebrows, angling up from the inner eye / nose to the temple. Next, Sebastian created green rectangular blocks under the eyes resembling eye black; sports players use eye black to deflect glare. Finally, Sebastian made a long, wide red mouth, "I feel like everyone thinks we're evil. It's just not true. It's something you can't seem to escape."

Inner mask: He added a single blue tear out of the left eye-opening and a single yellow star over the right eye. "The tear is here because it's just so sad how people view us. Not all of us are bad. You go into something because you want to help people. It's disheartening to get so much hatred. The star is the hope that things will get better."

Adwin

Outer mask: Adwin divided his outer mask up into six equal horizontal sections. Starting at the top, he added bands of color. He used orange across the top of the head, yellow over the forehead, green across the eyes, blue over the nose section, and purple laterally over the mouth. Finally, at the base of the chin, he added a small pot of gold. "The idea is if you are fair to everyone, you get a pot of gold at the end. I try to be respectful no matter what someone's background is."

Inner mask: Adwin divided the inside of his mask into three equal vertical sections. In the center section, he added four images to the forehead space:

• A flag with the "thin blue line."
• A lightning strike image "for responding confidently and accurately."
• An African flag, "for my heritage."
• An American flag, "for my love of this country."

Adwin added brown to the left vertical section and the right with pink. "This is the balance between masculine and feminine. All of these things connect you to what's important."

Lucas

Outer mask: Lucas drew three triangles that appeared to create a widow's peak across his forehead, pointing down. He colored them in using black, red, blue, and purple markers. "I feel like this is all the stuff that goes on in my head, but I have to keep it under control to do my job." Then, he created two thin black lines for eyebrows, which elicited curiosity/questioning. Next, he gave the mask nostrils and drew a goatee in black around the mouth.

Inner mask: The inside of his mask comprised a large red pyramid, broken into four sections. He added more red lines, which created roughly 20 more triangles, all pointing up. Next, Lucas added 21 yellow exclamation points inside the residual shapes. "The push and pull between what administration wants us to do and what's possible. You get mixed messages. A couple bad apples can ruin it for everybody. Most of us are just brothers and sisters trying our best." Finally, Lucas added a thick red rectangular block across the mouth referring to speaking up when something happens that he opposes: "You're damned if you do, damned if you don't. I just keep my mouth shut."

Shared Trauma from One of the Authors' Points of View

Told from the perspective of Aimee Jette, one of the authors of this chapter: I am a cis-gendered White woman (she/her) of European descent. My paternal grandparents, Ruth and Art Jette (also White) were social workers committed to raising the Black vote during Jim Crow. They lived in segregated communities of color in the South, which allowed them to meet regularly with community organizers and strategize. By the end of Reconstruction (1877), 90% of Black men were registered to vote; many held office. However, by 1940, this number had decreased to a mere 3% due to Jim Crow and the black codes. Southern municipalities made it nearly impossible to register through complex applications and intimidation (Constitutional Rights Foundation, 2021). Ruth and Art moved their small but growing family into deeply segregated Southern Black neighborhoods and aided in its reversal.

In the 1960s, they moved to New Haven, CT, and worked with Latinx communities fighting for equality in education, voting, housing, and employment. Thus, when I was a child, I was privy to narratives of confronting social injustice outside the home and inside. My dissenting grandmother promptly schooled dinner guests who held a patriarchal-colonialist mindset. I honestly thought all grandmothers behaved like this and I watched her closely. As I got older, my transition toward work with disempowered individuals felt urgent and necessary.

When Ann Goelitz asked me to co-author this chapter with Tina Sacks, I felt innervated and moderately hesitant since I'm far from scholarship in critical race theory. Still, I trusted Ann's vision and immediately connected with Tina. My initial view was: "police reform is attainable with sufficient attention to mental health and a lot of sensitivity training." I had just finished up a project educating officers about mental health and self-care, hoping that small changes from the inside would resonate beyond in the form of better care for oppressed populations. Looking back, I realize my view was not reality based; rather it was akin to dropping a penny in the center of the ocean and expecting the ripple to make it to shore.

While I have been candid in personal and professional settings on critical social justice initiatives, I found writing this chapter challenging on a personal and emotional level. Each piece of literature researched was hard to emotionally assimilate, revealing yet another layer of privilege as a cis-gendered non-BIP[W]OC (non-Black, Indigenous woman of color) person and a reckoning with inaction. I thought of Ruth and Art often, my respect for their life work intensified. I found that I could no longer drive or walk by a police officer without acute aversion and new underlying feelings of hostility; the interview with Khalon impacted me profoundly. Waves of shame and dislike arose for officers, for our history, for me. I considered quitting at times. Additionally, I couldn't figure out how my experience with law enforcement could fit into the chapter.

Tina and I had a pivotal conversation one day. We agreed that police brutality could not be a shared trauma between all social workers and clients; it felt like a gross miscalculation to say it was. Differentiation was mandatory. As a (White) clinician who does not share a history of violence against my body due to skin color or sexual preference, I cannot claim shared trauma. I may hear a person share about their experience with police brutality, but I have *no lived experience* growing up as a Black/Indigenous/female/person of color, an LGBTQIA+ or disabled individual. My privilege has been so entrenched that I rarely had to question who police were protecting me from in the first place. Even with an activist ancestry I hadn't fully examined the narrative that "police protect white communities from armed black men."

I grappled with having the right to write about the topics in this chapter. There were times when our conversations about the direction of the chapter were impassioned. I experienced displaced anger at our editor, which looking back was a response to my own discomfort and frustration. It's been a year since I worked with officers doing art therapy which I view as a personal marker more than anything else. I understand that there are officers who entered law enforcement to be of service or to extend a generational vocational calling. However, even for those who are motivated by altruism, without deeply examining privilege and unconscious prejudice, espousing a system historically rooted in terrorizing Black people serves to buttress enduring attitudinal stereotypes. As evidenced in a recent empirical analysis of fatal police shootings in *The Lancet*, this is an even larger issue than many considered it to be. The analysis showed that police violence is grossly underreported and that implicit bias and de-escalation interventions are largely ineffective (GBD 2019 Police Violence US Subnational Collaborators, 2021). As such, I no longer feel willing to continue that work. My hope is that this chapter will inspire you to do the difficult task of examining privilege, in whatever forms it takes, because unless scrutinized, it will continue to hide in plain sight.

Summary and Conclusion

The history of policing and social work in the US requires us to deeply consider how both professions have been used to control ethno-racial minorities. As a profession, social workers (along with other mental health providers) must reckon with their past with a particular focus on how we can redress these harms in the present. Working with survivors of police violence, for example, requires a deep sensitivity to how anti-Blackness disproportionately impacts communities of color and makes them systematically more vulnerable to police violence. Being vigilant about broadening our practice capacities to include trauma-informed modalities that carefully consider how police encounters may deepen feelings of helplessness, anger, and frustration is also important. The profession of social work must redouble its commitment to social justice as well. This includes fighting against systematic racism and police violence in all of its manifestations.

Although many social workers may be drawn to the profession because they have had life experiences similar to those they will eventually serve, we argue that the experience of police violence likely differs by the race, gender, and other statuses of the social worker and the client. Police violence may not necessarily lead to feelings of shared trauma between social worker and client. As the empirical evidence demonstrates, the victims of police violence are disproportionately Black, Indigenous, LGBTQIA+, and disabled people. Further, perceptions of culpability around instances of police violence are not necessarily shared by all people in the United States or abroad. For example, according to a 2020 Pew Research poll, 84% of Black adults noted that Black people were generally treated less fairly than White people; 63% of White people agreed. Almost 90% (87%) of Black people and 61% of White people said the US criminal justice system treats Black people less fairly (Horowitz et al., 2019). Although a majority of both Black and White people agree that police and the criminal justice system treat Black and White people differently, there is still a substantial racial gap in perceptions of fairness. Based on these data, and our own lived experience, we argue that there is likely great variation in the perception and experience of police trauma such that it cannot be discussed as a universally shared trauma between social worker and client. For some social workers, the experience of working with a client who has been traumatized by a police encounter may be similar to their own experience with police. However, for other social workers, a client's encounter with the police may be met with scrutiny, disbelief, or suspicion instead of empathy. Given that the perceptions of law enforcement often take precedence over the accounts of Black, Indigenous, Latinx, LGBTQIA+, and disabled people who are the targets of police violence, it is difficult to make the argument that any trauma will be universally shared. As such, we cannot assert that police violence engenders shared trauma between social worker and client unless the clinician shares a lived and/or generational history of police as human rights violator which includes but is not exclusive to those in the BIPOC, LGBTQIA+, and similar communities.

References

Abulhul, Z. (2021). Social work (social policy) used as a tool of social control. *Open Journal of Social Sciences*, 9, 249–262. doi:10.4236/jss.2021.91018.

American Psychiatric Association. (2013). *Diagnostic and statistical manual of mental disorders* (5th edn). American Psychiatric Association. https://doi.org/10.1176/appi.books.9780890425596.

Baum, N. (2010). Shared traumatic reality in communal disasters: Toward a conceptualization. *Psychotherapy: Theory, Research, Practice, Training*, 47(2), 249.

Bell, C. H., & Robinson, E. H., III (2013). Shared trauma in counseling: Information and implications for counselors. *Journal of Mental Health Counseling*, 35(4), 310–323.

Boulanger, G. (2013). Fearful symmetry: Shared trauma in New Orleans after hurricane Katrina. *Psychoanalytic Dialogues*, 23(1), 31–44.

Brown, D. L. (2020). "It was a modern-day lynching": Violent deaths reflect a brutal American legacy. *National Geographic*. www.nationalgeographic.com/his tory/article/history-of-lynching-violent-deaths-reflect-brutal-american-legacy.

Brown, S., McGriff, K., & Speedlin, S. (2018). Using relational-cultural theory to negotiate relational rebuilding in survivors of intimate partner violence. *Journal of Creativity in Mental Health*, 13(2), 136–147.

Burns, G. (2019, April 3). 11,000 untested rape kits: Detroit police "cut corners," blamed victims, report says. *Advance Local Media*. Retrieved from: www.mlive. com/news/detroit/2015/04/11000_untested_rape_kits_detro.html.

Campbell, R., Fehler-Cabral, G., Pierce, S. J., Sharma, D. B., Bybee, D., Shaw, J., & Feeney, B. A. (2015). *The Detroit sexual assault kit (SAK) action research project (ARP), executive summary*. US Department of Justice.

Carr, J. (2016). The lawlessness of law: Lynching and anti-lynching in the contemporary USA. *Settler Colonial Studies*, 6(2), 153–163.

Centers for Disease Control and Prevention. (2021, February 5). *Preventing sexual violence*. Retrieved from: www.cdc.gov/violenceprevention/sexualviolence/fastfa ct.html.

Connecticut Racial Profiling Prohibition Project. (2015, April 30). State of Connecticut traffic stop data analysis and findings. DataHaven. Retrieved from: www.ctdatahaven.org/data-resources/state-connecticut-traffic-stop-data-analysis-and-findings.

Constitutional Rights Foundation. (2021). *Race and voting in the segregated south*. Retrieved from: www.crf-usa.org/black-history-month/race-and-voting-in-the-se gregated-south.

Dekel, R., Nuttman-Shwartz, O., & Lavi, T. (2016). Shared traumatic reality and boundary theory: How mental health professionals cope with the home/work conflict during continuous security threats. *Journal of Couple & Relationship Therapy*, 15(2), 121–134.

Department of Justice. (2015). *Identifying and preventing gender bias in law enforcement response to sexual assault and domestic violence*. Retrieved from: www. justice.gov/opa/file/799366/download.

Department of Justice Office of Justice Programs. (n.d.). *Sexual assault kit initiative (SAKI)*. Retrieved from: https://bja.ojp.gov/program/sexual-assault-kit-ini tiative-saki/overview?Program_ID=117.

DeVylder, J. E. (2017). Donald Trump, the police, and mental health in US cities. *American Journal of Public Health*, 107(7), 1042. www.ncbi.nlm.nih.gov/pmc/a rticles/PMC5463226/.

DeVylder, J. E., Frey, J. J., Cogburn, C. D., Wilcox, H. C., Sharpe, T. L., Oh, H. Y., Nam, B., & Link, B. G. (2017). Elevated prevalence of suicide attempts among victims of police violence in the USA. *Journal of Urban Health*, 94(5), 629–636.

End the Backlog. (n.d.) *Detroit*. Retrieved from: www.endthebacklog.org/detroit.

Eskridge, W. N., & Eskridge, W. N. (2009). *Gaylaw: Challenging the apartheid of the closet*. Harvard University Press.

Figley, C. R. (Ed.). (1995). *Compassion fatigue: Coping with secondary traumatic stress disorder in those who treat the traumatized*. Psychology Press.

GBD 2019 Police Violence US Subnational Collaborators. (2021). Fatal police violence by race and state in the USA, 1980–2019: A network meta-regression. *The Lancet*, 398(10307), 1239–1255.

Glenn, E. N. (2015). Settler colonialism as structure: A framework for comparative studies of US race and gender formation. *Sociology of Race and Ethnicity*, 1(1), 52–72.

Hadden, S. E. (2003). *Slave patrols: Law and violence in Virginia and the Carolinas*. Harvard University Press.

Hartman, S. V. (1997). *Scenes of subjection: Terror, slavery, and self-making in nineteenth-century America*. Oxford University Press.

Hill, E., Tiefenthäler, A., Triebert, C., Jordan, D., Willis, H., & Stein, R. (2020, May 31). How George Floyd was killed in police custody. *The New York Times*. www.nytimes.com/2020/05/31/us/george-floyd-investigation.html.

Horowitz, J. M., Brown, A., & Cox, K. (2019). *Race in America 2019*. Pew Research Center. Retrieved from: www.pewresearch.org/social-trends/wp-con tent/uploads/sites/3/2019/04/Race-report_updated-4.29.19.pdf.

Hudson, R. (2014). Being a cop showed me just how racist and violent the police are. There's only one fix. *The Washington Post*. Retrieved from: www.washing tonpost.com/posteverything/wp/2014/12/06/i-was-a-st-louis-cop-my-peers-were-racist-and-violent-and-theres-only-one-fix/.

Jacobs, L. A., Kim, M. E., Whitfield, D. L., Gartner, R. E., Panichelli, M., Kattari, S. K., Downey, M. M., McQueen, S. S., & Mountz, S. E. (2021). Defund the police: Moving towards an anti-carceral social work. *Journal of Progressive Human Services*, 32(1), 37–62.

Katz, M. B. (1996). *In the shadow of the poorhouse: A social history of welfare in America*. Basic Books.

Lave, T., & Miller, E. (Eds.). (2019). *The Cambridge handbook of policing in the United States*. Cambridge University Press.

Mapping Police Violence. (2021). *2020 Police Violence Report*. Retrieved from https:// policeviolencereport.org/.

McClain, A. (2020). Social workers cooperate with police forces. *The Wall Street Journal*. Retrieved from: www.wsj.com/articles/social-workers-cooperate-with-police-forces-11592255480.

Mesic, A., Franklin, L., Cansever, A., Potter, F., Sharma, A., Knopov, A., & Siegel, M. (2018). The relationship between structural racism and black-white disparities in fatal police shootings at the state level. *Journal of the National Medical Association*, 110(2), 106–116.

Muhammad, K. G. (2019). *The condemnation of Blackness: Race, crime, and the making of modern urban America, with a new preface*. Harvard University Press.

Norman, S., & Maguen, S. (2020, May 19). *Moral injury*. National Center for PTSD. Retrieved from: www.ptsd.va.gov/professional/treat/cooccurring/moral_injury.asp.

Ogden, P., & Fisher, J. (2015). *Sensorimotor psychotherapy: Interventions for trauma and attachment*. Norton series on interpersonal neurobiology. W. W. Norton & Company.

Oklahoma City. (2020, March 9). US Supreme Court rejects ex-cop's appeal of rape convictions. *The Associated Press*. Retrieved from: https://apnews.com/a rticle/7e2b2a5d9561871d809f8819e40ed478.

Osborne, D. (2012, May 23). Queer youth of color complain of West Village stop and frisk. *Gay City News*. Retrieved from: www.gaycitynews.com/queer-youth-of-color-complain-of-west-village-stop-and-frisk/.

Papazoglou, K., Blumberg, D. M., Chiongbian, V. B., Tuttle, B. M., Kamkar, K., Chopko, B., Milliard, B., Aukhojee, P., & Koskelainen, M. (2020). The role of moral injury in PTSD among law enforcement officers: A brief report. *Frontiers in Psychology*, 11, 310.

Park, Y. (2020). *Facilitating injustice: The complicity of social workers in the forced removal and incarceration of Japanese Americans*. Oxford University Press.

Pierson, E., Simoiu, C., Overgoor, J., Corbett-Davies, S., Jenson, D., et al. (2020). A large-scale analysis of racial disparities in police stops across the United States. *Nature Human Behaviour*, 4(7), 736–745.

Piven, F. F., & Cloward, R. (2012). *Regulating the poor: The functions of public welfare*. Vintage.

Roberts, D. (2009). *Shattered bonds: The color of child welfare*. Civitas Books.

Ross, C. T. (2015). A multi-level Bayesian analysis of racial bias in police shootings at the county-level in the United States. *PloS one*, 10(11), e0141854. www.ncbi. nlm.nih.gov/pmc/articles/PMC4634878/.

Sedensky, M., & Merchant, N. (2015, November 1). Hundreds of officers lose licenses over sex misconduct. *The Associated Press*. Retrieved from: https://ap news.com/article/oklahoma-police-archive-oklahoma-city-fd1d4d05e561462a85a be50e7eaed4ec.

Smedley, A. (2003). *Race: The power of an illusion*. Retrieved from: www.pbs.org/ race/000_About/002_04-experts-02-01.htm.

Steadman, H. J., Deane, M. W., Borum, R., & Morrissey, J. P. (2000). Comparing outcomes of major models of police responses to mental health emergencies. *Psychiatric Services*, 51(5), 645–649.

Tosone, C., Nuttman-Shwartz, O., & Stephens, T. (2012). Shared trauma: When the professional is personal. *Clinical Social Work Journal*, 40(2), 231–239.

Walters, K. L., Mohammed, S. A., Evans-Campbell, T., Beltrán, R. E., Chae, D. H., & Duran, B. (2011). Bodies don't just tell stories, they tell histories: Embodiment of historical trauma among American Indians and Alaska Natives 1. *Du Bois Review: Social Science Research on Race*, 8(1), 179.

Wilderson, F. B., III (2010). *Red, white & black: Cinema and the structure of US antagonisms*. Duke University Press.

Zimering, R., Munroe, J., & Gulliver, S. (2003). Secondary traumatization in mental health care providers. *Psychiatric Times*, 20(4). Retrieved from: www.psychiatrictim es.com/view/secondary-traumatization-mental-health-care-providers.

Chapter 5

Social Resilience and Natural Disasters
Effective Social and Community Response to Shared Trauma

Ngoh Tiong Tan

Introduction

We all share experiences with others along life's journey. Shared traumatic experiences, however, are not as common. They are, nevertheless, relevant for therapeutic intervention and may either hinder or facilitate growth. Meeting at the middle focuses on the mental health aspects of the social worker's shared experience that can catalyze positive change. Members of the community sharing trauma experiences helps them to identify with and support each other as they face the crisis together. This process is critical to dealing effectively with trauma.

Social workers and other mental health professionals who both live with and practice within the traumatized community are 'doubly exposed' (Lavi et al., 2015). They are knowledgeable about the community and understand their clients better but are also coping with their own responses to the natural disaster. Fortuitously, their responses to shared trauma may be creatively applied as a therapeutic tool for helping individuals grow as well as for community intervention.

Collaborative practice where clients and workers work through shared trauma together may be empowering for both. This 'middle approach' involves identifying and owning the process as a way to facilitate healing and wholeness. In co-constructing the future, both clients and workers are strengthened by the relationship as they become more resilient individuals and community members. The unified building of hope can bring greater solidarity and cohesion to the people, the group and the community.

The development of social resilience and community resources are both needed for effective social and community response to crisis brought on by disasters. This chapter focuses directly and indirectly, personally and professionally and at individual, community and societal levels on working for growth and change, using a strengths-based social resilience perspective with trauma brought about by natural disasters.

Natural disaster, due to weather changes such as tidal waves, floods, fires or geo-thermal phenomena of earthquakes, volcanic eruptions, etc.,

DOI: 10.4324/9781003176947-7

disrupts the lives of individuals, communities and whole societies. A holistic approach involving community-based intervention has been effective in the disaster recovery and rehabilitation process. Climate change has resulted in increased weather hazards, as well as increases in the vulnerability of communities to natural disasters (World Meteorological Organization, 2021a). It is therefore essential to create mechanisms for coping with these kinds of shared traumas.

Conceptual Framework

Shared Trauma and the Community

The theory of shared trauma for therapeutic intervention provides an understanding of how workers' dual exposure to trauma may be impacted in their situation, both professionally and personally. Tosone et al. (2012) suggested that vicarious traumatization, stress, compassion fatigue and burnout may be some of the ramifications therapists experience while working with traumatized clients. Evidence shows that the possibility of shared trauma increases when mental health professionals and their clients are from the same environment, such as those affected by Hurricane Katrina (Tosone et al., 2017). In prolonged working situations, therapists may experience compassion fatigue (Tosone et al., 2012). Burnout can also occur and this may be symptomatic of a lack of coping strategies. Compassion fatigue and vicarious trauma may be experienced as well when social workers are immersed in trauma work, and are unable to effectively process their own traumatic events (Day et al., 2017).

There may also be unresolved feelings and subjective reactions of the worker to the client, and vice-versa, when both are members of the community experiencing shared trauma, especially with situations of natural disasters. Transference and countertransference may occur in this relationship as well. Social workers may respond positively or negatively with regards to the various traumatic situations (Boulanger, 2007). They should be self-aware and endeavor to keep their own experiences out of the therapeutic relationship. Otherwise, they may project their own experience onto the client or client system. Though the traumatic experience may be constructively shared with clients, care must be taken to differentiate the unique aspects 'owned' by clients.

Shared traumas suggest both unique as well as common elements in social workers' experience of the crisis (Tosone et al., 2012). Both opportunities for personal and professional growth as well as transformative change can take place when there is a realization of shared grief and appropriate community expression. Often, this is accompanied by an awareness that their own traumatic responses have affected the nature of their professional relationships (Tosone et al., 2012). This awareness is crucial for the therapeutic use of shared experience in bringing about insights and change. Illustrating this, Tosone, et al. (2012) cited studies which found that high levels of exposure to life threats and stresses can also coexist with good professional functioning and resilience.

Working through Shared Trauma

Working through shared trauma requires introspection and reflection that involves a meta-level analysis of the condition. Seeking supervision to gain insight and to ensure that professional boundaries are not crossed is advantageous. Supervision or consultation may provide the opportunity for professional growth, as well as access to resources within educational organizations and agency-based work settings. Over and above these, the personal support the workers receive from family and friends is also useful for their own personal coping.

Social resilience may be a mediating factor between the client's traumatic life events and shared traumatic stress of the worker. Bauwens and Tosone (2010) found that shared experiences may enhance the intervention, enabling workers to address real concerns and expressed needs. The workers' compassion and connection with their clients may increase and be enhanced. However, there may be also an extra sense of personal vulnerability in the relationship with clients. The worker's strong identifications with clients and communities impacted by the natural disaster are certainly a shared reality (Dekel & Baum, 2009).

Ethics in Shared Trauma Work

In *The Wounded Healer* (Nouwen, 1972) it is noted that setbacks of the worker may become a strength for working with clients who have similar experiences. It was surmised that it may be possible for the worker who has experienced a shared trauma to incorporate this into the helping process. However, while engaging in therapy and helping others, they may experience again their own wounds and fears (Seeley, 2003; Nouwen, 1972). Though they may have difficulty separating themselves from those they are 'healing' (Tosone et al., 2012), with support and appropriate reflection, the shared trauma can become powerful material for the change process. With clearer boundaries established, the workers as 'social physicians' should be better able to heal themselves and thus for them to together be healed. Therefore, with these safeguards, both clients and workers' resilience may be further developed as a result of shared trauma (Tosone et al., 2017).

Care must be taken for ethical practice such as when there is a blurring of boundaries so that clients may not receive the full service they deserve. Social workers must be careful not to mix their personal concerns and those of their families or loved ones with the client's issues. Therapists and professional helpers may need supervision should they experience anxiety, guilt or self-esteem issues. These and other variables that facilitate and impede the professionals' functioning need to be addressed as they arise (Lavi et al., 2015; Tosone et al., 2012).

Allison Rowlands, for example, while working on the frontline of disasters in Australia observed that in a situation of a

> major flood disaster where we funded and supported a community recovery support service, I worked with the local community development worker who very closely identified with her local community and its loss, and I noted how this identification with people she knew well impacted her own performance, judgment, and coping style—it was difficult for many people.
>
> (Rowlands, 2021, n.p.)

Social and Community Resilience

Conceptually, social resilience is a multilayered framework emphasizing the interactions between enabling factors and capacities operating at different levels of society. The theory of social resilience describes the capacity to cope with adverse conditions, enabling individuals to bounce back to normalcy utilizing a proactive rather than a reactive response. Resilience theories provide an understanding of how professionals who were exposed to potentially traumatizing events can develop optimal effectiveness (Horwitz, 1999).

Building resilience involves enhancing and increasing competence, whether in clients or workers or with individuals or communities (Obrist et al., 2010). Competence enables the solving of problems by applying both knowledge and skills to deal with the shared trauma brought about by disasters. The facilitation of resilience requires a sense of efficacy to 'achieve success' which in turn promotes self-esteem and pride.

Other factors may impact the ability to build the resiliency needed to cope with trauma. The mediating variables for resilience include insecure attachments and inability to deal with life stressors (Tosone et al., 2017). It is noted that this lowered resilience may not necessarily be due to shared traumatic life events or exposure to the traumatic situation itself. The shared traumatic episodes and social resources developed may, however, be instrumental in strengthening the therapeutic relationship and enhancing social resilience (Tosone et al., 2017).

Community resilience may be described as the development and engagement of community resources so the community can thrive in the midst of change and uncertainty (Berkes & Ross, 2012; Wilson, 2012). There are social and ecological aspects of community resilience which view the environment and its stress systemically, connecting both the social and ecological dimensions together. This results in resilient communities being more prepared for emergencies and recovering better after natural disasters (Sulaiman et al., 2019).

An integrative approach to working with trauma incorporates the systems and ecology models as well as the social strengths approach. The social connections are vital in building capacities (Magis, 2010; Sulaiman et al., 2019). Systems intervention views communities as either resilient or vulnerable and seeks to optimize personal as well as community resilience (Wilson, 2012). The ecological perspective offers the idea that coping and effective adaptation indicate resiliency and strength. The systems view provides concepts for intervention related to: 1) dealing with adaptive relationships and learning in social–ecological systems across different levels, 2) avoiding isolation within the community, 3) linking people and systems to resources, and 4) opening 'windows of opportunity' (Magis, 2010).

Community resilience is the result of effective and functioning social networks. In the nexus of social interface lies the 'in-between' space for the practice arena (Ross & Berkes, 2014). The building of social capital and social support networks is thus the community worker's practice space and social intervention. Another way of building community strengths is through reinforcing community agency or organizational focus on individual connections, agency networks and organizational culture.

For effective resilience, it is necessary to build capacity for both individuals and communities. For example, both need to be self-sufficient and sustainable, like individuals being able to self-help and communities having access to water and food sovereignty during natural disasters. The development of local capacities, resources, skills and people, as in asset-based community development, has been applied in the management of natural disasters. The assets and strengths of communities enable them to be resourceful in coping with calamities. In the midst of globalization, there is perhaps a need to 're-localize communities' so that self-sustainability can be achieved (Wilson, 2012). Community resilience, for example, could be enhanced if affected communities have 1) first responders and community volunteers trained to deal with natural disasters, and 2) local food sufficiency.

Building Social Resilience

Social resilience acts as a buffer to crises and shared trauma. Strengthening resilience, through shared experience in the social context, is an effective approach in coping with both current and future crises. To build resilience we need to consider both the appraisal and coping patterns with crises, like those brought about by natural disasters (Bonanno et al., 2011;

Tosone et al., 2017). As coping is dependent on both the trauma and internal/external resources and support, multiple factors need to be considered (Bonanno et al., 2011).

First off, there is a need to identify and understand the specific needs of communities and client groups so as to strengthen their coping and response to natural disasters. To strengthen community resilience and COVID-19 response through community actions, for example, the WHO European Healthy Cities Network provides needs assessment, technical support and guidance, as well as direct support to communities in need (Community Action Interventions, 2020).

Generally, there is a need for a coordinated societal response to natural disasters so that the right help can be given to the right people at the right time. Disaster preparedness and resilience is necessary to save lives, protect infrastructure and to preserve livelihoods (Combaz, 2014; Transitions, 2020a). The vulnerability of social systems and the environment can be reduced with planning and appropriate support. The worker as an insider within a community may be more effective in enabling individuals' and communities' capacities to cope with and adapt to the devastations and stresses associated with natural hazards (Combaz, 2014).

The building of disaster resilience is thus a more cost-effective and sustainable approach than resorting to disaster relief and developmental aid after the natural disaster. Illustrating this, in Singapore, the Resilience Fund was launched to support local activists, NGOs and others in helping their communities to build resilience. Building community resilience, before, during and after natural crisis is vital for effective coping (Hall, 2020; Sulaiman et al., 2019). People helping people and recognizing efforts for prevention and recovery are all important for resiliency. Community efforts for disaster relief and recovery show social cohesion and solidarity in times of disaster (Tan et al., 2006).

Natural Disasters: Nature and Impact

Climate Change and Natural Disasters

Climate change has impacted the world's weather and human living. *State of the Global Climate in 2020* provided the indicators of climate change based on greenhouse gas concentrations, the rise in ocean temperatures, melting ice, higher sea levels and extreme weather (World Meteorological Organization, 2021a). Rising temperatures on the global surface, brought about by the greenhouse effect, has affected wind patterns and brought about adverse weather conditions. Changes in precipitation patterns, with consequential strong winds, droughts, flooding and storms, have increased in various parts of the world (World Meteorological Organization, 2021a, 2021b). Deadly hurricanes and tornadoes, as well as other weather changes, have killed thousands all over the world. This is especially true with the tsunamis in Indonesia and Haiti (NO-AA, 2019). Devastating typhoons in the Philippines have forced mass evacuations and destroyed both homes and businesses.

Climate change directly or indirectly impacts polar ice melting, stunted vegetation, droughts and other extreme environmental conditions. Numerous earthquakes, typhoons, hurricanes, heavy rains, floods and wildfires have been reported in recent decades (World Meteorological Organization, 2021b). According to the United Nations, natural disasters are occurring three times more often than 50 years ago (UN News, 2021). The California wildfire season in 2018 and the Australian bushfires in 2020 were the deadliest and most destructive on record. Strong damaging earthquakes and tsunamis in Indonesia and Japan, and typhoons and floods in Thailand, China and the Philippines were also seen in recent years.

In a combination of homogenic and natural disasters, Japan's Fukushima experienced an earthquake and tsunami resulting in a man-made nuclear disaster. The breakdown of the nuclear facility impacted both social and economic life, as well as the housing and fishing industry. However, social resiliency was demonstrated by 1) the discipline of the frontline Japanese rescue corps, and 2) the volunteerism and civic mindedness of the people, both of which saved many a life and enabled the systematic rebuilding of the society (World Bank, 2017). Providing disaster preparedness training and developing effective first-responder systems helps with the overall recovery from natural disasters (Hall, 2020) and builds a resilient society, like that of Japan (World Bank, 2017).

Dealing with Natural Disasters

Although there may be some disagreement, many would include biogenic causes such as the bird flu, SARS and COVID-19 as natural disasters. These have brought major social and economic disruptions to the world, as we are all experiencing now with COVID-19. Compounding this, climate change has impacted not only the eco-system but also socio-economic development, migration and food security (World Meteorological Organization, 2021a).

Most natural and human-culpable disasters need intervention at various levels. At a national level, helpers are more likely to have shared traumatic experiences as both workers and clients come from if not the same community, then neighboring communities. At all levels, the shared experience of local and international organizations engenders a feeling of solidarity and comradeship and enables the provision of relevant and acceptable support.

Crisis intervention, disaster management and relief as well as recovery work are done by professionals who often share the traumatic experiences as they live amidst the societies impacted by natural disasters. International organizations like the United Nations Development Program, United Nations High Commission for Refugees, the United Nations International Disaster Risk Reduction, the Red Cross and Social Work Across Borders have also brought external resources when internal institutions and organizations are unable to cope due to the extensiveness of the disaster. Intervention and social work practices among these different types of disasters vary, e.g. depending on the scale of different types of natural disasters, be they fires, floods, earthquakes or hurricanes.

Social Work Intervention

Crisis occurs when coping resources are limited in the face of devastation. Crisis intervention can help return traumatized societies to a state of equilibrium at previous or even, hopefully, higher levels (Tan, 2004). The social work profession is particularly appropriate for this kind of disaster work because of its holistic epistemology at the generalist level (Dominelli, 2015).

The ecological framework and the emphasis on the person-in-environment, which are both tenets of social work, provide useful concepts for disaster work. Strengths-based interventions emphasize competence and capacity building in dealing with environmental stresses. In the intervention process, building disaster resilience involves supporting the capacity of individuals and communities to adapt and cope with crises, drawing on relevant personal and community resources. At the community level the focus is on enhancing clients' rights as well as addressing the socio-economic or even environmental inequalities that may exacerbate the problems brought about by the natural disaster (Ramsari, 2020), both of which are relevant areas of support for social workers.

Conceptual Framework for Social Intervention and Shared Trauma

A framework for practice needs to include key values and assumptions as well as principles, methods and processes of the intervention. Key social work values for trauma work include respect for diversity and empowerment, individuality, and for the dignity and worth of every person. The focus of social work on the role of relationship and on these values sets the stage for intervention within a shared traumatic experience. Valuing the experience of individuals and communities with respect to the natural disaster is crucial in co-creating solutions and interventions. During shared trauma brought about by natural hazards, workers can provide effective support by creatively applying these values throughout the intervention process.

A community-based disaster management approach would need to include working with the community to build resilience with facing natural disasters. Workers within the community would have experienced shared trauma at both the macro and micro levels. In macro practice the process includes the identification, analysis, treatment, monitoring and evaluation of disaster risks and vulnerabilities within the community. The goal in this process is to reduce community vulnerabilities and enhance capacities. A key in empowering communities is for people experiencing the disaster and trauma to be participating in the decision making and implementation at the various stages in the process of disaster management.

Using the systems concept for social work intervention provides us with the tools for fostering re-equilibrium at a higher level of functioning. In shared experience within a common environment, social workers, together with their clients, focus on enhancing resilience through the sharing of and linking to resources that provide social, environmental and economic resilience (Dominelli, 2015). It is suggested that natural disasters may expose and often 'magnify inequities' (Zwi et al., 2018). In order to reduce social inequities and vulnerabilities in the process of advocacy and planning, social workers must be mindful of the 'patterns of mortality, morbidity, loss, displacement, and recovery' that are present in the different disaster situations (Tierney, 2007, p. 515).

In the current raging COVID-19 pandemic, for example, an increase in inequality, exclusion, discrimination and global unemployment has been observed (Ramsari, 2020; WEF, 2021). Thus, there is a grave need for social protection systems and short-term food, shelter and income security provisions. In the long term there is the need for capacity building, job creation and structural interventions with disasters (WEF, 2021). Training and job restructuring is needed to enhance people's relevant work skills and added capacity to manage and overcome shocks and fallouts due to crises.

For crisis and crisis intervention the reference to the shared trauma experience seeks to build the strength of the client-worker relationship and to enable coping, resource mobilization and reorganization (Tosone et al., 2017). With relationships of trust the social work response to crisis and disaster at various levels can become more targeted. A research-based shared trauma framework can be applied to the process of working with individuals, groups and communities impacted by natural disasters.

Next, we will discuss the perspective of both social workers and other helping professionals with specific vignettes and case studies to illustrate coping and resilience, especially in shared trauma due to natural disasters.

Intervention with Specific Examples and Case Situations

Asian Tsunami and the FAST Project

In the immediate aftermath of the 2006 Indian Ocean Tsunami, the Family and Survivors of Tsunami (FAST) project was launched. The project acts as a catalyst in spearheading programs for the mental health and livelihoods of the survivors of the tsunami. Working with local organizations and local social workers, a number of sustainable projects were started. The training of both government and NGO welfare officials, in Aceh, Indonesia, for child protection, was conducted in collaboration with international organizations led by local workers (Tan et al., 2006).

In Sri Lanka, a micro-enterprise solution for financial support was developed by social workers from the FAST project, for women who had lost their husbands (Tan et al., 2006). Being in the community they were able to be a resource to the widows and to connect the home industries with the market. In a separate project the social workers from the tsunami-stricken community of Hambantota were able to connect with orphaned children through therapeutic support groups as well as other activities and programs dealing with trauma and social support of the mental health of the youths (Tan et al., 2006).

Mental health education for social work master's students for disaster preparedness in South India was another FAST-sponsored project (Tan et al., 2006). Mental health and community-based training were developed by students, practitioners and educators together with those affected by the tsunami, promoting resiliency and disaster preparedness in India and Thailand (Tan et al., 2006; Transitions, 2020a).

Sichuan Earthquake and Other Natural Disasters

Many international as well as local organizations responded to the devastating earthquake in Sichuan China in 2008. The author was involved with the training of social workers and volunteers working with a Non-Government Organization in Sichuan to support earthquake survivors. Key principles of grief therapy and counseling were covered in the training, but more importantly, the volunteer's shared experiences were utilized as case studies and illustrations of specific techniques and interventions for dealing with the trauma. In this way the volunteers were also able to process their own experiences of grief and trauma. Reflecting on their feelings of anxiety and depression, as well as the sense of hope and mastery workers developed, was a useful strategy that positively propelled therapeutic encounters (Tan et al., 2006).

Huang (2021) provided a reflection of shared trauma among social workers and survivors in the earthquake. In a post-earthquake social work project in Beichuan of Sichuan Province, about ten years ago, two local social workers were recruited to provide social services in a transitional community for homeless survivors. After a needs assessment of community residents, the two social workers were asked to enhance community resilience through organizing social groups to strengthen local residents' social network and social support.

The shared traumatic experiences of the earthquake helped the two social workers interact with community residents in a more empathetic manner and also contributed to the social workers' understanding of the importance of social networks and social support for earthquake survivors. They quickly established good rapport with community residents and organized social recreational groups, one for older adults and another for women. They promoted the smooth development of the two groups and the active participation of local residents. The planned outcomes of the project were achieved. Through participating in social recreational activities, older adults and women not only broadened their social networks and had more social support, but they also had improved physical and mental health.

The project showed that local social workers, with shared experience, can contribute to disaster survivors' recovery, enhancing their own as well as promoting their clients' social resilience. Social group work is likely to be a good way to enhance disaster survivors' support network given it provides participants with opportunities to interact and connect with each other, to understand and make friends and eventually to help each other. The success of the project also contributed significantly to the social workers' personal resilience and post-traumatic growth.

Illustrating this, Allison Rowlands (2021, n.p.) states: 'My experience as a local worker has helped me professionally in responding' to different disasters. For example, she lived in the Blue Mountains when there was a significant bushfire that destroyed homes and killed people. She was able to apply her shared experience, recounting that: 'Knowing the local community resources, interagency networks and demography, including vulnerable groups, aided needs assessment and working collaboratively across agencies, NGOs and emergent groups to support cohesion and re-build connectivity and resilience.'

Rowlands (2021, n.p.) also had experience with the Newcastle earthquake in Australia and said that although she did not lose family members, suffer property damage or need to flee, she was part of the local communities and she 'still felt the disruption and loss of familiar streetscapes,' especially after the earthquake. She could truly identify, in a psychological sense, with the impacted community, even though she was located away from the epicenter. In raising her own self-awareness of the impact of the natural disaster and her immediate reactions, including 'insight regarding one's current "fitness" to respond,' she advocated for the need of good supervision and consultation and a teamwork approach to effective intervention. Being part of the community she was able to advocate for the community and the individual need for resources and effective coping.

In a class on Disaster Management in Social Work at a university in Chengdu, China, the social work students, who had encountered firsthand earthquakes and tremors during the Great Wenchuan earthquake, were able to share and reflect on their experiences in class as well as in the assignments. This provided material to understand shared trauma and generated a high degree of empathy in working through issues and concerns arising from the sharing. Appropriate intervention, as in building personal and community resilience, was discussed and subsequently carried out by some of the student social workers.

In interviewing Yan, an earthquake survivor, in China, the researchers found that sense of community was vital for social recovery and rebuilding lives (Huang et al., 2016). This study found that social support and sense of community were negatively associated with depression, so that depression decreased as social support and sense of community increased. Therefore, the psychological wellbeing of the survivors of the earthquake was enhanced through social support, governmental support and especially through the sense of community or social resilience (Huang et al., 2016). Note that the building of social capital and support networks enhances social psychological recovery.

Thus, applying community resilience in training curriculums and practice research is important for the field of disaster management and trauma therapy. Research and training of social workers in crisis intervention and inter agency relief work in China included the key principles of community participation, self-help and planning. This was important because for continuity and sustainability, disaster management programs must include participation of the clients and the local counterparts.

Global and Macro Intervention Approaches

In the United Nations Development Plan's response to pandemics, building capacities and providing key resources are key (Obrist et al., 2010). Studies on the health and economic impact of COVID-19 indicated that disproportionately more poor people, especially the homeless, are exposed to the danger and need safe shelter. The poor also have barriers in accessing running water and nutritious food. In organizing disaster relief and recovery, vulnerable people, like refugees, migrants or displaced persons, who have limited movement and less employment opportunities have greater need of community resources and should have priority in receiving assistance and support (Obrist et al., 2010).

Illustrating this, Transitions, a non-profit grassroots organization, developed a working handbook: *Ready Together: A Neighborhood Emergency Preparedness Handbook* (Hall, 2020; Transitions, 2020b) as a strategic move towards disaster risk reduction. Organizational strategy for internet access and constructing a more informative and accessible website for information, referral and resource allocation are useful for communities in the face of natural disasters. The goals in this intervention were to connect with people and to provide mutual aid, as well as to provide a forum for sharing, support and learning from each other. The worker facilitates interactions between individuals, NGOs and other community groups for harnessing and disseminating key resources. This enhances recovery through providing an effective social support network and building capacity during crises or natural disasters (Transitions, 2020a).

Social Intervention in Emergencies and Natural Disasters

There are various observable phases in response to emergencies and disasters, whether natural or not. Comprehensive, professional intervention requires strategies for both a short-term response to the crisis, rescue or relief, as well as the long-term recovery and capacity building.

Whether supporting individuals or communities, one key assumption is to note that people are resilient and systems can be developed to serve and empower them. Resilience in the midst of disaster involves both physical and social resources. Though physical and environmental resilience are important, the building of community social resilience is vital. Recovery involves a sense of community and thus the development of an effective and caring social support network (Huang et al., 2016).

Building resilience means dealing with and reducing the problems faced by vulnerable groups: migrant workers, women, the elderly and children within the community. It is important not only to enhance individual resilience through enabling effective coping and extending social support, but also to empower and facilitate group decision making. People need to rebuild their lives, take control of their situations and participate together in rehabilitating their community, and social workers from within the community can help make this happen by effectively using their social capital to develop trust and social solidarity for effective social recovery.

In extending help to others, social workers' shared experience, systemic orientation and community-focused interventions are useful concepts to be considered. The sense of community is vital for good mental health and recovery from trauma and this is true for both social workers and the clients they work with. Social capital is thus as important, if not more so, as economic and physical resources (Huang et al., 2016).

Summary

Shared lived experience can be useful in working with trauma brought about by natural disasters at the individual, community and societal levels for positive growth. So, what are the specific implications and principles for social work practice with trauma?

Firstly, this chapter provided the conceptualization of crisis, social resilience and shared experience in personal as well as community intervention with natural disasters. Social resilience is vital in dealing with crisis and trauma.

Secondly, building of social resilience and solidarity with both individuals and communities is vital for effective coping and natural disaster management. This is based on shared social capital, trust and social cohesion in dealing with the crisis and building social solidarity.

Thirdly, applying social work values and ethics as well as community organization principles and strategies of participation in joint assessment and decision making, as well as empowerment in creative and collaborative intervention, is essential.

Fourthly, building social inclusion and social resilience responsibly with the shared experience of the worker and client can be a powerful way to deal with trauma, providing healing for them both.

Meeting in the middle thus highlights the joint ownership of the process of recovery that is effective for dealing with shared trauma brought about by natural disasters.

References

Bauwens, J., & Tosone, C. (2010). Professional posttraumatic growth after a shared traumatic experience: Manhattan clinicians' perspectives on post-9/11 practice. *Journal of Loss and Trauma*, 15(6), 498–517.

Berkes, F., & Ross, H. (2012). *Community resilience: Toward an integrated approach*. Retrieved from: https://doi.org/10.1080/08941920.2012.736605.

Bonanno, G. A., Westphal, M., & Mancini, A. D. (2011). Resilience to loss and potential trauma. *Annual Review of Clinical Psychology*, 7(1), 511–535.

Boulanger, G. (2007). Wounded by reality: Understanding and treating adult onset trauma. Taylor & Francis.

Combaz, E. (2014). *Disaster resilience: Topic guide*. GSDRC, University of Birmingham.

Day, K. W., Lawson, G., & Burge, P. (2017). Clinicians' experiences of shared trauma after the shootings at Virginia Tech. *Journal of Counseling & Development*, 95, 269–280.

Dekel, R., & Baum, N. (2009). Intervention in a shared traumatic reality: A new challenge for social workers. *The British Journal of Social Work*, 32, 1–18.

Dominelli, L. (2015). The opportunities and challenges of social work interventions in disaster situations. *International Social Work*, 58(5), 659–672.

Hall, D. (2020). *Building community resilience: Before, during, and after COVID-19*. Retrieved from: www.resilience.org/stories/2020-04-08/building-community-resilience-before-during-and-after-covid-19/.

Horwitz, M. (1999). Social worker trauma: building resilience in child protection social workers. *Smith College Studies in Social Work*, 68(3), 363–377.

Huang, Y. N. (2021). *A reflection of shared trauma among social workers and the Wenchuan earthquake survivors*. Personal communication.

Huang, Y. N., Tan, N. T., & Liu, J. Q. (2016). Support, sense of community, and psychological status in the survivors of the Yaan earthquake. *Journal of Community Psychology*, 44(7), 919–936. doi:10.1002/JCOP.21818.

Lavi, T., Nuttman-Shwartz, O., & Dekel, R. (2015). Therapeutic intervention in a continuous shared traumatic reality: An example from the Israeli–Palestinian conflict. *The British Journal of Social Work*, 47(3), 919–935. doi:10.1093/bjsw/bcv127.

Magis, K. (2010). Community resilience: An indicator of social sustainability. *Society and Natural Resources*, 23(5), 401–416. doi:10.1080/08941920903305674.

NO-AA. (2022) *Global Historical Tsunami Database*. Website of the National Oceanic and Atmospheric Administration. Retrieved from: www.ngdc.noaa.gov/hazard/tsu_db.shtml.

Nouwen, H. J. M. (1972). *The wounded healer: Ministry in contemporary society*. Image Books.

Obrist, B., Pfeiffer, C., & Henley, R. (2010). Multi-layered social resilience: A new approach in mitigation research. *Progress in Development Studies*, 10, 283–293. doi:10.1177/146499340901000402.

Ramsari, A. (2020). The rise of the COVID-19 pandemic and the decline of global citizenship. In J. M. Ryan (Ed.), *COVID-19: Global pandemic, societal responses, ideological solutions* (pp. 94–106). Routledge.

Ross, H., & Berkes, F. (2014). Research approaches for understanding, enhancing, and monitoring community resilience. *Society & Natural Resources*, 27(8), 787–804. doi:10.1080/08941920.2014.905668.

Rowlands, A. R. (2021). *My experience as a local worker*. Personal Communication.

Seeley, K. (2003). *The psychotherapy of trauma and the trauma of psychotherapy: Talking to therapists about 9–11*. Retrieved from: www.coi.columbia.edu/pdf/seeley_pot.pdf.

Sulaiman, N., Teo, W. S., & Fernando, T. (2019). Community resilience frameworks for building community resilient community in Malaysia. *Planning Malaysia: Journal of the Malaysian Institute of Planners*, 17(1), 94–103.

Tan, N. T. (2004). Crisis theory and SARS: Singapore's management of the epidemic. *Asia Pacific Journal of Social Work and Development*, 14(1), 7–17.

Tan, N. T., Rowlands, A., & Yuen, F. K. O. (Eds.). (2006). *Asian tsunami and social work practice: Recovery and rebuilding*. Routledge.

Tierney, K. (2007). From the margins to the mainstream? Disaster research at the crossroads. *Annual Review of Sociology*, 33, 503–525.

Tosone, C., Nuttman-Shwartz, O., & Stephens, T. (2012). Shared trauma: When the professional is personal. *Clinical Social Work Journal*, 40(2), 231–239.

Tosone, C., McTighe, J. P., & Bauwens, J. (2017). Shared traumatic stress among social workers in the aftermath of Hurricane. *The British Journal of Social Work*, 45(4), 1313–1329.

Transitions. (2020a, April 8). *Transitions: Building community resilience*. Retrieved from: www.resilience.org/stories/2020-2004-08/building-community-resilience-before-during-and-after-covid-19/.

Transitions. (2020b, April 30). *Ready together: A neighborhood emergency preparedness handbook*. Retrieved from: www.youtube.com/watch?v=MVwcOmFiYds.

UN News. (2021). *Natural disasters occurring three times more often than 50 years ago: New FAO report*. Retrieved from: https://news.un.org/en/story/2021/03/1087702.

WEF. (2021). *The global risks report 2021* (16th edn). Retrieved from: www3.weforum.org/docs/WEF_The_Global_Risks_Report_2021.pdf.

Wilson, G. A. (2012). *Community resilience, globalization, and transitional pathways of decision-making*. Retrieved from: https://doi.org/10.1016/j.geoforum.

World Bank. (2017). *Sharing Japanese expertise in emergency preparedness and response (EP&R) systems at national and local levels*. Retrieved from: www.

worldbank.org/en/news/feature/2017/10/12/sharing-japanese-expertise-in- em ergency-preparedness-and-response-systems-at-national-and-local-levels.

World Meteorological Organization. (2021a). *Climate change indicators and impacts worsened in 2020*. Retrieved from: https://public.wmo.int/en/media/press-release/ climate-change-indicators-and-impacts-worsened-2020.

World Meteorological Organization. (2021b). *State of the global climate 2020*. WMO-No. 1264. Retrieved from: https://library.wmo.int/doc_num.php?explnum_id=10618.

Zwi, A. B., Spurway, K., Marincowitz, R., Ranmuthugala, G., Hobday, K., & Thompson, L. (2018). *Do CBDRM initiatives impact on the social and economic costs of disasters?*EPPI-Centre. Retrieved from: https://eppi.ioe.ac.uk/cms/Portals/ 0/PDF%20reviews%20and%20summaries/CBRDM%20final%20report.pdf?ver= 2018–2011–22–120410–370.

Shared Reality as a Result of War and Terror

Orit Nuttman-Shwartz

Introduction[1]

Trauma workers, including social workers worldwide, are accustomed to being trained to work in adverse situations (Berger, 2012). This training is provided in accordance with the National Association of Social Workers' code of ethics (2017) which states that social workers must be cognizant of their obligation to "provide appropriate professional services in public emergencies to the greatest extent possible" (p. 29). Consistent with this idea, social workers acting as first responders have a considerable role to play during communal disasters (Bauwens & Naturale, 2017), and in war and terror situations (Nuttman-Shwartz & Sternberg, 2017).

When professionals *both live and work* in the same community as the people they serve, they are exposed to the very same traumatizing circumstances as their clients, and this phenomenon has been defined as "shared trauma" (Saakvitne, 2002; Altman & Davies, 2002; Tosone et al., 2003). Trauma workers working under such conditions are exposed to trauma on two levels. First, they are vicariously exposed via interactions with clients (e.g., hearing clients' traumatic stories). Second, they are themselves directly exposed, as they also belong to / live in the affected community (Baum, 2010, 2012a).

Given that the shared trauma phenomenon is applicable to a wide variety of traumatic events, I undertook a literature review of research that has been conducted in the context of war and terror attacks. War and terrorism, which are generally based in political conflict, can create a state of intense fear, destroy safe environments that are essential for healthy development and create despair for both trauma workers and clients. Volkan (1988) claimed that war and terror, which usually relate to a specific enemy, can become transformed over the years into a "chosen trauma," referring to the shared mental representation of massive trauma that the group's ancestors suffered at the hands of an enemy. Chosen trauma describes the collective memory of a disaster, the echoes of which become a paradigm that keeps the existential threat in the national

DOI: 10.4324/9781003176947-8

memory in order to ward off potential complacency. For example, we can say that in Israel every act of terror revives a primary threat to Jewish survival from the destruction of the second temple, the exile from Spain in 1492, the Holocaust, etc. (Volkan, 1997). When a group's chosen trauma is reactivated (i.e., when a new traumatic event is encountered), this reactivation may have destructive consequences for all group members, including a heightened sense of fear and grieving and even a reduced ability to regulate emotion; therefore, qualifying as a shared trauma (Weinberg & Nuttman-Shwartz, 2006). In order to provide emergency assistance, ongoing help and even healing, social workers and the people living in these situations must work together to make sense of the adverse event and find safety in the midst of shared trauma. As such, my aim is to explore the unique conceptual and practical challenges inherent to the trauma worker-client relationship in this shared war and terror context.

Procedure

In this review, the Google Scholar database was used systematically to locate peer-reviewed articles written in English and published between 1990 and 2020. The rationale for focusing on this period was that the "shared traumatic reality" (STR) paradigm was only fully conceptualized after the Gulf War (1991). The most straightforward search was conducted. Specifically, in the first search wave the terms searched for were: "shared traumatic reality," "shared war," "shared reality," "shared trauma," "shared experience," "double exposure" and "shared resilience." Conjugations and plural forms of these words were also included, along with "terror" and "trauma" in some cases. In the second search wave, I included articles that focused on specific war and terror attacks throughout the years such as: "North Ireland," "The Troubles," "Kosovo War," "war in Afghanistan," "Moscow theatre," "Iraq War," "Beslan school siege," "Madrid train bombings," "7 July London bombings," "2011 Norway attacks," "Charlie Hebdo," "Bataclan terror attack" and "Manchester terror attack." These events were searched for along with the terms "trauma," "shared trauma," "shared reality" and "social workers." In addition, the articles' reference lists were also scanned so as to extend the data found on Google Scholar.

The majority of the research that was related to STR in the shadow of war and terror was conducted in Israel. Of that research, 40% focused on one-time events, and 60% on events that could be referred to as "continuous traumatic stress" (CTS), "emergency routine" and "escalation." In comparison, 84% of the research conducted in the US focused on a single terror event. The literature review also revealed that trauma workers used a variety of interventions connected to STR, consisting of emergency assistance (15 articles), ongoing therapy after short one-time events (16 articles) as well as therapy during continuous traumatic situations.

Results

The Development of the Shared War and Terror Reality Concept

Looking at the development of the concept enables us to identify several traumatic events that have shaped our understanding of STR in the context of war and terror attacks. The STR concept started in Europe and can be traced back to a study published in the mid-20th century by Schmideberg (1942) on the impact of the London blitz, with its repeated bombings, on the civilian population. Although terror events still take place in Europe, the two main locations that are dominant in terms of the STR concept in the literature are (first) the US and (second) Israel.

In the US, early reports on professionals who provided emergency services following the 1995 bombing of the Federal Building in Oklahoma downplayed the implications of the professionals' personal exposure to STR. In their brief report, Krug et al. (1996) claimed that the event did not affect them as individuals but acknowledged that the attack was an experience shared by them (in their role as psychotherapists) and the victims. In their words: "The pressure of work is so constant and immediate that you forget you are part of this community and it's bereavement as much as you are its clinician..." (p. 103). It was only after September 11, 2001 that Wee and Myers (2002) reported findings showing that professionals who provided help after the Oklahoma bombing suffered very high levels of distress and, moreover, that the major predictor of their distress was intense worry about their families.

The 9/11 terror attack constituted a turning point in the consideration of situations during which psychotherapists and their clients were exposed to the same traumatic event. Most researchers who wrote about the impact of 9/11 on mental health professionals treated it as an unprecedented situation for them (e.g., Batten & Orsillo, 2002), in which client and therapist were both in the process of mourning actual and ambiguous losses (Tosone & Bialkin, 2003). Since that time, this topic has been investigated in a growing collection of articles and chapters, for instance in the context of ongoing wars, such as in Afghanistan and Iraq (e.g., Johnson et al., 2011; Tyson, 2007). The clinicians who had hitherto been the main writers on the subject were joined by a variety of researchers carrying out empirical studies, and the phenomenon became a new subcategory within trauma theory known as shared traumatic reality (or STR).

The Development of the Shared Reality Concept in the US

The STR concept was also brought up in the scientific literature related to Israel in the wake of the first Gulf War (1991). During that war the Israeli population was exposed to repeated Iraqi bombings and to the threat of chemical warfare. The Gulf War generated a fair number of studies—all by Israeli writers (e.g., Kretsch et al., 1997; Loewenberg, 1992). In addition, I identified several major wars in which it is clear that the STR phenomenon existed: the second Lebanon War in 2006 (Lev-Wisel et al., 2009) and the ongoing conflict between Israel and Gaza (Baum, 2012a, 2012b, 2014; Dekel & Baum, 2010; Nuttman-Shwartz, 2016), mainly during Operation Cast Lead (2008–2009) and Operation Protective Edge in 2014 (Freedman & Tuval-Mashiach, 2018). Furthermore, I identified several periods marked by continuous terror attacks such as the second Intifada uprisings (2000–2005) (Cohen et al., 2006; Somer et al., 2004), the two decades of ongoing exposure to threats at the border between Israel and Gaza and the forced evacuation from Gaza and North Samaria (2005) (Dekel, 2010; Nuttman-Shwartz & Dekel, 2009).

The Development of the Shared Reality Concept in Israel

The literature review revealed that a variety of expressions are used to describe shared traumatic experiences related to war and terror. Although after the Oklahoma bombing, Krug et al. (1996) termed their experience an "intense shared experience," the expression "shared trauma" was first used after 9/11, when psychotherapists and psychoanalysts wrote about the impact of that terrorist attack on them and their clients. The use of the term "shared trauma" reflects the shift in the phenomenon's conceptualization, now viewed from the perspective of trauma theory, as well as the feelings of the writers who underwent the experience. This new term was used, however, only in papers relating to the clinicians' professional experiences (i.e., mainly reflective works), not in empirical studies. Cabaniss et al. (2003) used "shared reality." Eidelson et al. (2003) used "shared tragedy." Others did not give the phenomenon a name at all (e.g., Adams et al., 2008; Seeley, 2003) but described the dramatic effects of being a trauma worker when the whole community was exposed simultaneously to a terror attack.

In Israel, the first term to be used to describe this kind of phenomenon was "shared reality," and it was used in relation to the first Gulf War (Kretsch et al., 1997). Afterwards, most of the expressions used to refer to STR included the words "war" or "trauma," to stress the context and the negative consequences of the event, for example "shared war experience" (Lev-Wiesel et al., 2009), "shared traumatic reality" (Dekel & Baum, 2010) and "shared war reality" (Peled Avram et al., 2021). In addition, as a result of CTS exposure, wording such as "shared the same stress" (Dekel

& Baum, 2010) and "double exposure" (Baum, 2014) became prevalently used. Combining the terms reality, war and trauma may have reflected the ongoing Israeli–Palestinian conflict encountered by the Israeli researchers.

Several researchers claimed that working in STR situations forced them to expand their theoretical–therapeutic perspective and, as such, came up with concepts such as "ongoing traumatic stress response" (OTSR) (Diamond et al., 2010). This concept describes a situation in which residents in an STR may display clinically significant anxiety symptoms which, although perhaps adaptive, are also stress reactions. These individuals do not have symptoms of PTSD; rather, their symptoms include a range of nonpathological responses that reflect an incipient or subthreshold syndrome along the PTSD spectrum. These responses can significantly impair everyday functioning and quality of life.

Unsurprisingly, and like posttraumatic stress, the shared trauma concept has mainly been viewed through a prism of pathology. Only recently has it also been viewed in other ways, allowing us to see the potentially positive aspects of working in shared continuous traumatic situations. The shared reality phenomenon has thus been broadened, with the addition of the "shared resilience in traumatic situations" conceptualization (Nuttman-Shwartz, 2015b). As can be seen, the current literature argues that STR's negative implications coexist with its positive ones, including resilience; thus, STR should not be seen as an either-or dichotomy (Bauwens & Tosone, 2010; Lavi et al., 2017; Nuttman-Shwartz, 2015b; Pruginin et al., 2017).

Theoretical Framework

Working "under fire" (i.e., in the context of terror attacks and war) poses special challenges for social workers, who are expected to function fully and professionally in a violent reality (e.g., Joseph & Murphy, 2014). In order to do so they need to explore in what way the current situation and being directly exposed to it affects them (e.g., they need to be able to distinguish between secondary traumatization, transference and reactivation of therapists' past traumas) (Shamai, 2005; Somer et al., 2004). Similar to what happens in other emergency situations (Shalev et al., 2012), specific protocols for intervention are also expected to be adopted in STR situations (Nuttman-Shwartz & Sternberg, 2017). Among experienced trauma workers such protocols were found to have been internalized, enabling them to carry out these trauma protocols in STR contexts, despite the stressfulness of these events. In shared reality situations, trauma workers must engage simultaneously in ongoing processes of decision-making and assessments of how the shared reality is affecting both them and the people they assist (Band-Winterstein & Koren, 2010; Baum, 2012b). The distinct knowledge required for interventions in these contexts has been addressed in the literature, where specific approaches are described (e.g., Lahad et al., 2014).

The Positive Implications of Working in a Shared Traumatic Reality

It is important to emphasize the positive findings related to professional growth as well as professional competence that were reported by trauma workers working in a continuous shared reality (Dekel et al., 2016). One of the unique concepts in this context is "shared resilience in a traumatic reality," which encompasses various manifestations of STR-related positive outcomes, both emotional and behavioral. It describes the mutual growth process between therapist and client as a result of reciprocal learning and shared experience, and even the exchange of roles in the relationship. The reciprocal learning, which is undertaken to find a creative solution to the shared threat, may accelerate the therapeutic alliance and process, for instance (Nuttman-Shwartz, 2015b). Therapists, supervisors and managers working in these situations referred to positive aspects of their STR-related training: gaining awareness of the manager's parental role; being supported by their team and developing suitable programs to promote workers' capacities to remain in a war zone out of a sense of moral obligation (Orbach-Avni, 2018); helping employees acquire a deep desire to fulfill their role in an emergency, not because they are bound to do so, but because of a sense of mission and an understanding of their importance (i.e., a commitment to their peer group in the organization that goes beyond a commitment to their supervisors and managers). To develop a sense of commitment in the context of war or terror, social workers must routinely work for it and then, in the event of an emergency, they can adjust and preserve what has already been achieved.

The Role of Social Policy

Part and parcel of the STR experience (resulting from war and terror) is the sudden loss of young people, family members, friends, colleagues, relatives and innocent civilians. Such losses can significantly heighten sensitivity and intensify the difficulty of coping with these situations when the stricken community and the social workers are disconnected from the greater society in which these events are occurring. As such, it is also critical to make a link between social policy and social recognition of the events taking place as well as the lifelong effects of their consequences on helpers, helpees and society as a whole. Just as trauma workers working in military and combat zones need to have extensive knowledge about human development (i.e., what typically happens over the course of the lifespan) and intervention methods, so too do trauma workers in civilian communities that suffer from recurrent war and terror attacks. In both contexts, many complex challenges need to be simultaneously addressed.

STR Assessment Instruments

Over the years, several tools have been developed in an attempt to capture the STR dynamic. It is important to note that the first two tools relate only to the effects of the therapeutic dynamic on the therapist. Both tools were developed in relation to war and terror events, with the first relating to one-time war / terror events and the second to ongoing situations (CTS). The first is the "shared traumatic and professional posttraumatic growth inventory" (STPPG scale; Tosone et al., 2016), which has been in use since post-9/11. The second is the "working in a shared traumatic reality" (Baum, 2014) instrument, which mainly relates to the therapeutic relationship. These instruments have already been elaborated upon in earlier chapters.

Recently a new index was developed, with the focus being on areas of concern that are shared by both therapist and client. This "shared concern measure," developed by Nuttman-Shwartz & Shaul (2021), was constructed on the basis of perceived symmetry between therapists and their clients in situations of a shared reality (Boulanger, 2013) and examines the similarities and differences in therapists' and clients' concerns.

These three tools, in addition to being useful for research purposes, may also be useful for assessing therapist-client relations during therapeutic sessions as well as for increasing therapists' awareness during their own supervision. The three tools in combination may better help to identify: 1) therapists' personal and professional as well as negative and positive responses, and the STR-specific techniques they use; 2) therapists' lack of awareness regarding their responses within the therapeutic relationship (such as intrusive anxiety, lapses in empathy, role expansion and professional immersion); and 3) areas of concern they share with their clients. Using all three measures in combination will help professionals in the field arrive at a better understanding of the STR phenomenon on multiple levels (therapist, client, dyadic relations), both separately and as a whole. That said, to date the tools at our disposal mainly measure the therapist's perspective (i.e., we have yet to "hear" the client's voice on these matters).

The Therapist, the Client and the Dyadic Relations

The majority of the reviewed articles examined the effects of STR situations on therapists; six articles were devoted to the therapeutic relationship; one article focused on supervision and, surprisingly, there were no articles devoted to understanding the STR phenomenon from the client's point of view.

Due to the nature of the STR situation for professional trauma workers (i.e., experiencing trauma via their clients' experiences and also as people who live in the affected community), clinicians may experience significant positive and negative changes in their personal and professional lives. These reactions have the potential to cause permanent changes in clinicians' existing mental schemas and worldviews. As such, it is important to ask how clinicians can be directly exposed to traumas first-hand and maintain their professionalism.

The STR experience causes therapists to become potentially more susceptible to posttraumatic stress and may lead to the blurring of professional and personal boundaries, as well as to increased self-disclosure (Tosone et al., 2012). It perhaps goes without saying that to deal with such blurring of roles requires considerable flexibility and professional maturity (Dekel & Baum, 2010). Research has shown that, unsurprisingly, STR affects trauma workers on the personal, family and professional level (Lavi et al., 2017).

As such, it is important to assess the trauma worker's basic life situation and take into consideration potential risk factors. Such factors include personal factors (e.g., being the parent of young children) (Pagorek-Eshel & Finklestein, 2019), professional factors (e.g., being inexperienced practitioners with little trauma and/or psychotherapy practice) and organizational factors (e.g., lack of supervisor or colleague support) (Nuttman-Shwartz, 2015a). Other relevant factors might include, for instance, being the parent of a soldier (Freedman & Tuval-Mashiach, 2018).

As alluded to earlier, in order to know how to create a therapeutic relationship, either in the acute or chronic phase of a war/terror event, social workers must be aware of both their own and their clients' direct exposure responses. They must have an understanding of the "shared concerns" concept, which is based on the very real physical danger posed by the concrete traumatic threat, and they must acknowledge that this shared situation creates a strong client-therapist symmetry. Such symmetry, of course, flies in the face of the fundamental premise of the treatment relationship, which is meant to be asymmetrical (Aron, 1996).

Furthermore, this symmetry is only likely to increase in certain contexts: if the therapist feels obliged to come to the client's home (e.g., if the home itself is close to the site of a bombing or has actually received a direct hit) or when offering teletherapy (e.g., if the clients live in the exposed area, the roads near their home have been closed by the army and the area has been declared a danger zone) (Nuttman-Shwartz & Shaul, 2021). The literature review showed that this symmetry increased trauma workers' sense of vulnerability and helplessness, affected both the helping relationship and the relationship's setting and impaired workers' ability to give clients their full attention or show empathy. It may also have lessened their ability to make assessments (Shamai, 2005).

In addition, therapists will likely find themselves feeling more preoccupied, anxious and defensive than they would under routine circumstances. Several researchers focused on the shared situation's impact on the ongoing therapeutic process, on the psychotherapist-client relationship and on themselves, both as professionals and as individual members of the threatened community. For example, the Gulf War studies focused on mental health professionals' inner conflict in dealing with this emergency situation. These studies explored the conflict between professional commitments and loyalty to family (as indicated by not having time for them, having difficulties attending to their needs and even experiencing dissociation) faced by social workers and psychologists who provided emergency mental health assistance to civilian victims whose homes were bombed (Keinan-Kon, 1998; Kogan, 2004; Miller-Florsheim, 2002). Similar findings regarding the effects of the symmetrical aspect of the relationship were reported by trauma workers who assisted civilians living in a continuous traumatic situation (Lavi et al., 2017) after more than a decade of the Israeli-Palestinian conflict. The shared nature of the experience may lead clients to lose confidence in the therapists' ability to help and contain them, may blur distinctions between therapists' roles (personal or family vs. therapeutic) and may even lead to temporary role exchanges (Baum, 2010).

These consequences can have both negative and positive effects on therapists' professional identity and professional efficacy (Baum, 2014; Dekel et al., 2016) and may even create shared resilience (Nuttman-Shwartz, 2015b). What practitioners retain from incidences of shared resilience is treasured by them and often perceived as a source of wisdom and inspiration. This is true because shared resilience is something that can be used as a source of professional growth (Baum, 2014) and is crucially important among those who give help in shared and chronic war or terror situations (Nuttman-Shwartz, 2015b).

"Gun Powder Settles Slowly, Penetrates and Causes Despair": A Close-Up Picture of the Therapy Room

The context: Since the end of March 2018, in addition to terror caused by the firing of missiles into Israel, residents on the Israeli side of the border with Gaza have been coping with explosive balloons and kites. Data from the regional resilience center show a substantial increase in the number of clients seeking help, starting from the year 2018, including those who approached the resilience center as a result of this threat (Resilience Center, 2018). What's more, it appears that the explosive balloons and kites in the Gaza envelope (as this area is called) constitute a new and unfamiliar type of threat that challenges existing perspectives among residents of the region, as well as among trauma workers and service providers who are accustomed to making treatment accessible in shared reality situations (e.g., Nuttman-Shwartz & Sternberg, 2017; Tosone et al., 2012).

The client: Miriam (fictitious name), a mother in her 40s who lived in the Gaza envelope area of Sderot, was the first client of Liat's (therapist) to mention the terror of kites and balloons during the therapeutic session. She had been referred for treatment due to depression, which was accompanied by anxiety that impaired her functioning. The security events that took place while she lived in Sderot and raised her children (i.e., missile attacks and military campaigns) affected both her and her children, particularly the younger ones. Her own life and the life of her family were characterized by tension and arousal in this continuous traumatic reality for many years. In the therapeutic sessions, she would share her feelings of anxiety and talk about her young children's avoidance. On several occasions, she would say:

> I'm okay, but what can I do about my children? How can I help them? One of them doesn't want to go to school; the other one started wetting his bed... not to mention that they don't want to go [grocery] shopping or help me.

When military tensions worsened and there were rocket attack sirens, these simple questions become more complex, and the therapeutic sessions became characterized by silences.

The therapeutic process: In theory, Miriam's therapy was supposed to have been short term, with cognitive and behavioral components. It had been based on a plan of gradual exposure to various avoidances, taking into consideration cognitive distortions that affected her depressive symptomatology as well as her anxiety reactions.

Lately, however, Miriam tended to share less, although she maintained contact with Liat and carried out tasks as requested. Nonetheless, she was now bringing to their sessions the threat that was just beginning to emerge: the terror of explosive kites and balloons. Miriam's description of her exposure to this threat included the following: "Gunpowder settles very slowly. It penetrates and causes despair."

Liat, for her part, related to the threat as low-intensity terror, certainly compared to the rockets which over the years had taken human lives and destroyed property. In fact, Liat viewed the explosive kites and balloons as somewhat ridiculous. In her view, they were a temporary type of terror which was not very likely to cause harm. Therefore, she viewed Miriam's terror as another type of intensified cognitive distortion. Based on the well-known children's book *The Story of Five Balloons*, Liat would refer lightly to this form of terror as *A Story of Too Many Balloons*. Initially, such nonchalant reactions were also fueled by the media. Radio broadcasters and journalists defined the new type of terror as a "threat that isn't serious," that wouldn't be too harmful. Maybe, like all types of terror, the terror would mainly end up causing harm only to people's morale.

In light of the way Liat devalued the threat, as well as the way she denied and reduced its severity in the therapeutic discourse, Miriam assumed the role of "responsible adult," and took it upon herself to explain to Liat that this was not "just any kite with fire." Repeatedly she would say to Liat: "It poses a real threat, you can smell the burning" and "You know, it causes real fires." Subsequently, the media started reporting on the damage that the kites caused to vast agricultural areas in the region.

Although no fires broke out in the city of Sderot, they were seen and felt in the open agricultural areas around the city, and this intensified Miriam's anxiety. In the therapeutic sessions, she shared her anxiety with Liat and said, "You can smell it." To reinforce her argument, she added: "My neighbor also mentioned a smell of burning; she even said that the laundry she'd hung outside had absorbed the smell." She explained why she was so afraid: Even though she had gained extensive experience in Sderot regarding how to behave when there was a missile attack, the kites and balloons were something new and different, and they had come without any warning. "Now I have to explain to the kids that they can't go near a kite or a balloon, just like they can't go near the remains of a shell or a rocket." In the past, of course, the kids had always associated kites and balloons with fun and happiness.

Therapist's reflection: Liat who, as mentioned, was surprised to discover the extent to which the new terror posed an unconscious threat (i.e., to Liat) in the initial stages, began to reevaluate. At first, she ignored the threat and tried to learn—on an intellectual level—about its characteristics and how it was reflected in the therapeutic sessions. In particular, she adopted an "omnipotent" perspective in an attempt to learn how to protect her client and herself. Whereas Miriam understood quickly that she needed new knowledge, Liat asked herself on several occasions, in a fairly casual way, "What's going on with these kites now?" It took time for her to realize that, in her words, "The threat of the explosive kites and balloons requires new knowledge as well as a deeper understanding in order for me to connect with the client's reality and with my own reality as a therapist."

The insight that "The kites, which are a symbol of innocence and freedom, have become a symbol of burning and horror" was intolerable at first. Over time, Liat felt that the new threat had penetrated the personal and interpersonal domains, and that this threat called for a new perspective, and even for an evaluation of the threat based on an internal observation of her own cognitive distortion: minimizing the significance of the threat, and faulty thinking about Miriam as someone who intensified the situation too much. In retrospect, Liat knew that like Miriam (notwithstanding Liat's efforts to the contrary), she was also beginning to perceive the explosive kites and balloons as a threat. This feeling of being threatened impaired her ability to consider the nature of the threat. In addition, the sense of threat had succeeded in penetrating the therapeutic room: it posed obstacles, led to confusion, made it difficult to create a safe therapeutic space and called for new evaluations and thinking. Furthermore,

Liat felt that she needed to struggle with herself to determine the extent to which she identified with Miriam's reactions regarding her inability to protect her children.

She also needed to determine the extent to which she was dedicated to continuing treatment with Miriam, or to allowing Miriam's perspective to take hold of the therapy (i.e., allowing Miriam to "manage the therapy"). She worried that Miriam's anxiety might color their relationship in terms of transference or other responses, such as secondary traumatization, that can emerge from empathy. Liat struggled with a range of dissociative reactions and identification, which at times reduced the "therapeutic space." She knew that, ordinarily, her goal would be to expand the therapeutic space (meaning the safe place in which the client can play, use metaphors and associations and be creative). However, the mutual concern, as well as the fear of future attacks, made it difficult for Liat to be present.

That said, she felt that in some ways she was making progress. While containing the shared reality, she also carried out a psychosocial evaluation of Miriam and her needs vis-à-vis the current threat, and she succeeded in evaluating these currently emerging needs, compared to needs that had emerged in light of exposure to other threats. This evaluation contributed to expanding the use of the classic cognitive-behavioral model, which focused on reducing symptoms related to somatic aspects of smells that were relevant to Miriam's distinctive responses to the latest form of terror (i.e., responses she had not had prior to the launching of the incendiary kites and balloons).

The more sessions they had, the more Liat learned about Miriam's terror of the kites and balloons, so that she was able to distinguish between exposure to that terror and exposure to other threats. This enabled her to help Miriam regulate her emotional responses and to separate those responses from her somatic responses, which were adversely affecting Miriam's well-being. In this way she was able to restore balance and bring the traditional client-therapist relationship back into the room.

It was only through the process of reflection and supervision that Liat was able to learn from her experience and move away from a position of vulnerability. In this process, she became aware of the personal meaning of exposure to danger both for her and for her client, so that she could find relevant professional skills and undergo a sense of professional growth despite the feeling of despair and lack of knowledge that characterized her immediate response.

Liat's professional growth was reflected in her ability to combine old and new knowledge, so that she could again conduct "professional" therapeutic interventions. Clearly, Miriam and Liat had shared a traumatic reality for many years prior to the appearance of the kites/balloons. But it took some time to understand that the launching of these incendiary kites/

balloons had also launched a new shared reality for them. This new threat assumed a different form that obligated both of them to re-acknowledge the shared reality, as well as to create an appropriate therapeutic space that allowed for discourse on the meaning of exposure to this threat and that promoted the development of adaptive coping strategies.

Discussion: What We Already Know and What We Still Need to Explore

Over the last 30 years, as war and terror-related traumatic events have become prevalent worldwide, the term "shared reality" has become frequently used to describe the unique therapeutic dynamic that reflects the therapist, the client and the dyadic relations. As mentioned, these understandings have been found to be crucially important when dealing with war and terror situations, whether acute one-time events or chronic ongoing situations. Looking at the literature review overall, it is clear that the experience of a shared war and terror reality gave rise to the STR concept and terminology.

As said, this terminology may reflect a "chosen trauma," which sheds light on the importance of knowing not just trauma theory but also the social meaning of a shared loss (Volkan, 1988). Findings have shown that in war and terror events, people often report an increased sense of solidarity, belonging, nationalism and sameness, all of which increase feelings of symmetry and identification between helpers and helpees. As a result of the feeling that "we are all in the same boat," people feel unified as a nation, a culture, etc. and are less attentive to the differences that exist between them.

Along these lines, given that in the US and Israel (and likely in many other places around the world) people tend to see war and terror events as national security threats, it is important to recognize the power that these events have to elicit memories of major traumatic events, such as World War II. Such chosen traumas can, in a pathological way, shape the therapist's and client's unconscious fear of annihilation, which is reconstructed during the therapeutic encounter in a shared reality situation resulting from new or ongoing war/terror events. These ancient events tend to be "social markers" for both client and therapist, strengthening the symmetry between them and diminishing the distinction between the here and now and the now and then. This unconscious dynamic within the therapist-client dyad abolishes the traditional asymmetry that forms the therapeutic relationship and helps to create the professional working alliance (Boulanger, 2013). Both partners are thus forced to find ways to create mutual and reciprocal relations, which have been found to promote strength and resilience (Nuttman-Shwartz, 2015b).

As mentioned, in addition to the direct and indirect exposure of both client and therapist, the shared nature of the trauma and all that it entails (e.g., the symmetry in the therapeutic relationship) has been found to have negative effects on therapists' ability to cope with the war and terror situation and also affects therapists' professional functioning and personal family life (Baum, 2014; Dekel, 2010). Trauma workers' families, in fact, have been found to be particularly vulnerable. The shared trauma prism, for this reason, may also be an effective construct for understanding family dynamics when the family as a whole is living in a shared reality situation.

Clearly, the traditional trauma perspective still prevails, meaning that trauma tends to be seen mostly through a prism of pathology. Few attempts have been made to identify the factors that facilitate coping and/ or promote growth, resilience and the positive dynamics that develop as a result of the client–therapist encounter in a shared reality (Nuttman-Shwartz, 2016). However, the establishment of a more reciprocal therapist-client relationship, increased empathic bonding, greater therapeutic flexibility and the exchange of therapist and client roles may be seen as positive STR outcomes, on both emotional and behavioral levels. In fact, the positive dimension of working in a shared reality situation is also reflected in the previously mentioned assessment tools which, for example, assess professional growth.

A key point to be gleaned from the literature is the importance of proper STR-specific training for therapists, beyond trauma theory, in order to better identify the differences between shared trauma responses and secondary traumatization, compassion fatigue, secondary trauma and vicarious trauma (Figley, 1995). Direct and indirect responses may occur simultaneously under STR conditions, and social workers must be keenly aware that their traumatic responses and their own dissociative processes may alter the nature of their relationships with their clients (Tosone et al., 2012), colleagues and even family members (Dekel et al., 2016). That said, they should also be mindful of the potentially positive outcomes of STR, including shared resilience and professional growth resulting from improved client-therapist reciprocal relations. Such reciprocity allows for the two dyad members to jointly reach a desired outcome (Tosone, 2021) and promotes the mental health of both parties. In addition, in terms of a shared traumatic reality resulting from political violence, a distinction must be made between working in the context of a one-time acute event vs. dealing with an ongoing traumatic situation, which includes vacillating between routine and emergency.

Despite the fact that the word "shared" figures so prominently in the literature on this topic, there is very little material, if any, on the client's perspective towards shared reality situations. Although it is possible that articles based solely on the client's point of view do exist, the search process that I personally conducted did not unveil any such articles, and none of the studies I identified used any type of shared measure to elicit clients' responses. As such, there is a still a missing link, preventing a full exploration and description of the shared reality experience, as well as impeding the tailoring of suitable interventions. Clearly, an ecological perspective must be adopted in the STR context, especially when this traumatic reality is a result of war and terror. With most of the data being based on therapists' points of view, it is imperative that clients be included in the next research agenda.

Another important point is that although over the years it has become clearer that shared trauma is one of the most important constructs in understanding the mental health consequences for mental health experts working with trauma survivors 1) in times of war, 2) as a result of terror attacks, and 3) as a result of a variety of recent adverse events worldwide, the shared reality perspective only seems to figure prominently in the US and Israel. Thus, several questions emerge: What about the missing data from other parts of the world that also suffer from shared trauma as a result of war and terror, such as Europe, Asia or Africa? Is the shared reality concept universal? Does STR as a result of war and trauma belong to a unique cultural domain? Is it related to the cultural, social or national agenda? Does it matter *where* the war and terror are taking place?

As of the time of this writing (April, 2021), Israel finally seems to be coming out of the COVID-19 pandemic, after a successful vaccination rollout. The pandemic represented yet another shared traumatic reality, but for some Israelis—those living on the border with Gaza—this trauma has been compounded by the trauma described throughout this chapter. During the past week, dozens of rockets were again launched from the other side of the border, and so instead of enjoying their newfound post-pandemic freedom, southern Israelis—after spending a year in lockdowns and quarantines—found themselves running back into shelters. Israeli children, in voices wise beyond their years, described to news reporters how they have been traumatized over and over again; unfortunately, they have never known anything *but* a traumatic reality.

Recommendations for Practice

Several practical recommendations have already been suggested by a number of scholars (Cohen et al., 2015; Joseph & Murphy, 2014; Nutt-man-Shwartz & Green, 2020; Nuttman-Shwartz & Sternberg, 2017; Orbach-Avni, 2018):

1   Trauma workers need to receive training and retraining. In the context of STR, there is a need for the organized provision of primary, inter-mediate and advanced training with regard to concepts such as shared resilience in traumatic situations, mitigation and preparedness and the importance of familiarity with the specific tools and skills that have

already been conceptualized, such as the previously mentioned assessment tools, and with the population receiving assistance.

2 Trauma workers must stay current, as knowledge in this area is constantly evolving. The STR concept is continually being fine-tuned and added to, with related ideas such as CTS (ongoing traumatic situations, typified by frequent shifts between routine and emergency) and OTSR (ongoing traumatic stress responses). Also, recent resilience research has emphasized the importance of using an ecological perspective, which aligns well with the social work profession, in a shared reality context.

3 Trauma workers' families have been found to have heightened vulnerability in times of STR. As such, based on a social work systems perspective, it is important to widen the shared trauma concept to include not only the therapist-client relationship but also the therapist-family dynamic. After all, therapists presumably live with their families and are therefore, during times of war/terror, experiencing yet another shared reality.

4 Regarding levels of intervention, it is important to consider the community as a whole, which is recognized today as an essential component for promoting resilience. In this regard, trauma workers, and especially social workers, play a key role in all stages of the intervention.

5 It is recommended that practitioners be permitted to work "from a distance" and, if they so choose, temporarily move with their families out of the danger zone, to someplace relatively close by. In this way they would be able to spend time with their families but also continue working.

6 Trauma workers need to allow themselves to oscillate between their personal and professional roles, as well as between their own experiences and their clients' experiences. The ability to oscillate in this way has been found to be effective in shared traumatic situations.

7 Staff members of social and psychological service agencies should have a good deal of professional experience and awareness. In addition, they must be able to focus on the needs of the population and put aside their own personal and familial needs when working. Clearly, this is a more difficult task for younger, more inexperienced workers who also tend to have young children at home.

8 Team managers and supervisors need to provide frequent supervision and encourage more interpersonal collegial support. For example, they could encourage workers to work together with a colleague as a team; they could suggest to less experienced workers that they work with those who have already been evacuated from the "war zone" rather than with those still inside it; they could encourage burned-out/stressed-out workers to take frequent breaks. Finally, supervisors and

managers should acknowledge and recognize (socially and professionally) the value of the work these workers are doing under
extremely difficult conditions.

9   Direct and indirect supervisors can play a key role in emotion regulation and in providing social workers with emotional containment
and support. Such support might enhance workers' sense of being an
integral part of the staff, post-event, and of feeling more competent.

10 Reflective work and work documentation have been found to be
effective ways to continue working in a shared reality, to better conceptualize the situation, to improve protocols and to receive recognition from other professionals in the field as well as society at large.

11 When implementing trauma-informed care during situations of war
and terror, trauma workers need to ensure the protection of people in
vulnerable situations, understand the pervasive nature of trauma and
promote an environment of healing (rather than practices that may
inadvertently retraumatize people) while always respecting the rights
of all involved. In addition to exploring whether shared resilience
processes, crisis resolution and reconciliation can be added to their
intervention "toolbox" in the STR context, they must first and foremost be mindful of core social work principles such as human rights,
human dignity, social justice and service to others, including offering
help to all who are in need. Finally, they must adhere to all of these
core principles, even in a war/terror context, as well as promoting
peace-related approaches.

Note

1   The author wishes to acknowledge Eve Horowitz Leibowitz's contribution to
the writing of this chapter.

References

Adams, R. E., Figley, C. R., & Boscarino, J. A. (2008). The compassion fatigue
scale: Its use with social workers following urban disaster. *Research on Social
Work Practice*, 18(3), 238–250. https://doi.org/10.1177/1049731507310190.

Altman, N., & Davies, J. M. (2002). Out of the blue: Reflections on a shared
trauma. *Psychoanalytic Dialogues*, 12(3), 359–360. https://doi.org/10.1080/
10481881209348672.

Aron, L. (1996). *A meeting of minds: Mutuality in psychoanalysis*. Analytic Press,
Inc.

Band-Winterstein, T., & Koren, C. (2010). "We take care of the older person, who
takes care of us?" Professionals working with older persons in a shared war
reality. *Journal of Applied Gerontology*, 29(6), 772–792. https://doi.org/10.1177/
0733464809357427.

Batten, S. V., & Orsillo, S. M. (2002). Therapist reactions in the context of collective trauma. *The Behavior Therapist*, 25(2), 36–40.

Baum, N. (2004). Social work students cope with terror. *Clinical Social Work Journal*, 32(4), 395–413. https://doi.org/10.1007/s10615–004–0539–y.

Baum, N. (2010). Shared traumatic reality in communal disasters: Toward a conceptualization. *Psychotherapy*, 47(2), 249–259. https://doi.org/10.1037/a0019784.

Baum, N. (2012a). "Emergency routine": The experience of professionals in a shared traumatic reality of war. *British Journal of Social Work*, 42(3), 424–442. https://doi.org/10.1093/bjsw/bcr032.

Baum, N. (2012b). Trap of conflicting needs: Helping professionals in the wake of a shared traumatic reality. *Clinical Social Work Journal*, 40(1), 37–45. https://doi.org/10.1007/s10615–011–0347–0.

Baum, N. (2014). Professionals' double exposure in the shared traumatic reality of wartime: Contributions to professional growth and stress. *The British Journal of Social Work*, 44(8), 2113–2134. https://doi.org/10.1093/bjsw/bct085.

Baum, N., & Ramon, S. (2010). Professional growth in turbulent times: An impact of political violence on social work practice in Israel. *Journal of Social Work*, 10 (2), 139–156. https://doi.org/10.1177/1468017310363636.

Bauwens, J., & Naturale, A. (2017). The role of social work in the aftermath of disasters and traumatic events. *Clinical Social Work Journal*, 45(2), 99–101. https://doi.org/10.1007/s10615–017–0623–8.

Bauwens, J., & Tosone, C. (2010). Professional posttraumatic growth after a shared traumatic experience: Manhattan clinicians' perspectives on post-9/11 practice. *Journal of Loss and Trauma*, 15(6), 498–517. https://doi.org/10.1080/15325024.2010.519267.

Berger, R. (2012). Trauma and social work practice. In C. R. Figley (Ed.), *The encyclopedia of trauma* (pp. 700–703). Sage.

Boulanger, G. (2013). Fearful symmetry: Shared trauma in New Orleans after Hurricane Katrina. *Psychoanalytic Dialogues*, 23(1), 31–44. https://doi.org/10.1080/10481885.2013.752700.

Cabaniss, D. L., Forand, N., & Roose, S. P. (2004). Conducting analysis after September 11: Implications for psychoanalytic technique. *Journal of the American Psychoanalytic Association*, 52(3), 717–734. https://doi.org/10.1177/00030651040520030401.

Cohen, E., Roer-Strier, D., Menachem, M., Fingher-Amitai, S., & Israeli, N. (2015). "Common–fate": Therapists' benefits and perils in conducting child therapy following the shared traumatic reality of war. *Clinical Social Work Journal*, 43(1), 77–88. https://doi.org/10.1007/s10615–014–0499–9.

Cohen, M., Gagin, R., & Peled-Avram, M. (2006). Multiple terrorist attacks: Compassion fatigue in Israeli social workers. *Traumatology*, 12(4), 293–301. https://doi.org/10.1177/1534765606297820.

Dekel, R. (2010). Mental health practitioners' experiences during the shared trauma of the forced relocation from Gush Katif. *Clinical Social Work Journal*, 38(4), 388–396. https://doi.org/10.1007/s10615–009–0258–5.

Dekel, R., & Baum, N. (2010). Intervention in a shared traumatic reality: A new challenge for social workers. *British Journal of Social Work*, 40(6), 1927–1944. doi:10.1093/bjsw/bcp137.

Dekel, R., Hantman, S., Ginzburg, K., & Solomon, Z. (2007). The cost of caring? Social workers in hospitals confront ongoing terrorism. *British Journal of Social Work*, 37(7), 1247–1261. https://doi.org/10.1093/bjsw/bcl081.

Dekel, R., Nuttman-Shwartz, O., & Lavi, T. (2016). Shared traumatic reality and boundary theory: How mental health professionals cope with the home/work conflict during continuous security threats. *Journal of Couple & Relationship Therapy*, 15(2), 121–134. https://doi.org/10.1080/15332691.2015.1068251.

Diamond, G. M., Lipsitz, J. D., Fajerman, Z., & Rozenblat, O. (2010). Ongoing traumatic stress response (OTSR) in Sderot, Israel. *Professional Psychology: Research and Practice*, 41(1), 19–25. https://doi.org/10.1037/a0017098.

Eidelson, R. J., D'Alessio, G. R., & Eidelson, J. I. (2003). The impact of September 11 on psychologists. *Professional Psychology: Research and Practice*, 34(2), 144–150. https://doi.org/10.1037/0735-7028.34.2.144.

Figley, C. R. (Ed.). (1995). *Compassion fatigue: Coping with secondary traumatic stress disorder in those who treat the traumatized*. Brunner/Mazel.

Finklestein, M., Stein, E., Greene, T., Bronstein, I., & Solomon, Z. (2015). Post-traumatic stress disorder and vicarious trauma in mental health professionals. *Health & Social Work*, 40(2), e25–e31. https://doi.org/10.1093/hsw/hlv026.

Freedman, S. A., & Tuval-Mashiach, R. (2018). Shared trauma reality in war: Mental health therapists' experience. *PloS one*, 13(2), e0191949. https://doi.org/10.1371/journal.pone.0191949.

Halpern, J. (2016). Maintaining helper wellness and competence in a shared trauma reality. *Israeli Journal of Health Policy Research*, 5, 38. https://doi.org/10.1186/s13584-016-0102-7.

Johnson, W. B., Johnson, S. J., Sullivan, G. R., Bongar, B., Miller, L., & Sammons, M. T. (2011). Psychology in extremis: Preventing problems of professional competence in dangerous practice settings. *Professional Psychology: Research and Practice*, 42(1), 94–104. https://doi.org/10.1037/a0022365.

Joseph, S., & Murphy, D. (2014). Trauma: A unifying concept for social work. *The British Journal of Social Work*, 44(5), 1094–1109. https://doi.org/10.1093/bjsw/bcs207.

Keinan-Kon, N. (1998). Internal reality, external reality, and denial in the Gulf War. *Journal of the American Academy of Psychoanalysis*, 26(3), 417–442.

Kogan, I. (2004). The role of the analyst in the analytic cure during times of chronic crises. *Journal of the American Psychoanalytic Association*, 52(3), 735–757. https://doi.org/10.1177/00030651040520031201.

Kretsch, R., Benyakar, M., Baruch, E., & Roth, M. (1997). A shared reality of therapists and survivors in a national crisis as illustrated by the Gulf War. *Psychotherapy: Theory, Research, Practice, Training*, 34(1), 28–33. https://doi.org/10.1037/h0087818.

Krug, R. S., Nixon, S. J., & Vincent, R. (1996). Psychological response to the Oklahoma City bombing. *Journal of Clinical Psychology*, 52(1), 103–105. https://doi.org/10.1002/(SICI)1097-4679(199601)52:1<103:AID-JCLP13>3.0.CO;2-Q.

Lahad, M., Leykin, D., Rozenblat, O., & Fajerman, Z. (2014). Exploring the efficacy of anxiety and PTSD therapeutic techniques and protocols in practice during ongoing terrorism: Evidence from a focus group research. *International Journal of Social Work*, 1(1), 49–69.

Lavi, T., Nuttman-Shwartz, O., & Dekel, R. (2017). Therapeutic intervention in a continuous shared traumatic reality: An example from the Israeli/Palestinian conflict. *British Journal of Social Work*, 47(3), 919–935. doi:10.10973/bjsw/bcv127.

Lester, P. B., Taylor, L. C., Hawkins, S. A., & Landry, L. (2015). Current directions in military health–care provider resilience. *Current Psychiatry Reports*, 17(2), 6. https://doi.org/10.1007/s11920–014–0539–8.

Lev-Wiesel, R., Goldblatt, H., Eisikovits, Z., & Admi, H. (2009). Growth in the shadow of war: The case of social workers and nurses working in a shared war reality. *British Journal of Social Work*, 39(6), 1154–1174. https://doi.org/10.1093/bjsw/bcn021.

Loewenberg, F. M. (1992). Notes on ethical dilemmas in wartime: Experiences of Israeli social workers during Operation Desert Shield. *International Social Work*, 35(4), 429–439. https://doi.org/10.1177/002087289203500405.

Miller-Florsheim, D. (2002). From containment to leakage, from the collective to the uniqe: therapist and patient in shared national trauma. In C. Covington, P. Williams, J. Arundale, J. Knox & J. Alderdice (Eds.), *Terrorism and war: Unconscious dynamics of political violence*. Routledge.

National Association of Social Workers. (2017). *Code of ethics*. NASW.

Nuttman-Shwartz, O. (2015a). Post-traumatic stress in social work. In J. Wright (Ed.), *The international encyclopedia of social & behavioural sciences* (2nd edn, Vol. 18, pp. 707–713). Elsevier.

Nuttman-Shwartz, O. (2015b). Shared resilience in a traumatic reality: A new concept for trauma workers exposed personally and professionally to collective disaster. *Trauma, Violence, & Abuse*, 16(4), 466–475. https://doi.org/10.1177/1524838014557287.

Nuttman-Shwartz, O. (2016). Research in a shared traumatic reality: Researchers in a disaster context. *Journal of Loss and Trauma*, 21(3), 179–191. https://doi.org/10.1080/15325024.2015.1084856.

Nuttman-Shwartz, O., & Dekel, R. (2009). Challenges for students working in a shared traumatic reality. *British Journal of Social Work*, 39(3), 522–538. https://doi.org/10.1093/bjsw/bcm121.

Nuttman-Shwartz, O., & Green, O. (2020). Resilience truths: Trauma resilience workers' points of view toward resilience in continuous traumatic situations. *International Journal of Stress Management*. https://doi.org/10.1037/str0000223.

Nuttman-Shwartz, O., & Shaul, K. (2020). Baloney nefetz veafifoney tavera bamerchav hatipuli [Explosive balloons and conflagration kites in the therapeutic setting]. *Society & Welfare*, 40(2–3), 295–318.

Nuttman-Shwartz, O., & Shaul, K. (2021). Online therapy in a shared reality: The coronavirus as a test case. *Traumatology*, 27(4), 365–374.

Nuttman-Shwartz, O., & Shay, S. (2006). Supervision groups at a time of violent social conflict in Israel. *Journal for Specialists in Group Work*, 31(4), 291–309. https://doi.org/10.1080/01933920600918741.

Nuttman-Shwartz, O., & Sternberg, R. (2017). Social work in the context of an ongoing security threat: Role description, personal experiences, and conceptualization. *British Journal of Social Work*, 47(3), 903–918. doi:10.1093/bjsw/bcw053.

Orbach-Avni, T. (2018). Merituk mishki lerituk rigshi—Model lrnihul ovdim behirum: Retrospectiva lemetziut habithonit beotef aza 2005–2018 [From economic paralysis to emotional grounding—A model for managing employees in an emergency: Retrosective to the conflicted reality of Ottef Gaza 2005–2008]. *Et HaSade,* 19, 169–187.

Pagorek-Eshel, S., & Finklestein, M. (2019). Family resilience among parent–adolescent dyads exposed to ongoing rocket fire. *Psychological Trauma: Theory, Research, Practice, and Policy,* 11(3), 283–291. https://doi.org/10.1037/tra0000397.

Peled Avram, M., Zrihan-Weitzman, A., Zilberberg, O., & Farchi, M. (2021). The lived experience of novice helpers as first responders in a shared war reality. *Journal of Evidence–Based Social Work,* 18(1), 85–100. https://doi.org/10.1080/26408066.2020.1814926.

Pruginin, I., Segal-Engelchin, D., Isralowitz, R., & Reznik, A. (2016). Shared war reality effects on the professional quality of life of mental health professionals. *Israeli Journal of Health Policy Research,* 5, 17. https://doi.org/10.1186/s13584–016–0075–6.

Pruginin, I., Findley, P., Isralowitz, R., & Reznik, A. (2017). Adaptation and resilience among clinicians under missile attack: Shared traumatic reality. *International Journal of Mental Health Addiction,* 15(3), 684–700. https://doi.org/10.1007/s11469–017–9748–9.

Pulido, M. L. (2012). The ripple effect: Lessons learned about secondary traumatic stress among clinicians responding to the September 11th terrorist attacks. *Clinical Social Work Journal,* 40(3), 307–315. https://doi.org/10.1007/s10615–012–0384–3.

Resilience Center. (2018). *Merkazey hosen—Sderot veyeshuvei ottef aza. Sikum shnat avoda—2018* [*Resilience Center—Sderot and Gaza envelope community. End of year review—2018*]. Resilience Center.

Saakvitne, K. W. (2002). Shared trauma: The therapist's increased vulnerability. *Psychoanalytic Dialogues,* 12(3), 443–449. https://doi.org/10.1080/10481881209348678.

Schiff, M., Dekel, R., Gilbar, O., & Benbenishty, R. (2018). Helping the helper: Posttraumatic distress and need for help among Israelis social workers in foster care agencies following armed conflict. *Child & Family Social Work,* 23(3), 466–474. https://doi.org/10.1111/cfs.12438.

Schmideberg, M. (1942). Some observations on individual reactions to air raids. *The International Journal of Psychoanalysis,* 23, 146–176.

Seeley, K. (2003). *The psychotherapy of trauma and the trauma of psychotherapy: Talking to therapists about 9–11.* Working Paper Series, Center on Organizational Innovation, Columbia University. Retrieved from: www.coi.columbia.edu/pdf/seeley_pot.pdf.

Segal-Engelchin, D., Achdut, N., Huss, E., & Sarid, O. (2020). CB–Art interventions implemented with mental health professionals working in a shared war reality: Transforming negative images and enhancing coping resources. *International Journal of Environmental Research and Public Health,* 17(7), 2287. https://doi.org/10.3390/ijerph17072287.

Shalev, A. Y., Ankri, Y., Israeli-Shalev, Y., Peleg, T., Adessky, R., & Freedman, S. (2012). Prevention of posttraumatic stress disorder by early treatment: Results from the Jerusalem Trauma Outreach and Prevention study. *Archives of General Psychiatry,* 69(2), 166–176. https://doi.org/10.1001/archgenpsychiatry.2011.127.

Shalvi, S., & Luzzatto, D. (2006). Lack of safe environment: Emotional difficulties and coping among clinicians treating traumatized patients within a terrorized society—Israel 2006. *Traumatology*, 12(4), 282–292. https://doi.org/10.1177/ 1534765606297818.

Shamai, M. (2005). Personal experience in professional narratives: The role of helpers' families in their work with terror victims. *Family Process*, 44(2), 203–215. https://doi.org/10.1111/j.1545-5300.2005.00054.x.

Shamai, M., & Ron, P. (2009). Helping direct and indirect victims of national terror: Experiences of Israeli social workers. *Qualitative Health Research*, 19(1), 42–54. https://doi.org/10.1177/1049732308327350.

Somer, E., Buchbinder, E., Peled Avram, M., & Ben-Yizhack, Y. (2004). The stress and coping of Israeli emergency room social workers following terrorist attacks. *Qualitative Health Research*, 14(8), 1077–1093. https://doi.org/10. 1177/1049732304267774.

Tosone, C. (2011). The legacy of September 11: Shared trauma, therapeutic intimacy, and professional posttraumatic growth. *Traumatology*, 17(3), 25–29. http s://doi.org/10.1177/1534765611421963.

Tosone, C. (2021) Introduction. In C. Tosone (Ed.) *Shared trauma, shared resilience during a pandemic* (pp. 1–11). Springer.

Tosone, C., & Bialkin, L. (2003). The impact of mass violence and secondary trauma in clinical practice. In L. A. Straussner & N. Phillips (Eds.), *Social work with victims of mass violence* (pp. 157–167). Jossey-Bass.

Tosone, C., Bialkin, L., Campbell, M., Charters, M., Gieri, K., Gross, S., Grounds, C., Johnson, K., Kitson, D., Lanzo, S., Lee, M., Martinez, A., Martinez, M. M., Milich, J., Riofrio, A., Rosenblatt, L., Sandler, J., Scali, M., Spiro, M., & Stefan, A. (2003). Shared trauma: Group reflections on the September 11th disaster. *Psychoanalytical Social Work*, 10(1), 57–77. https://doi.org/10.1300/J032v10n01_06.

Tosone, C., McTighe, J. P., Bauwens, J., & Naturale, A. (2011). Shared traumatic stress and the long–term impact of 9/11 on Manhattan clinicians. *Journal of Traumatic Stress*, 24(5), 546–552. https://doi.org/10.1002/jts.20686.

Tosone, C., Nuttman-Shwartz, O., & Stephens, T. (2012). Shared trauma: When the professional is personal. *Clinical Journal of Social Work*, 40(2), 231–239. doi:10.1007/s10615–10012–0395–0.

Tosone, C., Bauwens, J., & Glassman, M. (2016). The shared traumatic and professional posttraumatic growth inventory. *Research on Social Work Practice*, 26 (3), 286–294. https://doi.org/10.1177/1049731514549814.

Tyson, J. (2007). Compassion fatigue in the treatment of combat-related trauma during wartime. *Clinical Social Work Journal*, 35, 183–192. https://doi.org/10. 1007/s10615–007–0095–3.

Unger-Arnov, Y. (2009). *Metziut meshutefet shel milhama– Havayot haovdot haso-chyaliot bakirya harefuit Rambam bemilchemet levanon hashniya [Shared war reality: Female social workers experience's in Rambam Medical Center during 2006 Lebanon war]*. [Unpublished thesis dissertation]. Haifa University.

Volkan, V. D. (1988). *The need to have enemies and allies: From clinical practice to international relationships*. Jason Aronson.

Volkan, V. D. (1997). *Bloodlines: From ethnic pride to ethnic terrorism*. Farrar Straus and Giroux.

Wee, D. F., & Myers, D. (2002). Stress responses of mental health workers following disaster: The Oklahoma City bombing. In C. R. Figley (Ed.), *Treating compassion fatigue* (pp. 57–83), Psychosocial Stress Series, No. 24. Routledge.

Weinberg, H., & Nuttman-Shwartz, O. (2006). Group work and therapy in Israel—Mirroring a regressed–traumatized society. *The Journal Organizational and Social Dynamics*, 6(1), 95–110.

Part III

Battlegrounds of Shared Trauma: Social Work Modalities

DOI: 10.4324/9781003176947-9

Finding Our Way Together

Relational Therapy during a Global Pandemic

Johanna E. Barry and Jonathan B. Singer

Introduction

During the 134 years between Freud opening his clinical practice in 1886 and the US shutting down for the COVID-19 pandemic on March 13, 2020, psychotherapy was primarily an in-person endeavor. Whether you were in a comfortable office with soft couches and soothing lighting, or in the chaos of someone's double wide trailer in Central Texas, psychotherapy was face-to-face. Although a growing number of therapists were dipping their toes into the world of online therapy prior to the pandemic and scholars were establishing an evidence base for the effectiveness of online psychotherapy (Ahern et al., 2018; Andersson, 2016), there were attitudinal and functional barriers to widespread adoption of telemental health.

The COVID-19 pandemic brought two fundamental shifts to psychotherapy: online services and shared trauma. In many cases, both the client and therapist were figuring out at the same time how online therapy worked and how to live through the same catastrophe. Not since Freud decided to let his patients talk without interruption has there been such a seismic shift in the helping relationship. In this chapter, we discuss the shift in therapeutic interactions during the pandemic as well as the effectiveness of feminist relational therapeutic approaches in the face of shared trauma, brought to life through the descriptions of two case studies. We suggest that the concepts of shared resilience, trauma-informed care and accompaniment are useful in understanding how and why relational approaches are beneficial during a pandemic. We conclude by offering helpful tips to social workers practicing as therapists during the pandemic and after.

Shared Trauma

Shared trauma interrogates the assumption that the only person in the therapy room who has experienced a traumatic event is the client, or the assumption that practitioners may only be indirectly exposed to trauma through their clients' experiences. Instead, the concept of shared trauma

DOI: 10.4324/9781003176947-10

recognizes that there are times when practitioners are exposed to the same threats and disasters as their clients (Eidelson et al., 2003; Felsen, 2020; Tosone et al., 2016). During these times, therapists are responsible not only for shepherding clients through tragedy, but also for coping themselves. Often viewed from a negative vantage point, terms such as "shared trauma," "shared traumatic stress" and "shared tragedy" have proliferated within the professional literature.

Boulanger (2013) advanced our understanding of shared trauma through her detailed personal accounts of four therapists who, alongside their clients, survived the disaster of Hurricane Katrina in 2005. Years after the tragedy, three clinicians described the debilitating impact surviving the natural disaster had on their professional and personal lives. As one of the clinicians included in the longitudinal study attested, "It was the first time in my life that I ever felt incapacitated to work" (Boulanger, 2013, p. 33). Indeed, the widespread and long-term psychological and physical effects of shared trauma made it impossible for many therapists to do their jobs effectively due to the amount of support they also needed at that time. Perhaps the most striking difficulty the four clinicians report from this work was the insurmountable existential dread and inability to thwart the countertransference engendered from surviving the same tragedy as their clients. The therapeutic relationship, once characterized by its unique unidirectional offering of support, now involved blurred boundaries and the need for mutual healing.

In contrast to the negative repercussions of psychotherapy during collective trauma, Nuttman-Shwartz (2015) discussed positive consequences resulting from shared trauma through her work exploring the concept of "shared resilience in a traumatic reality." The author described the shared bonding and mutual empathic response generated from the client and therapist living in the same communities during traumatic events. Other scholars have noted that when resilience is experienced by both therapist and client, the therapist may in fact feel more confident and competent in providing support (Clemans, 2005). A great part of what affords resilience is the ability for therapists to be inspired by the capacity of the human condition and spirit through their clients' perseverance, resulting in a mutually beneficial and empowering relationship (Benatar, 2000). These feelings of empowerment and confidence have positive implications for the treatment therapists are then able to offer clients.

The Role of the Relational Therapy Model

During times of shared trauma, greater emphasis is often placed on the therapeutic relationship (Day et al., 2017). Relational therapy is a model that focuses on the power of the relationship between therapist and client to promote healing. Based on the idea that strong and fulfilling relationships with other individuals can help people maintain emotional well-being, this model may be especially helpful for those seeking therapy during times of trauma (Haskins & Appling, 2017).

Trauma is relational, resulting from a breach in the attachments to community and loved ones (Herman, 1992). Trauma is also a subjective experience (Tosone, 2021). During the COVID-19 pandemic, there are countless examples of isolation and disconnection from others which resemble trauma, could be perceived as traumatic and which could exacerbate the trauma responses clients bring to sessions. Centering therapy work on connection and relationship is one way of addressing these relational ruptures (Taylor, 2020).

When compared to some of the more manualized treatment models, such as cognitive behavior therapy (CBT), relational approaches and especially feminist relational techniques do well in contexts of shared trauma to account for the intersectionality of client identities and how these identities differentially impact clients' experiences in the face of catastrophe. Israeli and Santor (2000) explored the particularly effective aspects of feminist relational therapy and found the core component of consciousness raising and reflexivity to be particularly helpful in working with clients who were trauma survivors. Moreover, the effort feminist relational practitioners exert in understanding clients' experiences based on their identities and how these identities have shaped their worldview is fundamental to successful trauma treatment (Edwards et al., 2014).

During times of shared trauma, adhering to a feminist relational approach may further help therapists avoid over-identifying with a client and presuming to know their experience (Wolf et al., 2018). Feminist relational therapists practice reflexivity and constantly evaluate their positionality within the therapist-client dyad (Worthington & Stern, 1985). Positionality is defined as a concept in psychotherapy as well as social science research referring to how differences in social position and power shape identities and access to resources (Hesse-Biber, 2011). This idea is often discussed in the social work field due to the emphasis social workers place on understanding issues of power, privilege and oppression, and how one's positionality either bolsters or hinders an acknowledgement of such power differentials. By keeping diligent notes related to evaluating their positionality, feminist relational practitioners create the environment in which clients can have their own unique experiences in the safety of a relationship that honors such uniqueness. Feminist relational therapy can foster a mutually empathic relationship between therapist and client that results in their simultaneous growth and healing during shared trauma: dismantling the expert-client power differential and eschewing hierarchical forms of therapy (Matheson, 2004). Through a leveling of hierarchy, an important concept in the social work field as well as in trauma-informed care, there is an increased opportunity for the therapist to walk alongside their client and align with them during times of shared trauma.

Trauma-informed care (TIC) is an organizational framework that seeks to eliminate structures or processes present in many treatment settings that lead to clients being traumatized or retraumatized (McClatchey, 2020). Within the scope of TIC, it is understood that practitioners are sensitive to how environmental issues and past trauma impact the work and relationship. There are several key components for providing TIC, including: 1) meeting client needs in a safe, collaborative and compassionate manner; 2) preventing treatment practices that retraumatize people with histories of trauma who are seeking help or receiving services; 3) building on the strengths and resilience of clients in the context of their environments and communities; and 4) endorsing trauma-informed principles in agencies through support, consultation and supervision of staff (SAMHSA, 2014). TIC practitioners have a thorough understanding of the complex impact traumatic experiences have on the mind and body, and thus know that engaging in a relationship that models safety, security and the importance of moving at the client's own pace is paramount (Levine et al., 2021).

An understanding of TIC can also benefit the clinician during times of shared trauma (Tong et al., 2019). Tosone et al. (2012) describe the relational nature of trauma in their qualitative investigation of social workers' responses to shared trauma after two separate catastrophic events: the terrorist attacks of September 11th, 2001, and the Qassam rocket attacks on southern Israel from 2001–2006. As they discerned from case vignettes from therapists in both New York and Israel, therapists who were trauma-informed were better able to cope with the shared trauma evident in the therapeutic setting. From their training and knowledge about the impact of trauma, these clinicians knew the importance of increasing their personal self-care, writing their own trauma narratives to enhance cognitive processing of traumatic events and bolstering their supports through peer consultation and supervision (Tosone et al., 2014).

During shared trauma, it is possible and even likely that boundaries between the therapist and client may blur, making it difficult for the therapist to differentiate between the client's needs and their own countertransference (Tosone et al., 2012). As noted by previous research (LaPorte et al., 2010), therapists sometimes risk using self-disclosure too liberally or in ways that may not be in the best interest of the client. These potential pitfalls are accounted for in relational work due to the understanding that the therapeutic relationship is paramount to successful treatment and has been built to accommodate times when the therapist or client can openly discuss moments when sessions feel discordant (Edwards et al., 2014). Using a relational approach allows therapists and clients to co-create an understanding of traumatic events through dialogic processing and interaction. As the therapist and client work toward understanding the client's symptoms the therapist can also identify their own needs and work toward healing and growth.

Accompaniment during Shared Trauma

The concept of accompaniment, defined as going with, supporting and enhancing the therapeutic process (Finn & Jacobson, 2008), is a lesser known but equally important practice for therapists to consider during times of shared trauma (Novoa Palacios & Pirela Morillo, 2020). The accompaniment approach, developed by Canadian social workers Elizabeth Whitmore and Maureen Wilson from their experience providing direct practice care in Nicaragua, sees therapy as a partnership between two people to enable positive action. Whitmore and Wilson based their accompaniment model on feminist principles to create a concept that spoke to the importance of true partnership, fostered by a commitment to dignity, hope and trust in the therapeutic process (Finn & Jacobson, 2008; Whitmore & Wilson, 1997). The accompaniment principles mirror some of those of feminist relational components, with perhaps even greater emphasis placed on the critical nature of collaboration: 1) nonintrusive collaboration; 2) mutual trust and respect; 3) a common analysis of what the problem is; 4) a commitment to solidarity; 5) equality in the relationship; 6) an explicit focus on process; and 7) the importance of language (Wilson & Whitmore, 1995). When exploring the accompaniment principles of the therapeutic relationship during the COVID-19 pandemic, it is not difficult to see how an emphasis on partnership and equality may engender collective healing (Whitmore & Wilson, 1997). Moreover, accompaniment values fit closely with those of the social work profession and TIC.

Related to the concept of accompaniment, exposure to catastrophe necessitates that both parties in a therapeutic dyad interact and bear witness to one another even during times of ongoing uncertainty and stress, highlighting the concept of "being with." Worthington and Stern (1985), in describing the relationship process, asserted that the concept of "being with" involved: "Sharing in the experience with no attempt to change what the person is doing or believing" (Worthington & Stern, 1985, p. 148). A focus on the therapeutic relationship and mutual growth encourages us as therapists to engage in the process of bearing witness to the pain of another while also acknowledging the pain happening within ourselves. The relationship process can unfold in a way that the displays of empathy conveyed on behalf of both the client and therapist enable restoration.

The case studies below demonstrate the impact of the COVID-19 pandemic on the lives of two clients as well as the impact on therapist-client relationships. The case studies illustrate how both the focus of therapy and the approaches taken toward offering client support shifted in the face of shared trauma. Relational therapeutic and accompaniment approaches undertaken in both cases were ultimately what empowered both client and therapist to grow and heal.

Case Studies

The two case studies included in this chapter are from the clinical work of the first author, Johanna Barry. They illustrate how conceptualizations of psychotherapy shifted during the shared trauma inculcated by the COVID-19 pandemic. The clients, Lily and Emma (pseudonyms), were trauma survivors who experienced compounded trauma during the pandemic, albeit for different reasons. By exploring two disparate presentations of trauma, we hope to demonstrate how adhering to a relational therapeutic model can be helpful in promoting healing and growth for clients with differing presenting concerns. We begin here by exploring some of the theoretical work that helps to provide greater insight into the two cases.

The case of Lily exemplifies how the focus of therapy and the expectations and markers of therapeutic growth shifted during the pandemic. On a psychological level, much of the progress Lily made prior to the pandemic lockdown was overridden by fear from the thought that her mother might die from the COVID-19 virus. Lily had a complicated relationship with her mother which only heightened her anxiety that her mother would fall ill and die without the two of them mending their relationship. Further, Lily experienced trauma related to the religiosity in her upbringing that ultimately led to sexual and physical abuse. In her work with Johanna, they processed a great deal of the trauma incurred from the faith practice that was forced on her as a child. Yet, during the pandemic, Lily began to express her distress at moving away from the Church.

The psychological theory that helps to explain Lily's feeling is known as Terror Management Theory (TMT). TMT suggests that when one is reminded of the inevitability of death, it induces death anxiety which is often managed by attempts to cling more closely to family members and other loved ones, cultural beliefs and other belief systems that provide meaning and value (Soloman et al., 2015). Religious and spiritual practices and close family relationships have been found to moderate war-related trauma in Israeli youth and American military personnel deployed to war zones in Iraq and Afghanistan (Kick & McNitt, 2016; Laufer et al., 2010). The authors discerned that spirituality, when viewed as a way in which people connect with faith, family and the belief that there is a higher power, decreased PTSD symptoms and increased connection to their families. Importantly, even if one's daily life was relatively unaffected by the resulting quarantines and lockdowns of COVID-19, TMT suggests that the threat of mortality for oneself or loved ones weighs heavily on all people regardless of previous trauma history (Courtney et al., 2020).

The case of Emma highlights the importance of relational practice during times of shared trauma and addresses the concept of retraumatization (Smith, 2014). Emma was retraumatized when she lost her job during the COVID-19 pandemic and needed to live with her parents in their childhood home. When returning to this physical place, Emma was literally and mentally transported back to a time when she was abused. Keller-Dupree's (2013) work exploring the process of retraumatization provided a comprehensive review and list of helpful tips for providers to consider when working with individuals who have been traumatized. Among these guidelines, she noted the importance of providing safe, secure relationships within the therapeutic dyad and helping individuals prepare for the impact of returning to places where traumatic events occurred. Other scholars have commented on the importance of therapists being mindful of the retraumatization process when survivors are exposed to additional stressors (Schock et al., 2016). Emma was retraumatized by returning home and the destabilization caused by the pandemic and losing her job. The constantly changing external environment activated trauma responses that Emma and Johanna had worked on in therapy (i.e., flashbacks, feelings of hyperarousal) prior to the pandemic.

Each case study will begin with a description of the client's background and presenting concerns as well as a discussion of how the nature of therapeutic work with each changed considerably during the pandemic. In each case, the value of the relational therapeutic model is discussed.

Lily

At the time Lily and Johanna began working together in 2015, Lily identified as a white, cisgender, bisexual, able-bodied woman in her mid-30s. She had an extensive trauma history, predominantly involving the mind-control cult her mother belonged to throughout the entirety of Lily's youth. The cult leader, a man only ever identifying himself as "Tom" (pseudonym), manipulated Lily's mother into believing that she and her five children would go to hell if they did not follow his every order. This led to Lily's mother, Elaine (pseudonym), following Tom's every rule, including a starvation diet. Lily's father and mother divorced prior to Elaine's cult involvement and Lily's father apparently did not know the extent of the abuse that was taking place in his absence. Tom sexually and physically abused Lily and her four younger siblings, explaining this abuse as "God's will." Rationalizing his behavior by explaining that his acts would lead the family to Heaven, Tom eventually drained Elaine of all her financial savings, including the children's college funds.

Lily was able to escape to college in another state when she reached the age of 18. Four years later, Elaine left Tom's cult and began the arduous road to healing and recovery. However, a great deal of relational damage had already been done between Lily and Elaine, which prompted Lily to seek therapeutic support in her mid-20s. When Johanna met Lily, Lily experienced persistent PTSD symptoms ranging from graphic nightmares to unprompted physical sensations such as sweating and nausea. She was also diagnosed with severe obsessive-compulsive disorder (OCD), common among individuals who have suffered abuse during childhood (Griffiths et al., 2012). While Lily did not engage in visible compulsive behaviors, she suffered from mental obsessions classified as "scrupulosity." Scrupulosity OCD can assume several forms, but commonly involves obsessive thoughts about religion or god(s), harming oneself or others, or relationships. In Lily's case, she suffered from all three of these obsessive thoughts and the pervasiveness of these thoughts interfered considerably with her well-being and ability to engage fully in her life as a friend, journalist and sister.

In addition to engaging in CBT practices to help Lily avoid reassurance-seeking and mental rituals resulting from her obsessive thoughts, Johanna and Lily also practiced mindfulness techniques and discussed how to set healthy boundaries with Lily's mother. After leaving Tom's cult, Elaine's mental health suffered considerably. Elaine refused to see a professional psychotherapist and vacillated between lashing out at Lily verbally and relying solely on Lily for emotional support. As such, Johanna worked with Lily for several years around practicing the concept of separation-individuation (Saraiva & Matos, 2012). Separation-individuation is a developmental stage in which emerging adults develop autonomy within attachment relationships, most often with caregivers. The boundaries in Lily's relationship with her mother had become unhealthy, most often because Elaine treated Lily as a peer and relied on her heavily for emotional and financial support. Johanna and Lily worked together to practice setting boundaries with Elaine, helping Lily to feel confident engaging in healthy autonomous actions. Sometimes, such action took the form of not returning her mother's phone calls if Lily did not have the energy to speak to her mother, or in not visiting her mother during trips to her hometown if her mother was experiencing a mental health episode which often resulted in Elaine verbally abusing Lily.

When the COVID-19 pandemic hit the USA in March of 2020, existential fear and dread pervaded the therapy sessions between Johanna and Lily. Although Lily previously made great strides in attaining separation-individuation and setting healthy boundaries with her mother, the pandemic caused Lily to fear greatly that her mother, as an older adult, would catch the virus and die. This fear made it ultimately impossible for her to set the boundaries she had worked diligently to erect. Such fear also resulted in Lily feeling a great deal of guilt and shame for leaving behind the religion she practiced as a child. The church to which Elaine belonged is where she met Tom whose cult practices resulted in the physical and sexual abuse of her children. Prior to the COVID-19 pandemic, Lily was confident that her decision to eschew her religious beliefs was the right decision for her life, to leave behind the trauma engendered from the religion her mother embraced. Yet as TMT suggests (Courtney et al., 2020) during times of existential fear, Lily experienced a marked shift in how she thought about the religion of her childhood and expressed the need to adhere more closely to the teachings of the church she had left behind:

LILY: I just feel like I should go home and go to church with Mom. I know it's messed up, but what if she's right?
JOHANNA: ...right about what, Lily?
LILY: Right about all that fire and brimstone stuff. What if I have to go to church in order not to go to hell? Or for her to not go to hell?
JOHANNA: It sounds like you are feeling really frightened and uncertain about this COVID-19 virus. I feel really afraid because of it, too. And, we know it makes sense to want to cling to what's familiar when we are afraid.
LILY: No, no, it's more than that. I mean yeah, I feel terrified of the virus, but what if Mom's religion is the right thing and I messed it up by leaving the church?
JOHANNA: You had some incredibly valid reasons for ceasing to go to that church, Lily. That's where Tom came into your life and hurt you and your family for years.
LILY: [tearful] I know, but I just can't stop feeling like a bad daughter for not being there for my mom right now and showing her I care about her by going to church. I know she's been like, evil, but I still love her and I want her to be okay.

From this session excerpt, we can see how Lily's fear about what would happen both to her and her mother during the pandemic made it difficult to maintain distance from the church and from her mother. While the sect of religion to which Elaine belonged was ultimately too dangerous for Lily to reconnect with, Johanna and Lily together explored other faith and spirituality traditions that might provide the ability to believe in a higher power without needing to engage in a religious practice that might be retraumatizing.

The onset of the COVID-19 pandemic further shifted Lily's therapy sessions related to her OCD. Working on exposure to obsessive thoughts was too challenging for Lily to practice considering the compounded trauma the virus brought to her life. Rather than viewing successful sessions as only those in which Lily was able to practice exposure to harmful obsessive thoughts or healthy methods of attaining separateness, success was redefined as moments where both Lily and Johanna emerged feeling metaphorically held and comforted. This shift in how progress was measured in the therapy setting was profound and involved a great deal of transition in terms of what sessions looked like. Sessions involved more conversation and validation as well as increased focus on the importance of the therapeutic relationship and the steadfastness of that relationship in the moment. Rather than working on separateness from her mother, Johanna and Lily spent time brainstorming ways in which Lily could communicate with her mother regularly but in a way that kept her emotionally safe. This involved practicing such dialogues during session and focusing on ways in which positive elements from their working relationship (i.e., communication, mutual respect, appropriate boundaries), might be transferable to her relationship with her mother:

LILY: I just feel so bogged down. The anxiety about something bad happening to Mom... I can't get over it. But she was a monster, you know? How do I deal with that?

JOHANNA: I can hold the feeling of being bogged down by the fearful time we are living through. It is terribly difficult not to have the world be the same as it was. It definitely makes other stressors feel harder to deal with.

LILY: Right? I can't even see you in person. This sucks.

JOHANNA: It is really hard. I miss seeing you in person, but we can still hold space in real time together. Can I ask you, what are some of the things from the relationship you and I have that might be transferable to communicating with Mom?

LILY: I don't know. I don't think I can ever have an open conversation with her like I do with you. I feel stuck in my relationship with her.

JOHANNA: You feel stuck?

LILY: Because I want to talk to her and feel relaxed like I do with you, but I know that's never going to be the case. I'm just panicked something bad will happen to her or to me, especially that one of us will die, and we'll never make things right.

JOHANNA: What does "making things right" look like?

LILY: I don't know, having a semi-normal mother-daughter relationship, I guess. Having the opportunity to talk with her and not feel like I have to listen to all of her trauma and what that is like for her.

JOHANNA: That makes sense. Why don't we practice a way for you to call her and choose some topics that feel safe to you to talk to her about? How does that sound?

LILY: Yeah, I think it would help to practice here before doing that.

From this excerpt, we can see how Johanna and Lily used the therapeutic space for support and to practice bringing that support to Lily's relationship with her mother. Rather than focusing sessions on the work involved in separation-individuation or OCD, Johanna and Lily centered their time together on holding space and focusing on what was reasonable considering the circumstances engendered by the pandemic.

Emma

Johanna began working with Emma in 2018. Emma self-identified as a Black, cisgender, heterosexual, able-bodied woman who was in her mid-20s. Emma was a survivor of childhood incest perpetrated by her older brother, Daniel (pseudonym). From the ages of nine to 12 years, Daniel would engage in inappropriate behavior with Emma, molesting her and disguising these acts as play. Emma's family was extremely affluent and belonged to an echelon of society in which perfect outward appearances were expected and attending elite prep schools and colleges was the norm. Emma was provided for in every way financially during her upbringing but came of age as part of a family that was lacking in the provision of emotional support.

For many years, Emma dissociated from the incest. However, as a 16-year-old woman away at boarding school, she was bullied by classmates which incited flashbacks about her childhood trauma. Her trauma response coupled with the ongoing bullying caused her to leave school and return to her childhood home. Her parents put both Daniel and Emma in therapy but never spoke of the incest and told friends and neighbors Emma had returned home simply because she wanted to attend public school with her childhood friends. Around this same time, her mother attempted suicide and was hospitalized, another event that was never spoken about in the family. Her mother survived and was able to resume her life and career at a prestigious law firm shortly thereafter. When Johanna and Emma worked together, Emma often spoke about the depression she experienced and hypothesized that some of it was likely genetic.

Prior to the COVID-19 pandemic, Emma was employed at a stable job as a server at a restaurant, but she struggled with attachment and effective, interpersonal relationships. She would often begin dating men and want to escalate the relationship very quickly, often moving in with the other person after a matter of weeks. Johanna and Emma discussed attachment styles frequently and worked together in session to model healthy boundaries and safe, secure relationships. Despite Emma's parents being emotionally unavailable during most of her life, Emma spoke to them daily, often emerging from conversations feeling overwhelmed and depressed. Emma's parents had high expectations for Emma's performance as a student and in all her employment endeavors as an adult. She was frequently unable to meet these expectations which resulted in her parents chastising her and pressuring her to perform better in the future. School was especially difficult for Emma as a neurodiverse learner, or someone whose brain variations led to atypical learning styles, and she often struggled to hold onto jobs due to trauma responses (i.e., extreme fatigue, anxiety) interfering with her work performance.

Like Lily, Emma worked diligently in therapy to set boundaries with her parents and her older brother to maintain her emotional well-being. Emma was largely financially dependent on her parents, which made truly separating from them challenging. Like many people affected by the COVID-19 pandemic, Emma lost her job in the restaurant industry. Because she was no longer able to afford her rent at her apartment, she was forced to move back home with her parents. Her parents still lived in her childhood home and she was thus subjected to being back in the home where her brother abused her. Within the first few days of being back in her old bedroom, she began experiencing symptoms of retraumatization in the form of flashbacks, nightmares and overwhelmingly intense negative emotions (Smith, 2014; Butler et al., 2018). Similar to Lily's case, much of the therapeutic work Johanna and Emma engaged in needed to be reconceptualized due to the pandemic creating circumstances beyond anyone's control. Although her brother now lived in another state with his wife and daughter, Emma was faced with painful childhood memories related both to her brother's abuse and her parents' failure to protect her as a child. The following dialogic excerpt is derived from a telehealth therapy session after Emma had been back in her childhood home for several weeks:

JOHANNA: How are things feeling being there this week, Emma? Are any of the mindfulness exercises we practiced helping with the flashbacks?

EMMA: Honestly, I just can't practice them. I want to and I know it'll help, but when I get into my old bedroom I just get flooded and just… paralyzed.

JOHANNA: It makes sense you feel overwhelmed and even flooded. What happened to you was so unfair, Emma. And I'll remind you, what happened was not your fault.

EMMA: Yeah, but it was so many years ago! Seriously. Why can't I just get over it?

JOHANNA: What would you say to someone you love in a similar situation who said that?

EMMA: Um, I don't know. I'd probably say it wasn't their fault just like you told me, and that it's not possible to just white-knuckle trauma.

JOHANNA: I think that sounds like spot-on logic. Can you give some of that compassion to yourself?

EMMA: [laughs wryly] Ugh, I knew you would say that. I just feel frustrated with myself.

JOHANNA: When we are used to being able to do things on the first try, it is frustrating not to be able to fix something. But what happened to you is not something we can think our way out of.

EMMA: I just am worried I'm never going to get past it.

JOHANNA: I have every confidence we will be able to work through this, Emma. I am holding space and patience for this process, even when you can't. Remember, you're not alone. I am here holding this with you.

EMMA: [tearfully] I just worry that this will become too much for you to handle and you'll not be able to work with me. The pandemic has been hard on you, too.

JOHANNA: The pandemic has been tough, no doubt. But I want to remind you that our relationship is built on honesty and I will always communicate with you honestly. And I can hold space for you.

EMMA: It feels sad that my relationship with you is the only one that feels real sometimes.

JOHANNA: Can you say a bit more about that?

EMMA: Everything here is so fake. My parents don't ever communicate with me about anything that matters. All they care about is how things look to other people. I dunno, I feel like being one of the only super wealthy Black families in their area makes them feel like they have to put on some kind of show.

JOHANNA: I see. The ways our identities have been supported or oppressed by society certainly makes a difference in how we feel we need to present ourselves. I can't imagine how difficult it must be for them at times to be the only Black family in your neighborhood.

EMMA: …but they still need to be able to try and understand how hard it is being here. Getting some emotional support from them would be nice.

JOHANNA: And that is also true. What can you and I do together, apart from the specific strategies we talked about, that you think might be helpful?

EMMA: Honestly, just knowing you're here is enough. I know this is a crazy time for everyone but thank you for continuing to show up for me.

JOHANNA: You're showing up, too, Emma. And you keep fighting every single day. Don't underestimate how hard that is.

From this exchange, we see elements of both relational therapy and feminist relational therapy that were beneficial to Emma as she worked through retraumatization. Johanna validated and acknowledged the clients' family identity as a historically oppressed group, but still offered the space for Emma to be angry that her parents were so concerned about their image. Johanna also modeled a supportive, holding relationship for Emma to let Emma know she was not alone. Emma was able to verbalize what she needed and what was helpful in the moment, which also provided an entrée for Johanna to continue modeling the supportive relationship Emma needed. What should also be noted from this exchange is the way Johanna pivoted from encouraging Emma to practice the mindfulness skills they had discussed in prior sessions to merely listening and validating Emma's experience. Although it is difficult when a client is struggling with issues of retraumatization, Johanna noted that their work prior to the onset of the pandemic was not the most helpful to Emma. Reminding Emma that she had supportive relationships in her life during a challenging time was more warranted.

Relational Practice Revisited

Relational approaches focus on bearing witness and walking alongside clients rather than simply measuring and marking progress, the most basic aspect of behavioral therapies. The case studies presented in this chapter center on the client experience. However, relational therapeutic approaches can also benefit therapists during shared trauma. As the relational clinician seeks to understand and validate the client's experience, they can also experience inter- and intrapersonal growth (Tosone et al., 2014). When Johanna worked with Lily and Emma, the opportunity to walk alongside her clients during their trauma was undoubtedly challenging, but also forced her to practice bringing more of her humanity to their virtual sessions. Sometimes, simply having the opportunity to sit in company with another person provided reassurance and the opportunity to hold existential fear and dread together. Even though the therapeutic interactions described in this chapter occurred over telehealth, seeing each other's faces close and hearing each other's voices clearly helped to create an experience of togetherness that helped to relieve the some of the isolation brought forth by the lockdown (Ronen-Setter & Cohen, 2020).

A relational therapeutic approach can also be useful for initiating repair if the therapist inadvertently overidentifies with the client's struggle or uses self-disclosure too liberally. While working with Lily, there were two occasions when Johanna's own anxiety about the health of her aging parents was overwhelming and she shared her fears with Lily during session after Lily spoke once more about her concern for her mother. Realizing that this may not have been the moment to use self-disclosure, the following week Johanna apologized to Lily and asked to take time to process how that self-disclosure felt as a client. To Johanna's surprise, Lily found it helpful to hear about her struggles but noted that the disclosure caused her some anxiety and worry about the health of Johanna's parents. Johanna took the opportunity to remind Lily that while the therapeutic sessions were often mutually beneficial due to the changing nature of the world, they were ultimately times for Lily to receive support. They spoke openly about the boundaries needed for their relationship and identified ways to help maintain these boundaries. Within the relationship, Lily and Johanna decided that Johanna's self-disclosure would be better suited coming from her own experiences of fear from the pandemic and not mentioning her parents, at least for a time. Lily was a highly empathetic person. Talking about parents was too experience-near for Lily to process at the time. The tenets of the relational process allowed both therapist and client to navigate snags like the ineffective use of self-disclosure because of the emphasis on forging a secure, empathic, collaborative relationship that could withstand moments of disconnection (Grossmark, 2019). This process created more intimacy and authenticity in the relationship as it modeled how relationship snags can deepen bonds.

The feminist relational approach is evident in both case studies by the way Johanna aligned with the clients in their struggle and empowered them to engage in therapy and lead the course of the therapeutic process for themselves. Johanna sought to dismantle the traditional power differentials in the therapeutic process by treating Lily and Emma as equal partners and encouraging the realization that both clients already had the tools they needed to heal and recover (Haskins & Appling, 2017). Feminist relational therapy is explicitly referenced again in Emma's case when Johanna acknowledged the issues of power and privilege regarding Emma's family's race. Johanna acknowledged the struggle Emma's parents endured being one of the only families of color in their community and the differences in experiences of trauma based on one's race and positions of power (Matheson, 2004).

Considerations for Social Workers

Shared trauma experiences like those precipitated by living through the COVID-19 pandemic create the potential for increased intimacy and transformation on behalf of both client and therapist, but there are certain things therapists should consider when working with clients during these times. It is common for therapists to feel despairing and incompetent when they personally feel crushed by the same existential fear and dread (Tosone et al., 2014). However, if one can acknowledge their humanity and the struggle involved in providing support to others when their own fortitude is shaken, and engage in personally helpful practices, it can increase the positive outcomes of providing care to others during traumatic times. We offer three recommendations for social workers that are useful during disasters and non-disasters alike:

1) supervision/therapy; 2) writing a trauma narrative; and 3) radical self-care.

First, it is imperative that therapists engage in their own work around the catastrophe, seeking therapeutic support as well as professional and peer supervision. Supervision can be an especially helpful space to discuss and process the hardship involved in working with clients in shared trauma, as one may be able to learn from the strategies their supervisor utilizes (Englebrecht, 2019).

Writing one's own trauma narrative to process the impact of shared trauma can be helpful in reducing trauma symptoms and providing the therapist with a recent experience of doing something they are likely to do with the client (Levenson, 2020). The trauma narrative is written by trauma survivors to expose themselves to the traumatic event in a safe environment. Writing empowers survivors to reframe the experience and reclaim their autonomy. For therapists who are confronted with holding the trauma of their client in tandem with their own, a trauma narrative creates time and space for one to process their experience of double exposure through the written word.

In general, there are four parts to the process of writing a trauma narrative: 1) state the facts of what happened; 2) add thoughts and feelings about the event; 3) add more detail, slowly and as one is ready; 4) read and re-read the trauma narrative and add one paragraph about how one feels after the traumatic event as opposed to during the traumatic event (Levenson, 2020). The power of trauma narratives lies in their written form as this provides an additional avenue for cogitation apart from dialogue. Trauma narratives are meant to take time to complete and ought to occur in the context of supervision or therapy. Writing in the presence of a supportive other can help to aid any potential retraumatization that occurs. And, when a therapist discusses the process of what it was like for them to create the trauma narrative with their client, it can inspire the client to create their own narrative and empower them to feel like more of an equal within the therapeutic relationship (Evans, 2020). Thus, the trauma narrative is another example of a potentially mutually beneficial therapeutic technique.

The final suggestion is for therapists to engage in radical self-care (Dale et al., 2018). One must embrace the understanding that one has a responsibility to care for oneself before taking care of others (Powers & Engstrom, 2020). In the current professional climate, fraught with the need to provide too much care with too little time, self-care has become a concept that is often discussed in therapeutic and social work circles, but rarely practiced. Therapists who do not engage in self-care risk being emotionally constricted or dysregulated with clients, neither allowing for accompaniment. Self-care practices can assume myriad forms and must be individualized to the care provider to be successful. For example, while getting a massage or meditating may be self-care for some therapists, it is not necessarily effective for others. Identifying what self-care looks like for oneself and noting what practices result in calming relaxation is what makes self-care effective. In Johanna's case, using a combination of aromatherapy and reading novels during the pandemic allowed her the psychological space to engage in work with Lily and Emma. When Johanna shared that she engaged in radical self-care to help cope with the COVID-19 pandemic, this encouraged her clients to engage in their own variations of self-care.

Implications for Social Work

This chapter has discussed shared trauma practice for therapists in general, but there are specific implications for those working in direct practice as social workers. Although social work therapeutic practices must shift during shared trauma, the core values of the profession must remain the same and be upheld.

One of the six core values of the social work profession is the "importance of human relationships," highlighting through its very language the emphasis that ought to be placed on the connection between social workers and clients (NASW, 2018). Included within this core value is the social work axiom of meeting clients where they are. By focusing on the strength of the therapeutic relationship and moving away from previous therapeutic plans that might not be feasible during shared trauma, one demonstrates commitment to honoring the importance of human relationships. As evidenced in the case examples, Johanna did not focus on Lily engaging in exposure therapy for her OCD or working on separation-individuation, nor did she continue to encourage Emma to develop a mindfulness practice to help combat retraumatization. She listened to what both women were currently needing and pivoted to a format that would be more helpful in the moment. By focusing on the importance of human relationships, social workers by extension attend to another core value of "honoring the dignity and worth of all people." Treating clients as equal partners aids in them feeling their own value.

Finally, in times of shared trauma, it is also essential for social workers to uphold the core value of "service," even though the form service assumes may be different than initially conceptualized. Many social workers are accustomed to providing service such that there are clear markers of progress during sessions (Beresford et al., 2008). Providing service to clients may involve providing space in sessions to talk about something entirely unrelated to their presenting concern or using self-disclosure and sharing one's own struggles engendered from the catastrophe. Viewed from another vantage point, service to clients may look like therapists engaging in their own mindfulness practice as a form of self-care to help ensure they have the bandwidth to engage effectively during client sessions. Though it has become a somewhat hackneyed assertion that one must "put on your own life preserver before assisting others," such an adage is undeniably accurate when providing therapeutic services during traumatic events that impact all of us. Broadening the scope of how we view social work's core values, especially in terms of the importance of human relationships, honoring the dignity and worth of all people, and acts of service, is essential so that we maintain professional integrity in a way that is adaptive to the current milieu.

Conclusion

With the onset of the COVID-19 pandemic, therapists were thrust into the role of providing ongoing support for their clients as well as for themselves. The internal struggle many therapists face during such times can leave one feeling inadequate, hopeless and incompetent (Boulanger, 2013; Day et al., 2017). Yet, through shifting focus from previous markers of client progress to the all-important roles of relationship during tragic events, the power of the secure bond fostered between therapist and client can be sustaining for both parties (Beresford et al., 2008). The two clients discussed in this chapter, Lily and Emma, had each survived traumas prior to the COVID-19 pandemic. Although the lockdown affected each woman differently, what remained consistent was how much both women needed stable, nurturing therapeutic relationships.

While grappling with her own trauma caused by the pandemic, Johanna experienced feelings of sadness, incompetence, existential fear and isolation. Not only was it ineffective for her to continue to encourage her clients to stay their treatment courses by practicing exposures or mindfulness, but overseeing this type of therapeutic work was markedly difficult to do in the context of Johanna's own hardship. Providing a stable relationship base from which to assure clients that they were seen, heard and metaphorically held allowed Johanna to bear witness to her clients as a fellow human being and walk alongside them as equals. This shift in the context of the therapeutic relationship not only was manageable and beneficial to Johanna, but for Lily and Emma as well. Honoring the core tenets of accompaniment (Finn & Jacobson, 2005), which emphasize relationships and being present to one another over outcomes, has marked success in trauma work (Wilkinson & D'Angelo, 2019). Largely, this is due to the human need to feel supported and connected to others, particularly during and after trauma. Approaching sessions with her clients from a vantage point that honored the importance of relationship and connection was beneficial for her clients and also left Johanna feeling more capable and confident after sessions.

In seeking to discern the benefits of adhering to a relational practice style during shared trauma, understanding the core concepts of Terror Management Theory (Courtney et al., 2020) is useful. TMT suggests that when faced with mortality salience, a likely occurrence in the context of a global pandemic, one may experience a powerful need to adhere closely to loved ones and cultural beliefs. Relational practice allows for closeness in the therapeutic context that addresses one of the most devastating aspects of living through a catastrophe: isolation and loneliness (Haskins & Appling, 2017). By focusing on cultivating close, supportive relationships with clients, we can thwart the negative repercussions of mortality salience and engage together in supporting one another throughout times of uncertainty and strain (Courtney et al., 2020). In terms of cultural belief adherence, the tenets of relational practice also make space for the mutual sharing of such convictions and the ability to explore these needs in the context of a safe, supportive relationship (Laufer et al., 2010).

Adopting the relational approach to therapy allows providers to remain flexible in their work with clients because relationship-building is an essential component to healing. It also has the benefit of allowing us to respond more easily to interpersonal needs in pandemics, wars and natural disasters (Day et al., 2017; Eidelson et al., 2003). Research on therapist experiences during shared traumas such as 9/11 or Hurricane Katrina suggested that therapist flexibility and attention to relationships let clients know they were equal partners in their healing relationship, which allowed for mutual healing and growth (Faust et al., 2008; McTighe & Tosone, 2015).

Viewing clients as equal partners during shared trauma provides optimal care for clients, but also offers the chance for clinicians to grow from the openness and intimacy of the relationship (Grossmark, 2019). Traumatic events often lead therapists to maintain a sense of order and routine in therapy (Verma & Vijayakrishnan, 2018). The COVID-19 pandemic compelled many providers to reevaluate how they viewed progress and success. The desire to create order out of disorder and structure out of chaos presents therapists with the choice of doubling down on behavioral approaches and measurable outcomes, or the immeasurable qualities of a close and trusting relationship. For Lily, Johanna decided to forgo the structure and objectivity of exposure work in favor of deepening the therapeutic relationship and her own humanity so that Lily could process her fears about the pandemic and the complications generated from the lockdown and isolation.

The importance of therapists engaging in self-care cannot be underestimated, especially during shared trauma circumstances (Powers & Engstrom, 2020). Several studies have touted the importance of radical self-care during shared trauma and the positive effects felt on behalf of both clients and therapists. Other researchers on the topic have highlighted how reflexive self-care practices or learning about oneself and the routines that are helpful leads to strengthened, trusting relationships with others. Examining the social aspect of caring for oneself, Wong (2013) suggested that engaging in reflexive self-care leads to reciprocal relationships and an increased sense of freedom, autonomy and trust both in professional and personal contexts.

In both client cases illustrated in this chapter, Johanna also used a trauma-informed care approach to ensure the emotional and physical safety of Lily and Emma. By treating clients with compassion and acknowledging their resiliencies and strengths, as well as shifting her approach to better accommodate where her clients were at in their healing journeys, Johanna reduced the likelihood of retraumatization (Levine et al., 2021; McClatchey, 2020). A thorough understanding of the complex and relational nature of trauma is important during shared trauma both on behalf of client and therapist, which TIC training provides. Due to TIC's applicability to many traumatic contexts, direct practitioners would do well to receive such training (Tosone et al., 2014).

Although this chapter has argued for the importance of relational practice in times of shared trauma, the value of human relationships and the need for connection is omnipresent. Social workers are especially called to focus on the therapeutic relationship through their commitment to honoring the importance of human relationships in all the work they do. Emphasizing the importance of connection and bearing witness to the struggles of our fellow people must be evident during times of trauma and times of peace to ensure the bonds between therapist and client remain steadfast.

References

Ahern, E., Kinsella, S., & Semkovska, M. (2018). Clinical efficacy and economic evaluation of online cognitive behavioral therapy for major depressive disorder: A systematic review and meta-analysis. *Expert Review of Pharmacoeconomics & Outcomes Research*, 18(1), 25–41. https://doi.org/10.1080/14737167.2018.1407245.

Andersson, G. (2016). Internet-delivered psychological treatments. *Annual Review of Clinical Psychology*, 12(1), 157–179. https://doi.org/10.1146/annurev-clinpsy-021815-093006.

Benatar, M. (2000). A qualitative study of the effect of a history of childhood sexual abuse on therapists who treat survivors of sexual abuse. *Journal of Trauma & Dissociation*, 1, 9–28.

Beresford, P., Croft, S., & Adshead, L. (2008). 'We don't see her as a social worker': A service user case study of the importance of the social worker's relationship and humanity. *British Journal of Social Work*, 38(7), 1388–1407.

Boulanger, G. (2013). Fearful symmetry: Shared trauma in New Orleans after Hurricane Katrina. *Psychoanalytic Dialogues*, 23(1), 31–44. https://doi.org/10.1080/10481885.2013.752700.

Butler, L. D., Maguin, E., & Carello, J. (2018). Retraumatization mediates the effect of adverse childhood experiences on clinical training-related secondary traumatic stress symptoms. *Journal of Trauma & Dissociation*, 19(1), 25–38. http s://doi.org/10.1080/15299732.2017.1304488.

Clemans, S. E. (2005). Recognizing vicarious traumatization: A single session group model for trauma workers. *Social Work with Groups*, 27(2–3), 55–74.

Courtney, E. P., Goldenberg, J. L., & Boyd, P. (2020). The contagion of mortality: A terror management health model for pandemics. *British Journal of Social Psychology*, 59(3), 607–617. https://doi.org/10.1111/bjso.12392.

Dale, S. K., Pierre-Louis, C., Bogart, L. M., O'Cleirigh, C., & Safren, S. A. (2018). Still I rise: The need for self-validation and self-care in the midst of adversities faced by Black women with HIV. *Cultural Diversity & Ethnic Minority Psychology*, 24(1), 15–25. https://doi.org/10.1037/cdp0000165.

Day, K. W., Lawson, G., & Burge, P. (2017). Clinicians' experiences of shared trauma after the shootings at Virginia Tech. *Journal of Counseling & Development*, 95(3), 269–278. https://doi.org/10.1002/jcad.12141.

Edwards, L. L., Robertson, J. A., Smith, P. M., & O'Brien, N. B. (2014). Marriage and family training programs and their integration of lesbian, gay, and bisexual identities. *Journal of Feminist Family Therapy*, 26(1), 3–27. https://doi.org/10.1080/08952833.2014.872955.

Eidelson, R. J., D'Alessio, G. R., & Eidelson, J. I. (2003). The impact of September 11 on psychologists. *Professional Psychology: Research & Practice*, 34(2), 144. https://doi.org/10.1037/0735-7028.34.2.144.

Engelbrecht, L. K. (2019). Towards authentic supervision of social workers in South Africa. *Clinical Supervisor*, 38(2), 301–325. https://doi.org/10.1080/07325223.2019.1587728.

Evans, C. T. (2020). A fear come true: An autobiographical narrative inquiry of birth trauma through an Adlerian lens. *Journal of Individual Psychology*, 76(4), 361–371.

Faust, D. S., Black, F. W., Abrahams, J. P., Warner, M. S., & Bellando, B. J. (2008). After the storm: Katrina's impact on psychological practice in New Orleans. *Professional Psychology: Research & Practice*, 39(1), 1–6. https://doi.org/10.1037/0735-7028.39.1.1.

Felsen, I. (2020). Patient and psychotherapist meeting in shared intergenerational transmission of genocidal trauma. *Psychoanalysis: Self & Context*, 15(2), 170–186. https://doi.org/10.1080/24720038.2019.1612405.

Griffiths, J., Norris, E., Stallard, P., & Matthews, S. (2012). Living with parents with obsessive-compulsive disorder: Children's lives and experiences. *Psychology & Psychotherapy: Theory, Research & Practice*, 85(1), 68–82. https://doi.org/10.1111/j.2044-8341.2011.02016.x.

Grossmark, R. (2019). Difficult days: The continuing evolution of relational group analysis: Discussion of "Taking the Sting Out: Manifesting Aggression and Containing Difficult States in a Relational Group Psychotherapy." *Psychoanalytic Dialogues*, 29(2), 216–225. https://doi.org/10.1080/10481885.2019.1587991.

Haskins, N. H., & Appling, B. (2017). Relational-cultural theory and reality therapy: A culturally responsive integrative framework. *Journal of Counseling & Development*, 95(1), 87–99. https://doi.org/10.1002/jcad.12120.

Herman, J. L. (1992). Complex PTSD: A syndrome in survivors of prolonged and repeated trauma. *Journal of Traumatic Stress*, 5(3), 377–391.

Hesse-Biber, S. N. (2011). *Handbook of feminist research: Theory and praxis.* SAGE.

Israeli, A. L., & Santor, D. A. (2000). Reviewing effective components of feminist therapy. *Counselling Psychology Quarterly*, 13, 233–247.

Keller-Dupree, E. A. (2013). Understanding childhood trauma: Ten reminders for preventing retraumatization. *Practitioner Scholar: Journal of Counseling & Professional Psychology*, 2(1), 1–11.

Kick, K. A., & McNitt, M. (2016). Trauma, spirituality, and mindfulness: Finding hope. *Social Work & Christianity*, 43(3), 97–108.

LaPorte, H. H., Sweifach, J., & Linzer, N. (2010). Sharing the trauma: Guidelines for therapist self disclosure following a catastrophic event. *Best Practice in Mental Health*, 6(2), 39–56.

Laufer, A., Solomon, Z., & Levine, S. Z. (2010). Elaboration on posttraumatic growth in youth exposed to terror: The role of religiosity and political ideology. *Social Psychiatry & Psychiatric Epidemiology*, 45(6), 647–653. https://doi.org/10.1007/s00127-009-0106-5.

Levenson, J. (2020). Translating trauma-informed principles into social work practice. *Social Work*, 65(3), 288–298. https://doi.org/10.1093/sw/swaa020.

Levine, S., Varcoe, C., & Browne, A. J. (2021). "We went as a team closer to the truth": impacts of interprofessional education on trauma- and violence-informed care for staff in primary care settings. *Journal of Interprofessional Care*, 35(1), 46–54. https://doi.org/10.1080/13561820.2019.1708871.

Matheson, J. L. (2004). Flattening the hierarchy: The co-creation of an advanced, doctoral-level course in feminist-informed family therapy. *Journal of Feminist Family Therapy*, 15(4), 45–74. https://doi.org/10.1300/J086v15n04_03.

McClatchey, I. S. (2020). Trauma-informed care and posttraumatic growth among bereaved youth: A pilot study. *Omega: Journal of Death & Dying*, 82(2), 196–213. https://doi.org/10.1177/0030222818804629.

McTighe, J. P., & Tosone, C. (2015). Narrative and meaning-making among Manhattan social workers in the wake of September 11, 2001. *Social Work in Mental Health*, 13(4), 299–317. https://doi.org/10.1080/15332985.2014.977420.

National Association of Social Workers. (2018). *NASW Code of Ethics.* www.socialworkers.org/About/Ethics/Code-of-Ethics/Code-of-Ethics-English.

Novoa Palacios, A., & Pirela Morillo, J. (2020). Acompañamiento desde una ética de la vida: Para educar en tiempos de pandemia. *Utopia y Praxis Latinoamericana*, 25, 11–24. https://doi.org/10.5281/zenodo.3931040.

Nuttman-Shwartz, O. (2015). Shared resilience in a traumatic reality: A new concept for trauma workers exposed personally and professionally to collective disaster. *Trauma Violence Abuse*, 16(4), 466–475. doi:10.1177/1524838014557287.

Powers, M. C. F., & Engstrom, S. (2020). Radical self-care for social workers in the global climate crisis. *Social Work*, 65(1), 29–37. https://doi.org/10.1093/sw/swz043.

Ronen-Setter, I. H., & Cohen, E. (2020). Becoming "teletherapeutic": Harnessing accelerated experiential dynamic psychotherapy (AEDP) for challenges of the Covid-19 era. *Journal of Contemporary Psychotherapy*, 50, 265–273. https://doi.org/10.1007/s10879-020-09462-8.

Saraiva, L., & Matos, P. (2012). Separation-individuation of Portuguese emerging adults in relation to parents and to the romantic partner. *Journal of Youth Studies*, 15(4), 499–517. https://doi.org/10.1080/13676261.2012.663889.

Schock, K., Böttche, M., Rosner, R., Wenk-Ansohn, M., & Knaevelsrud, C. (2016). Impact of new traumatic or stressful life events on pre-existing PTSD in traumatized refugees: results of a longitudinal study. *European Journal of Psychotraumatology*, 7, 32106. https://doi.org/10.3402/ejpt.v7.32106.

Smith, C. (2014). *Retraumatization: Assessment, treatment, and prevention*, edited by M. P. Duckworth and V. M. Follette. *Journal of Trauma & Dissociation*, 15 (1), 108–110. https://doi.org/10.1080/15299732.2013.835652.

Solomon, S., Greenberg, J., & Pyszczynski, T. (2015). *The worm at the core: On the role of death in life*. Random House.

Substance Abuse and Mental Health Services Administration. (2014). *SAMHSA's concept of trauma and guidance for a trauma-informed approach*. HHS Publication No. (SMA) 14-4884. Substance Abuse and Mental Health Services Administration.

Taylor, M. (2020). Collective trauma and the relational field. *Humanistic Psychologist*, 48(4), 382–388. https://doi.org/10.1037/hum0000215.

Tong, J., Simpson, K., Alvarez, J. M., & Bendall, S. (2019). Talking about trauma in therapy: Perspectives from young people with post-traumatic stress symptoms and first episode psychosis. *Early Intervention in Psychiatry*, 13(5), 1236–1244. https://doi.org/10.1111/eip.12761.

Tosone, C. (2021). Introduction. In C. Tosone (Ed.), *Shared Trauma, Shared Resilience During a Pandemic: Social Work in the Time of COVID-19* (pp. 1–11). Springer International Publishing. https://doi.org/10.1007/978-3-030-61442-3_1.

Tosone, C., Nuttman-Shwartz, O., & Stephens, T. (2012). Shared trauma: When the professional is personal. *Clinical Social Work Journal*, 40(2), 231–239. https://doi.org/10.1007/s10615-012-0395-0.

Verma, M., & Vijayakrishnan, A. (2018). Psychoanalytic psychotherapy in addictive disorders. *Indian Journal of Psychiatry*, 60, S485–S489. https://doi.org/10.4103/psychiatry.IndianJPsychiatry_16_18.

Whitmore, E., & Wilson, M. (1997). Accompanying the process: social work and international development practice. *International Social Work*, 40(1), 57–74. https://doi.org/10.1177/002087289704000105.

Wilkinson, M. T., & D'Angelo, K. A. (2019). Community-based accompaniment & social work—A complementary approach to social action. *Journal of Community Practice*, 27(2), 151–167. https://doi.org/10.1080/10705422.2019.161664.

Wilson, M. G., & Whitmore, E. (1995). Accompanying the process: Principles for international development practice. *Canadian Journal of Development Studies*, 16, 61–77.

Wolf, J., Williams, E. N., Darby, M., Herald, J., & Schultz, C. (2018). Just for women? Feminist multicultural therapy with male clients. *Sex Roles*, 78(5–6), 439–450. https://doi.org/10.1007/s11199-017-0819-y.

Wong, J. (2013). Self and others: The work of 'care' in Foucault's care of the self. *Philosophy Today*, 57(1): 99–113. doi:10.5840/philtoday20135717.

Worthington, E. L., & Stern, A. (1985). Effects of supervisor and supervisee degree level and gender on the supervisory relationship. *Journal of Counseling Psychology*, 32(2), 252.

Chapter 8

Shared Trauma in a Group Context

Carolyn Knight and Alex Gitterman

In this chapter, the authors discuss shared trauma and the implications this phenomenon has when the social worker is engaged in group work practice. They begin by summarizing the clinical, theoretical, and empirical literature on shared trauma. The authors then elaborate upon the implications that shared trauma has for group work practice. The authors identify social work practice skills that lessen the risk that shared trauma will surface in the first place and assist the worker in managing its manifestations when they appear. This discussion is grounded in two conceptual frameworks which the authors briefly summarize: the mutual aid model of group work and the trauma-informed perspective.

Shared Trauma

The phenomenon of shared trauma received increased attention from clinicians and researchers in the wake of the terrorist attacks of 2001 in the United States, the ongoing conflicts and terrorist attacks in Israel, and the many natural and human-made disasters that have occurred around the world (Tosone, 2021). Authors indicate a preference for the term "shared traumatic reality" to refer to "the affective, behavioral, cognitive, spiritual, and multi-modal responses that clinicians experience as a result of dual exposure to the same collective trauma as their clients" (Tosone et al., 2016, p. 233). The authors of this chapter favor the term "shared traumatic exposure."

Consistent with the trauma-informed formulation discussed later, trauma "is in the eyes of the beholder" (Boals, 2018). Individuals may be exposed to the same potentially traumatic event (shared *exposure*). However, whether they experience it as traumatic—their traumatic *reality*—depends upon factors and characteristics unique to them.

Baum (2010) identifies four defining features of shared trauma:

1   The event has the potential to traumatize an entire community
2   The event is recent

DOI: 10.4324/9781003176947-11

3   Clients and practitioners are members of the community exposed to the event
4   Practitioners experience "double exposure" in their roles as both community members impacted by the event and professionals assisting clients impacted by the same event.

Authors focus on two circumstances that lead to shared trauma (Branson, 2019; Day et al., 2017). The first scenario occurs when professional intervention is initiated *in response* to a communal disaster. Intervention generally is crisis oriented and short term. In the second scenario, a communal disaster occurs *after a professional relationship has been established*. The distinguishing feature of both is that workers and clients are *simultaneously* exposed to the same communal event.

Blurred Boundaries

Professional boundaries easily become blurred when crisis services are provided in the immediate aftermath of communal trauma at the site of— or in close proximity to—the event. Social workers also may have to assume tasks not typically associated with their roles and with which they may be unfamiliar (Adamson, 2018). In their study of shared trauma among social workers practicing during the Israeli-Palestinian conflict, Lavi and colleagues found that these "breaches" in the typical ways of conducting their work "threatened [clinicians'] sense of coherence, security, and trust in the intervention process" (Lavi et al., 2017, p. 11).

In all instances of communal trauma, "the boundaries between the professional and personal realms may be blurred by both the intrusion of the personal world into the professional world and the intrusion of the professional world into the personal world" (Baum, 2010, pp. 252–253). Practitioners may have difficulty being affectively and cognitively present in their work due to their own exposure to the event. Clinicians' concerns can disrupt the "inner dialogue" they employ to continually analyze their and their clients' responses to one another which undermines their ability to accurately assess and attend to important interpersonal dynamics and therapeutic material (Baum, 2010). Practitioners may manage their reactions by adopting distancing strategies—more rigid boundaries—that protect them but reduce their ability to connect and empathize with their clients (Baum, 2010).

Practitioners may struggle to "leave work at the door" as demands on their time and energy increase. Lines between their professional and personal lives may become further blurred as the content of their discussions with clients mirror the experiences they are having in their personal lives and the experiences in their personal lives mirror those of their clients' (Tosone et al., 2012). Clients, in turn, may be ambivalent about accepting—or continuing to accept—help from the helping professional knowing—or worrying—that this individual, too, has been impacted by the communal trauma.

Mutual Aid Model of Group Work: A Brief Summary

To understand the implications that shared trauma has on group work practice, one must first appreciate what it is about this modality that is unique. The source of help in group work lies with the members, themselves, and the multiplicity of helping relationships that exist.

Four interdependent benefits distinguish group work from other modalities (Gitterman et al., 2021). First, once members discover they are not alone—that others also are "in the same boat"—they are empowered to work on the challenges they face. Second, members' sense of self-efficacy is enhanced when they are afforded the opportunity to help others, rather than solely being the recipients of help. Third, while members may learn from the group worker, their most valuable lessons come from one another, leading to greater self-understanding and a more realistic perception of themselves and the challenges they face. Fourth, members' connection to and acceptance of one another enhances self-esteem and self-worth.

The primary role of the group worker is to help members create a system of mutual aid that allows them to accomplish their collective goals. A distinctive aspect of the modality is that the worker's inner dialogue has a dual focus: The group-as-a-whole and each individual member. The worker constantly monitors members' individual and collective behaviors and, when needed, intervenes to modify those that may undermine the group's work.

The Trauma-Informed Formulation: A Brief Summary

The literature examining the implications that shared trauma has on clinical intervention, generally, is limited and largely anecdotal. In contrast, the trauma-informed orientation and its application to practice has received a great deal of attention and is suggestive of the impact that shared trauma has on workers and clients—which in this chapter refers to the group and its members.

In 2001, Harris and Fallot introduced the term "trauma-informed" (TI) to refer to a comprehensive practice approach to helping people exposed to traumatic life events. A TI orientation provides survivors with a therapeutic experience that counters—and begins to correct—the consequences of their experience (Hales et al., 2017). Harris and Fallot's TI formulation (2001) relied upon five principles: safety, trust, collaboration, choice, and empowerment. This perspective has been expanded upon by the United States Substance Abuse Mental Health Services Administration (SAMHSA) (2014).

Whether an event is experienced as traumatic depends upon various factors—particularly sociocultural—that are unique to those exposed to it (Boals, 2018; Montagner Rigoli et al., 2019; Pressley & Smith, 2017). Trauma exposure results in a range of social, psychiatric, emotional, and physical and somatic problems including substance abuse, depression, suicidal ideation, self-injury/harm, and psychiatric problems like stress, anxiety, and dissociative disorders (Copeland et al., 2018; Dye, 2018).

Trauma also often distorts survivors' core beliefs about self and others, leading to a worldview characterized by a lack of safety and a heightened sense of powerlessness (Currier et al., 2017). Mistrust of self and others also is common. Survivors' "self-capacities"—including the ability to self-soothe, manage affect, and trust one's judgment—may be compromised or remain undeveloped, undermining feelings of self-efficacy (Diehle et al., 2014).

In cases of shared trauma, clinicians are likely to experience the social, emotional, behavioral, and physical problems and distortions in thinking about self and others that are common to trauma survivors, generally. Research indicates that professionals directly impacted by communal trauma often experience heightened feelings of vulnerability and exhibit stress reactions consistent with PTSD (Finklestein et al., 2015; Freedman & Tuval Mashiach, 2018). Further, the more directly workers are exposed to the communal traumatic event, the more difficulty they will have managing its impact (Adamson, 2014; Rao & Mehra, 2015).

Trauma-Informed Practice

TI practice embodies and is reflective of core skills and values of social work practice (Gitterman et al., 2021; Levenson, 2020). A TI lens helps social workers engage with clients in ways that: Help them manage the stressors they face; lessen feelings of powerlessness; enhance trust in self and others; and reduce the likelihood of re-traumatization. The TI social worker also understands the need to help clients identify strengths that allowed them to bounce back from their experience—resilience—and the ways in which they have grown from their experience—adversarial growth.

TI practice has been found to be associated with clients' increased satisfaction with the therapeutic relationship and reduced rates of dropout (Bailey et al., 2019; Fondren et al., 2020; Jankowski et al., 2019). Direct benefits to clients include: enhanced feelings of self-efficacy and resilience; more rapid reduction in presenting problems; and reduced feelings of social isolation, depression, and anxiety.

Promoting safety and trust. The working relationship itself can counter the impact that trauma has on survivors' core beliefs about self and others. In addition, social workers who operate from a TI orientation (Knight, 2021a, 2021b):

1   Maintain clear boundaries and hold clear expectations
2   Establish and maintain open lines of communication
3   Protect client confidentiality to the extent that is possible
4   Reach for the unique meaning of clients' experiences
5   Demonstrate sensitivity to and respect for diversity and cultural humility
6   Provide clients with both physical and emotional safety
7   Assist clients in managing affect by helping them express and/or contain feelings.

Implied in these characteristics is the need for worker transparency, which is included in the SAMHSA formulation (2014).

Promoting choice, collaboration, and empowerment. The skills that operationalize these practice principles complement trust and safety and are consistent with the strengths-based orientation in social work practice. Workers assist clients in developing their self-capacities and successfully managing stressors-in-living. The SAMSHA formulation includes additional principles: Voice and sensitivity to historical, cultural, and gender issues (2014). Practitioners who adopt a TI orientation (Knight, 2021a, 2021b):

1   Ensure informed consent
2   Treat clients as experts in their own lives
3   Respect clients' cultural identities
4   View the working relationship as a partnership
5   Identify and build upon clients' strengths
6   Acknowledge, normalize, and validate clients' concerns
7   Help clients see the connection between life stressors and past trauma
8   Help clients recognize the ways in which their traumatic experiences reflect broader social forces like marginalization and oppression

Resilience and adversarial growth. While resilience and adversarial growth are not explicitly identified in the TI formulation, the perspective's defining principles promote both. Theorists and researchers have identified the ways in which survivors grow from their exposure to trauma and factors that assist survivors in bouncing back from it. Social support is the most influential variable and can either promote or undermine resilience and includes: availability of resources both at the time of and long after trauma exposure; validation and/or acknowledgement of the trauma; and reactions from significant others that convey either acceptance and understanding or blame and accusation (Pressley & Smith, 2017). Aspects of adversarial growth that have been observed include: a reordering of priorities; a new or renewed sense of spirituality; and enhanced feelings of empathy, concern for others, and self-efficacy (Bonanno et al., 2015).

Indirect Trauma

Practitioners who work with trauma survivors will be indirectly traumatized by their work (Knight, 2013). Indirect trauma is not the same as burnout or countertransference, but it can lead to both (Barros et al., 2020; Branson, 2019). Three distinct manifestations of indirect trauma have been identified, two of which mirror the reactions exhibited by those directly exposed to it (Barros et al., 2020).

Vicarious trauma refers to changes in practitioners' belief systems analogous to the changes in survivors' core beliefs about self and others (Blome & Safadi, 2016; Pearlman & Saakvitne, 1995). Clinicians also are likely to experience secondary traumatic stress and struggle with reactions analogous to PTSD (Bercier & Maynard, 2015). While compassion fatigue is not unique to clinicians who work with trauma survivors, they are at particular risk of experiencing it (Figley, 1995; Lee et al., 2018). Survivors of trauma may be difficult to engage in a working relationship and often present with numerous chronic stressors that they feel helpless to resolve, which can frustrate practitioners.

A noteworthy aspect of shared trauma is that social workers are "doubly exposed" to trauma through their own experiences with the event and through those of their clients (Baum, 2012; Tosone, 2021). Research substantiates that practitioners who respond to natural and human-made disasters are at heightened risk of experiencing all three manifestations of indirect trauma relative to clinicians who work with trauma survivors in other contexts (Gonzalez et al., 2019; Shannonhouse et al., 2016).

Vicarious post-traumatic growth and resilience. Risk and protective factors can lessen or exacerbate the impact of indirect trauma. The presence or absence of an organizational climate that acknowledges and normalizes social workers' experience with indirect trauma and provides opportunities for and encourages self-care is an especially influential factor (Dombo & Blome, 2016; Sprang et al., 2017). This type of organizational environment reflects TI care, but research continues to reveal that it is not the norm (Berliner & Kolko, 2016).

Exposure to indirect trauma provides clinicians with the opportunity for personal and professional growth. The organizational risk and protective factors noted previously contribute to (or thwart) vicarious post-traumatic growth and resilience (Frey et al., 2017; Killian et al., 2017). Supervision either exacerbates or diminishes the impact of indirect trauma and promotes or undermines resilience and vicarious post-traumatic growth. Research highlights the benefits of supervisors assisting supervisees with the clinical aspects of their work *as well as* their affective reactions to it (Bassuk et al., 2017; Collins-Camargo & Antle, 2018).

Trauma-Informed Care

TI practice requires an organizational context that models, supports, and reinforces it. Trauma-informed organizations normalize and validate clients' experiences and workers' affective reactions to their work. TI principles guide: staff interactions with one another and with clients; the physical layout and spatial arrangements of an organization; and decision- and policymaking (Berliner & Kolko, 2016; Lang et al., 2016).

Clinical supervision is an essential feature of TI care (Knight, 2021a, 2021b). When supervisors adopt a trauma-informed orientation, they create a learning environment that promotes supervisees' professional growth and self-understanding. The interpersonal dynamics that surface in the supervisory relationship mirror those that occur in supervisees' working relationships with clients (Shulman, 2010). Therefore, the TI supervisor is a powerful role model of TI practice, reflecting the parallel process (O'Donoghue, 2014).

It is essential that employing organizations adopt a TI orientation in a shared trauma context to: support and guide practitioners in their practice; promote post-traumatic adversarial growth among clinicians; and reduce the likelihood that practitioners will be indirectly traumatized. While scant, research on shared trauma affirms the advantages of TI care. An agency environment that assists practitioners with their clinical practice *and* with their affective reactions to their work and/or their own experience with trauma has been found to mitigate the impact of shared trauma and enhance clinical expertise and vicarious post-traumatic growth (Gonzalez et al., 2019; Kusmaul, 2021; Tosone et al., 2016; Tullberg & Boothe, 2019).

The Intersection of Trauma-Informed Practice and Group Work

The mutual aid model is consistent with and epitomizes the principles of the TI practice. Members help one another to address common life stressors which is empowering to all. Members' connections to one another promotes trust in others while their awareness that they are not alone enhances trust in self (Gitterman et al., 2021). The stigma and isolation that often are associated with adversity are reduced in a group as members discover they are not alone in their struggles. Therefore, group membership promotes resilience and adversarial growth consistent with the principles of the TI orientation (Baird & Alaggia, 2021; Huang & Wong, 2013). Both conceptual models lay the foundation for the social work skills needed to minimize the intrusive influence that shared trauma has on workers, clients, and their practice and to address its impact when it surfaces.

Addressing Shared Trauma in Group Work: Core Skills

Most of the shared trauma literature focuses on individual counseling. This is surprising since groups often are the modality of choice when services are offered in the wake of communal trauma and for survivors of past trauma. Groups also have been promoted as a resource for social workers on the frontline of disaster work (Sampson, 2016; Smith et al., 2015).

The dual focus that distinguishes group work means that group workers must attend to three different sets of transactions: interactions between members; between individual members and the worker; and between the group-as-a-whole and the worker (Gitterman et al., 2021). Manifestations of shared trauma can surface in all three of them. This fact, coupled with blurred boundaries and double exposure, means that managing shared trauma in groups is more complicated than it is in individual work.

The discussion that follows is organized around phases of work, paying particular attention to the beginning and middle—or work—phases since it is in these phases that the implications of shared trauma are likely to be most evident. The authors identify group work skills that lessen the intrusive impact of shared trauma on the group-as-a-whole, the worker, and the members, and allow the worker to proactively address its manifestations. Composite case examples reflect groups formed in response to the COVID-19 pandemic and ongoing groups impacted by it. The dynamics and skills that are described are applicable in *any* instance of shared trauma.

Preparatory and Beginning Phases of Group Work

A core social work practice skill—anticipatory empathy—sensitizes the worker in advance to the concerns and questions clients may have as they contemplate entering into a working relationship (Gitterman et al., 2021). When applied to group work, this means that social workers are prepared to address the question potential members are likely to have prior to entering the group which is, "How will being with others like me *possibly* be helpful?" This requires the worker to put into words the meaning and benefits of mutual aid.

In agency-based practice, social workers also must garner the support of their agency and create a responsive organizational climate in advance of the group's start (Gitterman et al., 2021). The group worker often must rely upon agency personnel for referrals. Equally important, the agency must provide a space for group members to meet that is comfortable and private and allows for honest conversations.

An essential formation task in the beginning phase is partnering with members to establish an internal environment that promotes their work.

The worker helps members create a culture that facilitates open discussion and encourages members to learn from and help one another.

Lessening the intrusive impact of shared trauma. Groups that are formed in response to a communal traumatic event typically focus on helping members manage life stressors and affective reactions associated with the event. Emphasis is placed upon reducing member stress and enhancing resilience and feelings of self-efficacy, consistent with the TI model (Maheshwari et al., 2010; West-Olatunji et al., 2015).

Three core group work skills in the beginning phase lessen the risk that shared trauma will undermine the group's work and enhance workers' and clients' ability to manage their trauma exposure (Gitterman et al., 2021). Research indicates that advance preparation for members' group work experience enhances commitment and motivation and lessens the risk of dropout. Therefore, in the preparatory phase, the worker should make the decisions upon which these skills are based and convey this information to potential members:

1   Clarify the worker's role and the purpose of the group
2   Clarify role and responsibilities of the worker and members
3   Establish guidelines and mutually established rules that promote TI principles

When the practitioner offers members a clear sense of group purpose, this provides much needed structure and decreases feelings of being overwhelmed and powerless. Crisis-oriented groups quickly develop a culture for work, given members' sense of urgency. This requires the worker to directly address members' heightened feelings of distress. Mutually developed protective guidelines and ground rules help members manage stressful feelings and reactions, minimizing the risk of re-traumatization. These skills also establish boundaries, thereby reducing the likelihood that they will become blurred.

Because the social worker has been exposed to the same traumatic event, judicious and informed use of another skill—self-disclosure—may be necessary to reinforce boundaries. Specific disclosures will depend upon the circumstances of the crisis group but are likely to include:

1   The impact the event has had on the worker
2   The challenges that the event may have on the group as members do their work
3   The possibility that the worker's personal reactions could surface in the group.

Social workers' transparency addresses and reduces the "elephant in the room" created by the shared trauma between group members and them.

Disclosures also normalize and validate members' concerns. To reinforce and affirm boundaries, the group worker also invites members to provide their reactions to the worker's revelations and clarifies that the group's emphasis will be on the *members*, not the worker.

Consider the following comments provided by a medical social worker, Candace, who offered a weekly support group for frontline workers on her critical care unit in a large teaching hospital. After she explained the purpose of the group and clarified expectations around issues such as confidentiality, Candace said:

> We're all really struggling with this pandemic. I don't know about you, but I go from feeling energized and proud to be on the frontline to being exhausted, pissed off that people aren't taking this seriously enough, and feeling guilty that I'm not doing enough to help patients and my colleagues. I hope this group allows you to support one other as we all do this stressful work and provides a place where you can let off some steam and let go of stress and help each other continue to do the great work you're doing. I do want to be clear: this is *your* group not mine. My job here is help you support and help one another. I promise you that I have my own system of support and my own way of managing the stress, and I want to be sure that when I'm here with you, the focus stays on you and what you all are going through. So, you have my permission to call me out if it sounds like we are focusing on *my* stuff, not yours.

The findings of research in group work generally and group work and trauma specifically indicate that the leader's genuineness and willingness to share thoughts and feelings promotes cohesiveness, members' comfort with one another, and their commitment to the group (Baird & Alaggia, 2021; Leszcz, 2018). The worker's expression of feelings encourages member self-disclosure and challenges coping mechanisms they may have adopted to defend against their own affective responses (Brownell et al., 2015; Phillips, 2013).

In another example, the social worker and his student clearly distinguish their reactions from those of the group members as a way of opening up a discussion about members' experiences with communal trauma. The social work student, Cheri, and her field instructor, Matthew, met with a group for the first time after a break of almost five months due to the pandemic. The setting is a violence prevention program. Members had been referred to the group after having been patients in the trauma unit in an inner-city hospital. Most had been in the unit due to a gunshot wound, and all had prior involvement with the criminal justice system. The purpose of the group was threefold, and was designed to help members help one another: identify nonviolent ways to resolve conflicts; avoid criminal behavior and the criminal justice system; and take steps to finish their education, find employment and stable housing, and the like.

The session included five members who had been in the group prior to the shutdown. The field instructor previously led the group, but this was the student's first experience with members. Members were able to meet— masked—in person outside in a relatively quiet and comfortable space. After initial introductions and clarification of expectations, Matthew began:

MATTHEW: It's hard to believe it's been almost five months since we've seen or spoken to one another. I'm sorry we ended so abruptly. Once we went into lockdown, we spent all our time dealing with patients who came into the ER. There might be a pandemic, but people kept getting shot. It's been crazy. A lot has changed (*members nodded their agreement*). I'm sure you guys want to hear how each other are doing. But let's start with the obvious. How's life been treating you through this pandemic?

Members remained silent and fidgeted

MATTHEW: How about I start? It's been rough. I lost two friends to the virus, my kids are driving me crazy at home, my wife is a frontline hospital worker, I'm worried about my grandmother who's ninety and lives by herself. It's like a whole new reality, and it's hard to adjust to it. But I am sure it's even a lot tougher for you guys.

Several members briefly disclosed challenges they were facing.
This was followed by silence

MATTHEW: Cheri, how about you let the group know how it's been for you?
CHERI: I live with my grandparents, so I worry about their health. And I lost my job, but I think I'm pretty lucky. From what Matt tells me, life was pretty tough before the pandemic for you guys. So, we gotta think that things have probably gotten even tougher since the pandemic and the lockdown?

Members began to discuss in more detail what the last several months have been like for them including homelessness, loss of employment, and substance abuse.

Matthew and Cheri discussed in advance how they should start this session. Matthew explained that even though the members had been in group together, the passage of time and their natural reluctance to talk about sensitive subjects made it likely that they would have difficulty talking about how they were coping with the stressors associated with the pandemic. Matthew suggested Cheri and he might have to "get the ball rolling" and share their experiences first to encourage members to do the same. The workers' comments were brief and general, and both quickly turned the focus back on the members. Matthew also explained to Cheri that he was prepared to remind members of professional boundaries, if needed, but did not anticipate this would be necessary given his prior relationship with the group.

Middle/Work and Ending Phases of Group Work

The social worker continually assesses whether the group's culture—defined by the expectations that govern members' interactions with one another—is supporting its work (Gitterman et al., 2021). At the outset, worker and members will have established guidelines—explicit expectations—for how they will work together. Group norms evolve naturally over time and are the implicit expectations that members come to hold about one another. Inconsistencies between group norms and explicit expectations create confusion and undermine the group's work. Of the two sets of expectations, norms will exert the more powerful influence on members' actions.

The worker also continually attends to internal group processes to ensure they are fostering mutual aid and the group's work (Gitterman et al., 2021). The worker looks for indications that dynamics like scapegoating, factionalism, monopolization, and individual or collective defensiveness are occurring and addresses them directly with members when they surface.

Addressing shared trauma between members. Nine group work skills associated with the middle/work phase address the impact that shared trauma can have on the group's culture and can come into play whether the group is formed in response to or pre-exists communal trauma (Gitterman et al., 2021):

Monitoring group culture:

1   Scan and monitor members' reactions and interactions
2   Put into words members' reactions to one another
3   Identify and focus on common themes
4   Renegotiate expectations for participation

Monitoring interpersonal dynamics:

1   Adopt a transactional definition of maladaptive processes
2   Identify maladaptive patterns for group members
3   Challenge avoidance
4   Hold members to agreed-upon focus
5   Search for and sustain expression of strong feelings

When shared trauma is manifested in the interactions that occur between members, they are likely to be unaware of its existence. Therefore, social workers help members identify and address the dynamics they have observed, as is evident in the next example.

The worker, Janae, works in a shelter for homeless women. The group meets weekly and is mandatory for any resident who is in the shelter at the time it is offered. The group is designed to help residents find employment and stable housing and provides them with a place to talk about the many stressors they face—including experiences with past trauma—and work through disagreements that occur in their communal living arrangement. The group was suspended for six weeks in the early stage of the lockdown and then resumed virtually. Residents were together in one space at the shelter, and Janae met with them virtually from her home.

In the initial session after the lockdown, Janae invited members to share how they were doing, acknowledged the challenges associated with meeting virtually, and invited them to provide suggestions for how she could make their time together more helpful. In the first several sessions, members expressed frustration with the restrictions placed upon them by the shelter to limit their outside contacts and their inability to work on leaving the shelter. As the group progressed, Janae noted that members' focus increasingly turned to religion and God. Two of the seven members in attendance were quite religious and their views dominated the discussion as the following excerpt illustrates.

TANYA (GROUP MEMBER): Like I keep saying, I just trust that the Lord will provide for me. I put my faith in Him and know He'll get me out of this shithole [the shelter] one way or the other.

CELESTE (GROUP MEMBER): Praise the Lord. I know He's looking out for me, so even though I'm stuck right now, I know he'll lead me out of here.

PAULA (GROUP MEMBER): I've been trying to read the Bible more to find guidance. But I'm not getting it like you ladies.

CHARMAINE (GROUP MEMBER): You just ain't trying hard enough.

PAULA: (*raising her voice*) That ain't true! I got nothing to do all day but read the Good Book. But it ain't giving me any help or guidance. We're all still stuck here with no way out.

Several members forcefully tell Paula she just "has to have faith"

JANAE (WORKER): Hold up! Let's talk about what's happening here. It seems like most of you believe that God will get you out of here and get you back on a path to being independent again. So, when Paula says that's not working for her, it's upsetting.

Members nod and voice their assent

JANAE: I want to give you something to think about. Even before this pandemic, many of you were feeling frustrated and pretty pessimistic about your future. And already struggling with a lot of trauma. The pandemic has just made it harder *and* you all are just stuck here with one another. You're worried about your future, your kids you can't see, your family members who might get the virus and still dealing with past hurts. It's all too much sometimes, maybe?

Several members nod their heads

JANAE: Maybe it all seems so overwhelming that you just want to throw up your hands and say, "Why bother?" You just hope and pray that things will just get better somehow. The Bible and your beliefs in the Lord can be really good sources of support and help you keep moving forward. But the reality is that it's you who has to do the work, and doing that work is a whole lot harder now. But the group and our staff are still here to help you do what you need to do to move on.

After some initial silence, members began to talk about their feelings of helplessness, fears related to the pandemic, and sadness and guilt that they could not be with their children

The group's emphasis on faith allowed members to avoid dealing with the reality of their situation and indicated their sense of helplessness and despair. Janae skillfully addressed interpersonal dynamics that reflected shared trauma and threatened to undermine members' work. Janae does not discount members' faith; rather, she reframes it as a source of support that will help them continue to take the steps needed to leave the shelter despite the pandemic.

Janae also recognizes that Paula was transitioning into the role of scapegoat. Paula voices the powerlessness that others feel but are trying to avoid. Janae provides members with a transactional interpretation of this dynamic. The worker neither protects nor defends Paula nor does she censor other members for their anger. She gives voice to members' sense of powerlessness and encourages them to persevere, despite the barriers that they face, barriers that have been exacerbated by the pandemic and its restrictions.

Emotional contagion. In addition to monitoring members' interactions with one another and with them, group workers attend to the possibility that individual members' feelings and reactions may become blurred. In groups in which there is intense affective expression, a phenomenon known as emotional contagion may occur (Barsade, 2002; Knight, 2009). Individual members' affective reactions "spread" to others, which obscures boundaries and intensifies the impact that shared trauma has on members. Group contagion is particularly likely to occur in response to traumatic events (Gill-Emerson, 2015; Trautmann et al., 2018).

Four group work skills—coupled with practice skills that assist clients in managing affect—address group contagion and reduce its impact (Gitterman et al., 2021):

1　Legitimize differences in perceptions and behaviors
2　Invite expressions of differences
3　Attend to each member's verbal and nonverbal communication
4　Invite members to build upon one another's contributions.

Contagion can become self-reinforcing and amplify members' feelings of powerlessness. The worker can capitalize upon emotional contagion to prompt members to engage in deeper exploration of their affective reactions. Consider the following two examples:

Case 1: One session of Candace's drop-in group for hospital personnel followed an especially difficult period in which many patients died from complications from COVID. She commented on this as she began the session, sharing her own sadness and frustration about the number of deaths she had been handling. Initially, the discussion was superficial, with members critiquing the measures that were taken to preserve patients' lives.

Candace pointed this out and suggested members might be avoiding talking about how they were feeling. She observed one member, Jeff, had become teary-eyed, and commented, "Jeff, it seems like all these deaths have really hit you hard." With that, Jeff, and everyone else in attendance that day, began to express intense feelings of grief, anger, frustration, and hopelessness.

Candace monitored members' reactions as they—for one of the first times since the group had started meeting—disclosed what the day-to-day reality was like for them. She determined that while members *were* very upset, the emotional contagion validated and normalized their feelings and assisted them in better managing them.

Candace reported she struggled to stay present in the group. However, prior to this session, she had processed with a colleague how she would approach it and what she would do should she become triggered. After the meeting, Candace again met with her colleague, vented *her* feelings both about the death of her patients (direct trauma exposure) and the impact this powerful group session had on her (indirect trauma exposure). Candace's ability to understand the interpersonal processes that surfaced in the group and use them to deepen the group's work depended upon this supportive and trauma-informed supervision.

Case 2: A group was offered by a transitional housing program for women who have problems with substance abuse. The group focused on helping members maintain their sobriety to prepare them for living independently in the community. After a four month break due to the pandemic, the group resumed and was conducted virtually for three months and then in person with social distancing in place and masks required. All the members continued to work during the pandemic, most at low wage jobs considered to be "essential." A common theme in the meetings was members' fears about contracting the virus but also their worry that losing their job would slow down their transition to independence.

The worker, Naomi, described a recent session that in her words, "erupted in chaos," leading her to end the meeting early. Members learned that another member, Beatrice, tested positive for COVID-19. They were angry because they believed she knowingly brought the virus into their housing and that she contracted it by being careless and flaunting shelter rules.

The discussion became more and more heated with members talking over and ultimately shouting at one another. Much of the anger was directed at Beatrice, although some members came to her defense. Eventually, members began to express anger at, according to Naomi, "everyone and everything." Naomi acknowledged afterwards that she was overwhelmed, angry—at herself and the members—and "ready to just give up." She ended the group by saying that members just needed to "suck it up" and "deal with it."

In this example, emotional contagion undermines members' resilience and compromises self-capacities. The worker needed to actively intervene and employ practice skills that help clients contain feelings in order to de-escalate the shared trauma they were experiencing. Unfortunately, Naomi was not provided with TI supervision and therefore had little to no understanding of what had happened in this session, why it happened, and what to do about it. Naomi, herself, was triggered by members' shared trauma which further undermined her ability to recognize and help members manage their intense emotional affect.

Managing shared trauma between worker and members and the group-as-a-whole. These two scenarios reflect the impact that shared trauma has on clinicians and by extension their ability to be helpful to the group. Through their inner dialogue, social workers continually assess what role *they* play when disruptions occur in their interactions with the group. Four group work skills address shared trauma when it surfaces in these interactions (Gitterman et al., 2021):

1   Adopt a transactional perspective to identify the maladaptive dynamic
2   Directly acknowledge maladaptive pattern
3   Point out transference
4   Acknowledge worker's reactions and response, including countertransference.

Naomi processed this session afterwards and, with much ambivalence and some guilt, she acknowledged that, like the group members, she was angry with Beatrice for putting her at risk for contracting the virus. Naomi also expressed anger at the agency director—her supervisor—who, she believed, had prematurely required staff to return to in-person work with clients. Naomi described a work environment that was dismissive of staff concerns about safety and other stressors associated with the pandemic. She also expressed frustration that she had not been provided with guidance on how to work with clients remotely or how to help them with any concerns they had about the pandemic.

Renegotiating with members their expectations for the group. The group worker may need to directly address with members the expectations they hold for one another and for the group, particularly in groups formed prior to a communal traumatic event. For example, Matthew's and Cheri's group—which had been formed prior to the pandemic—originally focused on helping members develop nonviolent ways to manage conflicts and their anger as well as help them secure employment, stable housing, and the like. In the first session that followed the five-month hiatus, the workers quickly learned that the pandemic was creating intense stress and anxiety for members, which increased the risk that they would engage in violent behaviors. Therefore, in this first session, the workers contracted with members to shift their focus to managing their affective reactions to the pandemic as well as assisting them in overcoming the obstacles the pandemic and lockdown created that impeded their efforts to become self-sufficient and heightened the likelihood that they would resort to criminal behavior.

In contrast, Naomi continued to direct her group to focus on the goals and purpose that existed prior to the pandemic, despite the obvious impact it was having on members. Reflecting on her group experience later, Naomi acknowledged that she was "torn," believing that members needed to discuss the impact that the pandemic and lockdown was having on them but also needing to adhere to the agency director's dictate that the group should remain focused on helping the women remain sober and transition out of the shelter.

Naomi's inability to recontract with members contributed to the "chaos" described in the previous example. Members clearly were distressed by the communal trauma they all were experiencing. Yet Naomi was unsure how to handle this "elephant in the room" which was even bigger and more distracting because Naomi never addressed how members would work together remotely. She reported that the virtual nature of the initial sessions was awkward for members and her, as were the in-person sessions in which members were masked and sat far apart from one another. Rather than discussing with members how they would work together despite the challenges created by social distancing, Naomi assumed that they would continue as they had before.

Instead of dismissing or ignoring the impact that the pandemic was having on the group members and her, consider this hypothetical observation Naomi could have made in the session that followed the one previously described:

I want to start by apologizing for getting out of patience with everyone last week. The pandemic is stressful for all of us, and that sure includes me. I realized that my reactions last week were more about *my* stress rather than anything to do with you guys. What I also realized is that the agency and I have been acting like the pandemic is no big deal and expecting you all to just carry on as usual. The problem is that it is a *very* big deal. I think that our group would be a lot more helpful to you if it could be a place where you could talk about of all the stress you are experiencing and support one another as you try—despite all the barriers the pandemic has created—to stay clean and transition out of the program. So, how about we talk about how this "new" group might work and how we can make it more helpful to you?

The worker's transparency, coupled with her emphasis on partnering with members to make the group more helpful, epitomizes trauma-informed practice.

Promoting resilience and growth in the ending phase. Whether a group has been formed in response to communal trauma or precedes it, group workers employ seven skills that assist members in ending with one another and with them (Gitterman et al., 2021):

1   Invite review of work together
2   Emphasize strengths and gains
3   Elicit discussion of remaining areas of difficulty, if needed
4   Review work and experience
5   Consider next steps: transfer, referral, or termination
6   Develop plans to carry out next step(s)
7   Provide opportunity for final goodbye.

When the group has been impacted by or formed to respond to communal trauma, the worker will need to pay particular attention to helping members reflect on the gains they have made, consistent with a trauma-informed perspective. Since the worker has been exposed to the same communal traumatic event as group members and boundaries may have become blurred, inviting members to provide feedback about the worker's leadership—what worked, what did not; what was helpful and what was not—takes on added significance.

The Need for Trauma-Informed Care

Returning once again to Naomi's group, the picture she painted was of an organization that was in chaos and ill-equipped to deal with the rapidly changing reality of the pandemic and its consequences. Naomi said that the director frequently admonished both workers and clients by saying, "We can't let the virus control us," a statement that was often repeated by staff to clients. This organizational climate stands in stark contrast to a trauma-informed one. Naomi and her colleagues were left to fend for themselves, which exacerbated the stress they were experiencing in response to the pandemic. With no outlet for or validation of Naomi's feelings, it is not surprising that they surfaced in the group. When this session is viewed through a trauma-informed lens and with an understanding of group dynamics and shared trauma, three issues become clear:

1   Members' fears about the virus—which were heightened because they worked in high-risk settings including health care—and their feelings of powerlessness and anger initially were directed at one member, Beatrice, placing her in the role of scapegoat
2   Members' feelings closely mirrored Naomi's, which led to a blurring of boundaries
3   The lack of guidance from the organization breached Naomi's sense of security leading to feelings of powerlessness and undermining her ability to do her job.

The skills the authors have described provide social workers with the tools they need to effectively manage shared trauma. *However*, clinicians cannot successfully employ them if they do not have trauma-informed support and guidance. If one contrasts Naomi's situation with Candace's, it is readily apparent that Candace had a support system—one that she developed for herself—that provided her with a place to process her thoughts about and reactions to her group as well as the stress she was experiencing due to the pandemic.

In one final example, the importance of a trauma-informed workplace is evident and illustrates the recontracting skill (Gitterman et al., 2021) that has much relevance for managing shared trauma. The setting is a residential facility for youth aging out of foster care. The worker, Jermain, leads a weekly group for residents who have had problems in the past with drugs and alcohol. The group has a dual focus on helping members help each other stay clean and preparing them for the transition to independence. Members range in age between 18 and 20, and all are young adults of color. By state law, they must leave the facility once they turn 21. Jermain relied upon a curriculum developed by his agency to facilitate the group. Each session focused on a specific topic staff felt would help members successfully transition to independent living. The sessions always began with a brief check-in where members could talk about anything that might be bothering them.

After the state went into lockdown, members gathered in the usual meeting space at the facility, and Jermain interacted with them virtually. Membership remained consistent throughout the pandemic; two members were to be discharged because they turned 21, but this was delayed due to the pandemic. Jermain reported that it "took some getting used to" for both the members and him, but he thought the group "went about as well as it could, at least for a while." Jermain reported that "things started to go downhill" after about five sessions. While members continued to attend since the group was mandatory, they became "apathetic." Jermain stated that he was "confused" and "pissed off" when he initiated a discussion about the Black Live Matter protests, and members were "indifferent." Prior to the pandemic, members often brought up issues associated with racial justice during the initial group check-in, and as a Black man himself, Jermain encouraged these discussions.

Jermain described a typical exchange he found frustrating. This occurred after an initial check-in when members made superficial comments about "being trapped in jail":

JERMAIN: So today, we thought it would be helpful to talk about how you set up a banking account, get a credit card, things like that. We want to make sure you know how to budget your money, so you don't run out of it. Does that sound okay? (*Members nodded in agreement.*) Okay, so take a look at this handout I have about money. Who wants to start?

Members look away and fidget

JERMAIN: Come on guys. This is important! We're working on completing your education, getting jobs. But if you can't manage your money, you're screwed.

Members remain silent

JERMAIN: Okay, well, how about I go over the handout and you can ask questions?

Jermain reported that the rest of the session "dragged on" with him doing much of the talking.

Afterwards, Jermain sought guidance from his supervisor, Anthony, worrying he had "lost the group." He came to understand the following:

1   Jermain confused his sense of urgency with that of his client's (the group)
2   Through their behavior—including their silence—group members were telling Jermain that the group was not helpful to them
3   Members were not interested in what *he* wanted them to talk about. What members *were* interested in and what was uppermost in their minds was what was going to happen to them once they had to leave the program. The lockdown exacerbated their worries about their future. Even though two members had been allowed to remain in the program after they turned 21, staff made it clear that this was only temporary

4   Jermain was experiencing a great deal of stress himself due to the pandemic. His girlfriend—with whom he lived—lost her job so they were living solely on his income. She had been unable to collect unemployment insurance, and he was worried that they would lose their apartment. Jermain's mother had contracted COVID-19. While she was home from the hospital, she remained seriously ill. His parents were very worried about how they would pay the medical bills since they had both lost their jobs due to the pandemic

5   Jermain's personal struggles associated with the pandemic prevented him from hearing what the group members were telling him.

Armed with this heightened understanding, Anthony helped Jermain decide how he should approach his next session.

Jermain began the next session by renegotiating with members how they would work together moving forward:

I owe you guys an apology. You've been telling me for a while now that this group isn't helping you, and I haven't been listening. I've been so caught up in my own worries about the pandemic that I haven't been able to see that it's stressing you out, too. I think that it's probably stressing you out even more. You're stuck in our facility; you can't really look for work. You can continue your education, but maybe you're feeling like what's the point. So how about for *this* check-in and from now on, we *always* start with that: Your worries about how the pandemic—and anything else—might affect your being able to leave here with somewhere to go?

Jermain's willingness to acknowledge his mistakes and the challenges he faced and to modify how the members and he would work together led to far more productive meetings.

This case clearly illustrates the benefits of addressing and directly working with shared trauma. Anthony explored without judgment Jermain's personal reactions to the communal trauma to which both he and the group members were exposed. His approach epitomized trauma-informed supervision. Anthony created an environment in which Jermain felt safe to discuss his concerns. He also provided Jermain with the tools and knowledge he needed to better understand and be more responsive to his client's—the group's—needs, which was empowering.

Conclusion

In this chapter, the authors integrate what have been two divergent bodies of empirical and conceptual inquiry: one that examines the shared trauma phenomenon and the other that elaborates upon the trauma-informed formulation. This integrated approach is required for *all* practice modalities impacted by shared trauma to ensure that resilience and adversarial growth are promoted for clients and workers, while the risk of re-traumatization and indirect trauma is reduced.

Relying upon the mutual aid model, the authors identify skills that workers can employ to address manifestations of shared trauma that surface in the group modality. These skills are not unique to a shared trauma context, but rather are part of the worker's larger repertoire of group work practice skills.

In the preparatory and beginning phases, five skills lessen the likelihood that shared trauma will surface when the worker forms a group in response to a communal traumatic event. In the middle/work phase, the worker can employ 13 skills to address shared trauma that occurs between group members. Five skills provide workers with the tools needed to manage shared trauma that surfaces in their interactions with group members and the group-as-a-whole. A final skill, recontracting, helps members refine their focus and the nature of their work together in response to their collective exposure to trauma. As the group comes to an end—or individual members leave—group work skills that encourage members to reflect on the gains they have made and to provide constructive feedback about the worker's facilitation of the group take on added significance.

Each of these basic group work skills allow social workers facilitating groups to address and manage manifestations of shared trauma. However, if social workers are going to effectively employ these skills, they need the support and guidance that comes from a trauma-informed perspective.

References

Adamson, C. (2014). A social work lens for a disaster-informed curriculum. *Advances in Social Work and Welfare Education*, 16, 7–22.

Adamson, C. (2018). Trauma-informed supervision in the disaster context. *Clinical Supervisor*, 37, 221–240.

Bailey, K., Trevillion, K., & Gilchrist, G. (2019). What works for whom and why: A narrative systematic review of interventions for reducing post-traumatic stress disorder and problematic substance use among women with experiences of interpersonal violence. *Journal of Substance Abuse Treatment*, 99, 88–103.

Baird, S. L., & Alaggia, R. (2021). Trauma-informed groups: Recommendations for group workers. *Clinical Social Work Journal*, 49, 10–19.

Barros, A. J., Teche, S. P., Padoan, C., Laskoski, P., Hauck, S., & Eizirik, C. L. (2020). Countertransference, defense mechanisms, and vicarious trauma in work with sexual offenders. *Journal of the American Academy of Psychiatry and the Law*, 48, 1–13.

Barsade, S. G. (2002). The ripple effect: Emotional contagion and its influence on group behavior. *Administrative Science Quarterly*, 47, 644–675.

Bassuk, E. L., Unick, G. J., Paquette, K., & Richard, M. K. (2017). Developing an instrument to measure organizational trauma-informed care in human services: The TICOMETER. *Psychology of Violence*, 7, 150–157.

Baum, N. (2010). Shared traumatic reality in communal disasters: Toward a conceptualization. *Psychotherapy: Theory, Research, Practice, Training*, 47, 249–259.

Baum, N. (2012). Trap of conflicting needs: Helping professionals in the wake of a shared traumatic reality. *Clinical Social Work Journal*, 40, 37–45.

Bercier, M. L., & Maynard, B. R. (2015). Interventions for secondary traumatic stress with mental health workers: A systematic review. *Research on Social Work Practice*, 25(1), 81–89.

Berliner, L., & Kolko, D. J. (2016). Trauma informed care: A commentary and critique. *Child Maltreatment*, 21, 168–172.

Berzoff, J., & Kita, E. (2010). Compassion fatigue and countertransference: Two different concepts. *Clinical Social Work Journal*, 38, 341–349.

Blome, W. W., & Safadi, N. S. (2016). Shared vicarious trauma and the effects on Palestinian social workers. *Illness, Crisis, and Loss*, 24, 236–260.

Boals, A. (2018). Trauma in the eye of the beholder: Objective and subjective definitions of trauma. *Journal of Psychotherapy Integration*, 28, 77–89.

Bonanno, G. A., Romero, S. A., & Klein, S. I. (2015). The temporal elements of psychological resilience: An integrative framework for the study of individuals, families, and communities. *Psychological Inquiry*, 26, 139–169.

Branson, D. C. (2019). Vicarious trauma, themes in research, and terminology: A review of literature. *Traumatology*, 25, 2–10.

Brownell, T., Schrank, B., Jakaite, Z., Larkin, C., & Slade, M. (2015). Mental health service user experience of positive psychotherapy. *Journal of Clinical Psychology*, 71, 85–92.

Collins-Camargo, C., & Antle, B. (2018). Child welfare supervision: Special issues related to trauma-trauma informed care in a unique environment. *The Clinical Supervisor*, 37, 64–82.

Copeland, W. E., Shanahan, L., Hinesley, J., Chan, R. F., Aberg, K. A., Fairbank, J. A., van de Oord, E. J. C. G., & Costello, E. J. (2018). Association of childhood trauma exposure with adult psychiatric disorders and functional outcomes. *JAMA Network Open*, 1(7), e184493–e184493.

Currier, J. M., Stefurak, T., Carroll, T. D., & Shatto, E. H. (2017). Applying trauma-informed care to community-based mental health services for military veterans. *Best Practices in Mental Health: An International Journal*, 13, 47–64.

Day, K. W., Lawson, G., & Burge, P. (2017). Clinicians' experiences of shared trauma after the shootings at Virginia Tech. *Journal of Counseling & Development*, 95, 269–278.

Diehle, J., Schmitt, K., Daams, J. G., Boer, F., & Lindauer, R. J. L. (2014). Effects of psychotherapy on trauma-related cognitions in posttraumatic stress disorder: A meta-analysis. *Journal of Traumatic Stress*, 27, 257–264.

Dombo, E. A., & Blome, W. (2016). Vicarious trauma in child welfare workers: A study of organizational responses. *Journal of Public Child Welfare*, 10, 505–523.

Dye, H. (2018). The impact and long-term effects of childhood trauma. *Journal of Human Behavior in the Social Environment*, 28, 381–392.

Figley, C. (1995). Compassion fatigue: Toward a new understanding of the costs of caring. In B. Stamm (Ed.), *Secondary traumatic stress: Self-care issues for clinicians, researchers, and educators* (pp. 3–28). Sidran Press.

Finklestein, M., Stein, E., Greene, T., Bronstein, I., & Solomon, Z. (2015). Post-traumatic stress disorder and vicarious trauma in mental health professionals. *Health and Social Work*, 40, 25–31.

Fondren, K., Lawson, M., Speidel, R., McDonnell, C. G., & Valentino, K. (2020). Buffering the effects of childhood trauma within the school setting: A systematic review of trauma-informed and trauma-responsive interventions among trauma-affected youth. *Children and Youth Services Review*, 109, 1–17.

Freedman, S. A., & Tuval Mashiach, R. (2018). Shared trauma reality in war: Mental health therapists' experience. *PLoS one*, 13, 1–13.

Frey, L. L., Beesley, D., Abbott, D., & Kendrick, E. (2017). Vicarious resilience in sexual assault and domestic violence advocates. *Psychological Trauma: Theory, Research, Practice, and Policy*, 9, 44–51.

Gill-Emerson, G. (2015). The trauma contagion. *Trauma*, 15, 8–11.

Gitterman, A., Knight, C., & Germain, C. (2021). *The life model of social work practice* (4th edn). Columbia University Press.

Gonzalez, T. C., Helm, H., & Edwards, L. I. (2019). An examination of resilience, compassion fatigue, burnout, and compassion satisfaction between men and women among trauma responders. *North American Journal of Psychology*, 21, 1–20.

Hales, T., Kusmaul, N., & Nochajski, T. (2017). Exploring the dimensionality of trauma-informed care: Implications for theory and practice. *Human Service Organizations: Management, Leadership & Governance*, 41, 317–325.

Harris, M., & Fallot, R. (2001). *Using trauma theory to design service systems: New directions for mental health services.* Jossey Bass.

Huang, Y., & Wong, H. (2013). Effects of social group work with survivors of the Wenchuan earthquake in a transitional community. *Health and Social Care in the Community*, 21, 327–337.

Jankowski, M. K., Barnett, E. R., Schifferdecker, K. E., Butcher, R. L., & Foster-Johnson, L. (2019). Effectiveness of a trauma-informed care initiative in a state child welfare system: A randomized study. *Child Maltreatment*, 24(1), 86–97.

Killian, K., Hernandez-Wolfe, P., Engstrom, D., & Gangsei, D. (2017). Development of the vicarious resilience scale (VRS): A measure of positive effects of working with trauma survivors. *Psychological Trauma: Theory, Research, Practice, and Policy*, 9, 23–31.

Knight, C. (2009). *Introduction to working with adult survivors of childhood trauma: Strategies and techniques for helping professionals.* Thomson/Brooks-Cole.

Knight, C. (2013). Indirect trauma: Implications for supervision, the organization, and the academic institution. *The Clinical Supervisor*, 32, 224–243.

Knight, C. (2021a). Trauma-informed field instruction from an international perspective. In R. Baikady, S. M. Sajid, J. Gal, & V. Nadesan (Eds.), *The Routledge international handbook of field work education in social work*. Routledge/Taylor & Francis.

Knight, C. (2021b). Trauma-informed supervision. In K. O'Donoghue & L. Engelbrecht (Eds.), *International Handbook of Social Work Supervision*. Routledge/Taylor & Francis.

Kusmaul, N. (2021). Role of trauma-informed care in disasters. In K. E. Cherry & A. Gibson (Eds.), *The Intersection of Trauma and Disaster Behavioral Health* (pp. 145–162). Springer.

Lang, J. M., Campbell, K., Shanley, P., Crusto, C. A., & Connell, C. M. (2016). Building capacity for trauma-informed care in the child welfare system: Initial results of a statewide implementation. *Child Maltreatment*, 21, 113–124.

Lavi, T., Nuttman-Shwartz, O., & Dekel, R. (2017). Therapeutic intervention in a continuous shared traumatic reality: An example from the Israeli–Palestinian conflict. *British Journal of Social Work*, 47(3), 919–935.

Lee, J. J., Gottfried, R., & Bride, B. E. (2018). Exposure to client trauma, secondary traumatic stress, and the health of clinical social workers: A mediation analysis. *Clinical Social Work Journal*, 46(3), 228–235.

Leszcz, M. (2018). The evidence-based group psychotherapist. *Psychoanalytic Inquiry*, 38, 285–298.

Levenson, J. (2020). Translating trauma-informed principles into social work practice. *Social Work*, 65, 288–298.

Maheshwari, N., Yadav, R., & Singh, N. (2010). Group counseling: A silver lining in the psychological management of disaster trauma. *Journal of Pharmacy & Bioallied Sciences*, 2, 267–274.

Manderscheid, R. W. (2009). Trauma-informed leadership. *International Journal of Mental Health*, 38, 78–86.

McCann, I., & Pearlman, L. (1990). *Psychological trauma and the adult survivor.* Brunner/Mazel.

Montagner Rigoli, M., Rainho de Oliveira, F., Klock Bujak, M., Volkmann, N. M., & Haag Kristensen, C. (2019). Psychological trauma in clinical practice and research: An evolutionary concept analysis. *Journal of Loss and Trauma*, 24, 595–608.

O'Donoghue, K. B. (2014). Towards an interactional map of the supervision session: An exploration of supervisees' and supervisors' experiences. *Practice: Social Work in Action*, 26, 53–70.

Pearlman, L., & Saakvitne, K. (1995). *Trauma and the therapist: Counter-transference and vicarious traumatization in psychotherapy with incest survivors.* Norton.

Phillips, S. B. (2013). From immersion to formulation and integration: The complicated journey of the trauma group leader. *Group*, 37, 31–39.

Pressley, J., & Smith, R. (2017). No ordinary life: Complex narratives of trauma and resilience in under-resourced communities. *Journal of Aggression, Maltreatment & Trauma*, 2, 137–154.

Rao, N., & Mehra, A. (2015). Hurricane Sandy: Shared trauma and therapist self-disclosure. *Psychiatry: Interpersonal & Biological Processes*, 78, 65–74.

Sampson, K. (2016). Shared trauma: Time to think. *Transactional Analysis Journal*, 46, 343–354.

Schmidt, R. W., & Cohen, S. L. (2020). *Disaster mental health community planning: A manual for trauma-informed collaboration.* Routledge.

Shannonhouse, L., Barden, S., Jones, E., Gonzalez, L., & Murphy, A. (2016). Secondary traumatic stress for trauma researchers: A mixed methods research design. *Journal of Mental Health Counseling*, 38, 201–216.

Shulman, L. (2010). *Interactional supervision* (3rd edn). NASW Press.

Smith, A. J., Abeyta, A. A., Hughes, M., & Jones, R. T. (2015). Persistent grief in the aftermath of mass violence: The predictive roles of posttraumatic stress symptoms, self-efficacy, and disrupted worldview. *Psychological Trauma: Theory, Research, Practice, and Policy*, 7, 179–186.

Sprang, G., Ross, L., Miller, B. C., Blackshear, K., & Ascienzo, S. (2017). Psychometric properties of the secondary traumatic stress-informed organizational assessment. *Traumatology*, 23, 65–171.

Substance Abuse and Mental Health Service Administration (SAMSHA). (2014). *SAMHSA's concept of trauma and guidance for a trauma-informed approach.* Retrieved from: https://ncsacw.samhsa.gov/userfiles/files/SAMHSA_Trauma.pdf.

Tosone, C. (2021). Introduction. In C. Tosone (Ed.), *Shared trauma, shared resilience during a pandemic: Social work in the time of COVID-19* (pp. 1–14). Springer.

Tosone, C., Nuttman-Shwartz, O., & Stephens, T. (2012). Shared trauma: When the professional is personal. *Clinical Social Work Journal*, 40, 231–239.

Tosone, C., Bauwens, J., & Glassman, M. (2016). The shared traumatic and professional posttraumatic growth inventory. *Research on Social Work Practice*, 26, 286–294.

Trautmann, S., Reineboth, M., Trikojat, K., Richter, J., Hagenaars, M. A., Kanske, P., & Schäfer, J. (2018). Susceptibility to others' emotions moderates immediate self-reported and biological stress responses to witnessing trauma. *Behaviour Research and Therapy*, 110, 55–63.

Tullberg, E., & Boothe, G. (2019). Taking an organizational approach to addressing secondary trauma in child welfare settings. *Journal of Public Child Welfare*, 13, 345–367.

Weinberg, H. (2020). Online group psychotherapy: Challenges and possibilities during COVID-19: A practice review. *Group Dynamics: Theory, Research, and Practice*, 24, 201–211.

West-Olatunji, C., Henesy, R., & Varney, M. (2015). Group work during international disaster outreach projects: A model to advance cultural competence. *Journal for Specialists in Group Work*, 40(1), 38–54.

Chapter 9

Shared Trauma and Community Organizing

Ozy Aloziem and JaLisa Williams

Introduction

Presently we are at a precarious point in history—a history which in the United States includes the genocide of the Indigenous and the enslavement of Black people. This ugly and traumatic history has bled into a strange present that includes two pandemics that disproportionately plague Black people—the COVID-19 pandemic and the ever-present pandemic that is systemic state-sanctioned racism and racial inequity. If that is our past and if this is our present, what kind of future is possible for us? And, as social workers, what is our role in this?

As Black female social workers who are deeply involved and invested in our community, we have noticed a particular kind of pain that lives in community organizers and leaders. The authors of this chapter started as community organizers before they became social workers. We know what it is like to show up to rallies and protests, to put our bodies on the line in demand of justice. We're very familiar with the emotional energy that takes and how it can degrade a body. Because of this, we both made the decision to stop attending protests and shift our attention elsewhere—to responding and tending to the shared trauma that often lives in the community organizing space.

Shared trauma is the "affective, behavioral, cognitive, spiritual, and multimodal responses that mental health professionals experience as a result of primary and secondary exposure to the same collective trauma as their clients" (Tosone, 2012, p. 625). While the limited research and writing about shared trauma has mostly been situated in the community of mental health practitioners, this phenomenon can be applied to community organizers as well.

Shared traumatic reality is a concept used to describe an experience of collective trauma in which health care professionals live in the same community as their clients and are exposed to traumatic events at various levels (Baum, 2010; Dekel & Baum, 2010). Shared trauma can be experienced on multiple levels (psychological, interpersonal, community, and societal) and can impact social workers personally and professionally in a

DOI: 10.4324/9781003176947-12

multitude of ways (Tosone et al., 2012). Shared trauma does not mean that individuals "share" the same experience in relation to collective trauma. Rather, the term acknowledges that we—as Black women, social workers, and community organizers—have reactions to the trauma histories of communities we serve, COVID-19 discussions and racial injustice in community organizing spaces, and we also have to contend with our own independent reactions to the intersection of these two pandemics.

The last year and a half of navigating a global pandemic and uprisings for racial and social justice have exacerbated the pervasiveness of shared trauma which necessitates attention and interventions. There is so much urgency at this moment; so much so that each morning seems to greet us with a new crisis to attend to. Both nationally and locally, community organizers have been getting swept up in the energy of emergency. An adrenalized body can provide—we feel the urgency and take immediate action. This can be incredibly powerful when organizing for social change but it cannot be the only state we exist in. Constant adrenal activation drains and degrades the body and spirit. So many of us are activated at this moment. So many are committing our lives to radical social change. An important lesson these last 18 months has been the revelation that we must pay deeper attention to healing as well.

We believe what is missing in community organizing spaces is a focus on preserving our spirits. We must center our healing as we do the work. Healing is an act of resistance. It is political action. It is what must occur alongside all of the dismantlings. We must create a praxis of healing in order to build as we break down—otherwise what will remain of us? We have to be able to heal inside of movements and in order to do that, we need to create a culture that can support that healing. Can we organize around trauma and healing simultaneously? This chapter explores the impact of shared trauma on community organizers and both poses and attempts to answer a question more pressing than ever before: How do we deconstruct systems of oppression while simultaneously reconstructing systems of support that cultivate individual and community well-being? As Black women who have been consistently exposed to racism and now the COVID-19 pandemic, we have our own trauma narratives to tell. Deriving from our own lived experiences of shared trauma and healing, the authors attempt to situate the impacts of shared trauma in the community organizing context in order to make necessary and relevant recommendations for community organizers and social workers organizing for change.

> How do we remain intact as we do significant work, but it's not either/or, but what will it take? What's the pace, what's the rhythm, what's the kind of care around us? What's the care for ourselves? That allows us to do the work that we're here to do without taking such a significant toll on our bodies and our spirits.
>
> (Prentis Hemphill, 2020, n.p.)

Our Positionality

Positionality refers to how one is positioned in society and where one positions oneself because of their various identities. It is where you stand in relation to your social and political contexts; in other words, "one's location within a given social reality" (Sanchez, 2006, p. 38). It is both structurally determined and relational. One is always positioned in reference to another's location, which can lead to a pitting of one group against another. On the other hand, positionality is defined as one's "imagined relation or standpoint in relation to one's structural positioning" (Sanchez, 2006, p. 38). In other words, it is an individuals' perspective on their structurally defined social location. For example: What is your proximity to privilege and oppression? Where are you in relation to systems of power? It is also how your identity shapes your stance or belief system and your overall take on the world. Your positionality shifts in response to the room you are in, its geographical and temporal location as well as in response to the other people in that room. Positionality also speaks to how our identities shape how we "read" a room and the people in it and how that lens informs our ways of knowing, ways of being, ways of valuing, and ways of believing (Sanchez, 2006).

The authors' positionality begins with our female Blackness. There will never be a day in our lives when our identification as Black women does not factor into how we are perceived or into how we perceive ourselves. It's not enough for us to simply lay claim to that identity, we are also dedicated to defending it. Our various experiences undoubtedly shape the way we think and write. This is actually the reality of all writing. There is no such thing as a neutral space. We all carry some degree of bias and socialization that we bring into whatever endeavor we embark on. We choose to be upfront and honest about how our identities and socialization impact us as social workers while also acknowledging how your identities and socialization will impact how you make meaning of the words we share.

Aligned with the Indigenist liberatory scholarship principle of relational accountability (Wilson, 2008) we begin with our positionality statement to ground our roles as insiders and outsiders to the study of shared trauma and community organizing. Wilson (2008) details the importance of relational accountability in research. Relational accountability refers to the ways in which a researcher forms a reciprocal and respectful relationship with the people and ideas being studied. We are relationally accountable to the Black women we work for and with as well as to our own ancestors. As such, it's important for us to place ourselves within the context of this writing and make our intentions and approach transparent.

Ozy

I identify as both an African American and an African. I was born on the land of the Omaha people, also known as Omaha, NE in the US but have been a visitor on the lands of the Cheyenne, Ute and Arapahoe people, also known as Denver, CO (also in the US) since 2015. I claim membership to multiple communities. I am an Igbo scholar situated at the intersection of multiple ways of knowing. The Igbos are one of the largest ethnic groups in Africa and are native to south central and southeastern Nigeria where my family and ancestral homes still reside. My full name is Ozioma Nkechi Aloziem. Ozioma means "good news." Nkechi means "God's gift or gift from God." Aloziem was my great-grandfather's first name. For us Igbos, our names carry great significance. They embody a collective of our rich history and provide insight into our value systems and life philosophies. In Igbo ontology, humans are relational, not static, and our identity is better defined and understood in relation to our families and community. We find meaning and identity in the idea and the reality of the other, and without others, we lose value. Meaning, community, and connection are paramount to our Indigenous culture.

I am a social worker deeply committed to radical imagination, community healing, transformational education, collective liberation, and creative expression. I have degrees in psychology and anthropology as well as a master's degree in social work. As a psycho-anthropological researcher and critical Black feminist, I am specifically committed to diminishing historical legacies of racial and gender oppression in the personal, economic, political, and social spheres. My scholarly activism is informed by Black women's liberatory pedagogies and shaped by Critical Race Theory and Black Feminist Thought. These theoretical frameworks shape my onto-epistemologies. As an educator, I take a transformational and embodied approach to teaching and learning.

These are just some of my various identifiers. I share them with you because they shape my positionality. I start by naming this because it is why I am who I am and also why I do the work that I do. And in order for me to show up fully, I wanted to first name my relation to this work and why it matters to me. I also share this to provide context for my specific kind of Blackness. I think that sometimes Blackness can be collapsed in a way that ignores or minimizes the variety of experiences that are beautifully textured and distinctly different. African American is not always synonymous with Black American, and as Dr. Bianca Williams states, "while historical and contemporary African American experiences make up a portion of Black experiences, they do not encompass all of what Blackness is" (Williams, 2016, p. 71).

JaLisa

As a badass Black woman, when asked what I do, I love to tell folks that I teach my people how to rest. I started graduate school in August 2014, about a week after the Mike Brown murder and the Ferguson protests began. That semester was this messy balance of being Black and being one of the youngest students in my cohort. I went to yoga teacher training as a part of my internship and really honed in on learning the depths of how our breathing can control our nervous system. I fell into imagining the possibilities for trauma survivors using these techniques—Black people who have experienced violence, who grew up around it, and even ones who thought they were the violence. At this time, "trauma-informed" was a key phrase in the social work world, Dianne Bondy was getting love for Yoga for Everybody, and I started to see more Black girls in holistic spaces I would participate in.

As a yoga instructor, I position myself as a healer—showing my people how to slow down, rest, breathe, move, give gratitude, and let go. As a lecturer, I position myself as a beacon of possibility, showing students ways to use imagination in radical ways to create change in our communities and in the systems that we function within. As a clinician, I position myself as a companion on the journey to healing ourselves and our environments. As a facilitator of intentional experiences, I have seen my community hurting and seeking healing, peace and connection. My people deserve rest and ease for the generations of harm. My research, imagination, and experience position me to believe that centering radical healing builds the capacity for individuals to fight for social change.

Critically Understanding the Issue: Causes and Effects of Shared Trauma in Community Organizers

Defining Collective Trauma

Recently, there has been a shift from understanding trauma primarily at the individual level to also including the community level, known as collective trauma (Pinderhughes et al., 2015). Researchers have defined collective trauma as the psychological reactions of an entire group after a large event that shifts the fabric of their reality (Saul, 2013; Watson et al., 2020; Hirschberger, 2018). This can be either a combination of trauma experienced by community members or an event that impacts a few people but has structural and societal traumatic consequences (Pinderhughes et al., 2015). These experiences include natural and human-caused disasters as well as the cumulative effects of poverty, oppression, illness, and displacement. (Saul, 2013). Trauma can be both acute and chronic. Acute trauma refers to a single instance of fear for one's safety, such as a car accident, experiencing an environmental disaster, or an assault. Recent examples include the murder of Breonna Taylor and Hurricane Ida. While these events happened to specific individuals and communities, Black people across the US and the world experienced a psychological reaction to these events. Chronic trauma refers to an ongoing perceived threat to one's safety, such as long-term housing instability or childhood abuse/neglect. Examples of chronic trauma include the effects of pervasive racism at all levels (individual, interpersonal, institutional, and systemic) which impact Black communities worldwide as well as the COVID-19 pandemic, which is disproportionately negatively impacting Black communities (Khazanchi et al., 2020).

The authors of *Trauma Informed Community Building* note:

> Ongoing trauma can have lasting adverse effects that compromise an individual's mental health and overall well-being. Moreover, trauma manifests at the family and community level by altering social networks and reducing community capacity to collectively identify and address its problems and plan for its future. Trauma can also undermine "readiness" for individual and community change—the extent to which community is prepared and inclined to take collective action on an issue.
>
> (Weinstein et al., 2014, p. 7)

As a result, experiencing prolonged trauma at all levels (individual, family, and community) impacts community organizing work. We can address this by incorporating trauma awareness and healing that is built upon a strengths-based, person-first foundation into our community organizing model. Community organizing and development work must therefore include practices that acknowledge and address the shared trauma of community members and their collective communities.

Trauma responses vary between groups and events but common responses are increased anxiety, insomnia, flashbacks, and other PTSD characteristics. Research indicates that collective trauma allows for something called collective memory. Jack Saul, author of *Collective Trauma, Collective Healing: Promoting Community Resilience in the Aftermath of Disaster*, states collective memory is constructed, shaped, and shared within groups of people such as nations, generations, and communities and is a social representation of history (Saul, 2013).

Defining Historical Trauma

Historical trauma refers to the collective and cumulative emotional wounding across generations that results from cataclysmic events targeting a community. This trauma is held both personally and collectively and is transmitted across generations (Brave Heart, 1998). As a result, individuals who have not directly experienced the trauma are able to feel the effects of the event several generations later. Historical trauma is an experience people have collectively and it accumulates intergenerationally (Ortega-Williams et al., 2021; Mohatt et al., 2014). Historic trauma is multigenerational and is experienced by demographics, groups, and families who have been impoverished, displaced, or otherwise oppressed over long periods of time. Examples include the Trail of Tears, slavery, the Holocaust, and Japanese internment camps. Historic trauma is about both what happened in the past and what is still happening. Scholars have broken historical trauma down to three elements—1) a traumatic event, 2) the shared experience of the trauma by a group of people, and 3) the multigenerational impact of such trauma (Mohatt et al., 2014)— and have introduced concepts like soul wounds (Duran, 2006) and post-traumatic slavery syndrome to the psychological world, that "captures the collective experiences of trauma across generations" (Mohatt et al., 2014, p. 128).

Charged traumatic stressors are transmitted from one generation to the next. For example, research shows that the descendants of Holocausts survivors have an increased vulnerability to developing psychological disturbances and stressors related to Holocaust loss (Dashorst et al., 2019). The research also shows that vulnerability is directly related to the negative life experience of the previous generation. Indigenous communities in North America, for example, have faced numerous historical traumatic events. These include planned phenomena by government and government-sponsored institutions (i.e. boarding schools), communally based incidents that cause catastrophic upheaval or high levels of community distress among and within communities, environmental trauma, and spiritual trauma, to name a few (Brave Heart, 2000). Historical trauma can make one predisposed to further trauma. Today, Indigenous and Native Americans continue to have high rates of unemployment, dependence on substances, diabetes, and depression correlated to the psychological impact of trauma (Designer, 2014). The suicide rates in Native and Indigenous populations are 3.5 times higher than the racial groups with the lowest rates (Leavitt et al., 2018). Not only this, but 1) lack of cultural competence in therapy training for social workers and other practitioners serving Indigenous and Native American communities has negative impacts, 2) geographical isolation has also created barriers to providing appropriate mental health resources, and 3) catastrophic events often open up or exacerbate previously existing fault lines of racism and other forms of discrimination, social and economic inequalities, and prior historical traumas (Saul, 2013). Each of these issues further complicates the impact of trauma on Indigenous and Native American communities.

Community Organizing and Shared Trauma

Community organizing is when a community that shares the same space, or in some cases a community that shares the same identities, comes together to organize for systemic change (Siddiqui, 1997; Simon, 1982). Community organizing is synonymous with grassroots action and entails using collective action to create social change. Community leaders fight for change and as they do, they also experience their own symptomatic responses to communities that suffer from shared trauma.

Shared trauma differs from compassion fatigue, secondary trauma, and vicarious traumatization in that these terms refer to trauma exposure responses and describe the damaging effects of working with survivors of trauma but do not consider the dual impacts of also experiencing a shared traumatic event (Tosone, 2021). Trauma exposure responses include chronic exhaustion, feeling helpless or hopeless, fear, guilt, and an inability to empathize, or a need to numb to get through the day-to-day. Shared trauma includes a trauma exposure response as well as a response to interacting directly with a traumatic experience (Tosone, 2021).

Clinical social workers serve as witnesses to the trauma narratives of their clients while experiencing the same collective trauma first hand, which can result in the blurring of professional and personal boundaries and the development of post-traumatic stress (Tosone, 2021). We suggest the same thing can be found in community organizers. Risk factors for shared traumatic stress include exposure to potentially traumatic life events such as instances of racism or racial oppression. Greater exposure to potentially traumatic life events can predict higher levels of shared traumatic stress (Tosone et al., 2015).

Health Outcomes

Shared trauma also takes a toll on the physical body, as illuminated by the COVID-19 pandemic. Race-based trauma refers to the mental and emotional injury caused by encounters with racial bias and ethnic discrimination, racism, and hate crimes (Helms et al., 2010). Racism can lead to chronic and toxic stress and shape social and economic factors that put some people from racial and ethnic minority groups at increased risk for COVID-19 (Garcia et al., 2021). It even impacts systems meant to protect well-being. Examples of such systems include those related to health care, housing, education, criminal justice, and finance.

Encountering threats like racism triggers the body to release stress hormones. These hormones increase heart rate and raise blood pressure, change the immune response, and suppress the digestive system, reproductive system, and growth processes. They also affect the brain, causing changes in mood, motivation, and fear. When an individual experiences continuous stress, such as repeated exposure to racial insults, attacks, and microaggressions, these stress responses can lead to serious health problems and premature aging. This is chronic or toxic stress. Moreover, stress from racial discrimination and other sources has been tied to heart disease, hypertension, and obesity. Studies have shown that long-term discrimination can lead to a disruption in the stress hormone cortisol, leaving people with less biological energy and more fatigue. It can also take a significant toll on mental health (Goosby & Heidbrink, 2013).

Critical race theorist William A. Smith first conceptualized Racial Battle Fatigue (RBF) which is the cumulative impact of race-related stress that results in physical, mental, and emotional fatigue. Constantly experiencing triggering situations related to race and racism in everyday life can cause racial battle fatigue to occur. Symptoms can include, but are not limited to, physiological effects like gastric distress, high blood pressure, headaches, and difficulty sleeping; psychological effects like irritability, helplessness, disbelief, and fear; and behavioral effects like increase in alcohol or drug use, impatience, loss of appetite, and high-effort coping (Smith et al., 2011). For us Black, Brown, Indigenous, and other organizers of color, the fight for racial justice has been both continuous and damaging to our bodies.

Impact on Personal and Professional Lives

The shared trauma experience shifts the way organizers show up as their full and professional selves. As Boulanger observes:

> In the case of shared trauma, when clinicians are struggling with these same grim realities, with memories that will not stay in the past, with ongoing disbelief about their own experiences, psychic equivalence is doubly powerful. It's like working in an echo-chamber.
>
> (2013, p. 37)

This is a multilayer experience. Boulanger later discusses how shared trauma shifts the patient-client relationship from asymmetrical—with the clinician being the one to seemingly have it together—to being more symmetrical. Clinicians also mentioned post-shared trauma that there had been an increase in self-disclosure and difficulty in maintaining boundaries during shared trauma events (Boulanger, 2013; Tosone et al., 2012).

Experiencing shared trauma can also result in the emergence or re-emergence of maladaptive mechanisms for coping. Crisis can cause people to relapse or self-indulge. Indeed, when thinking of our own experience navigating shared trauma and discussing it with colleagues and fellow organizers alike, many of us expressed similar sentiments and found ourselves reverting to negative coping mechanisms and vices we had been previously avoiding.

Trauma and Black Female Community Organizers

Trauma, of all kinds, produces the necessary conditions that make the premature death of Black women possible as well as the erasure and silencing that occurs in the hereafter. We are focusing on Black women specifically in this chapter because of our positionality. Our intention is to make visible the experiences of Black women, as shaped and perpetuated by shared and historical trauma.

As previously mentioned, long-term exposure to stress from racism and discrimination can lead to the decay of the cardiovascular, metabolic, and immune systems which can make an individual more susceptible to illness or early death. For Black women, this means a predisposition or vulnerability to "weathering," a term coined by Geronimus et al. (2006) to describe the long-term physical, emotional, mental, and psychological effects of racism and white supremacy. Demonstrating this, Black women have the highest allostatic load scores—a measurement of stress-associated body chemicals and their cumulative effects on the body's systems (Villarosa, 2018). Societal and systemic racism create toxic physiological stress in Black women, resulting in other stress-related conditions like hypertension and pre-eclampsia that directly lead to higher rates of infant and maternal death. This is further exacerbated by racial bias in health care (Villarosa, 2018).

Trauma responses are not necessarily negative. Beautiful things have been birthed from trauma, including: new cultural practices, the creation of art and music, deeper community connection and solidarity, as well as enhanced cultural pride. The difference between post-traumatic stress and post-traumatic growth—a theory that explains the positive kind of transformation that happens following a traumatic event (Tedeschi & Calhoun, 2004)—is often due to how the community responds and the resources it has access to.

Tending to Trauma in our Communities and Ourselves

Tending to Community Trauma

Many of those utilizing health supports and services have experienced trauma, as have many of the individuals organizing for justice. Ongoing trauma can have lasting adverse effects that compromise an individual's mental health and overall well-being. When social workers / community organizers avoid, overlook, or misunderstand trauma, we can be retraumatizing and interfere with the healing process. On the community level, trauma can reduce our capacity to collectively identify and address problems and plan for the future. Trauma can also undermine "readiness" for individual and community change—the extent to which the community is prepared and inclined to take collective action on an issue. Consequently, the experience of prolonged trauma—at the individual, family, and community levels—can pose a variety of challenges to community-building work.

Research suggests that the causes of community trauma lie in the historic and ongoing root causes of social inequities, including poverty, racism, sexism, oppression and power dynamics, and erasure of culture and communities (Falkenburger et al., 2018). This means that the trauma we are collectively experiencing as a result of the two aforementioned pandemics is exacerbated by these social inequities—all the more reason to be talking about this. Community building and development work must include practices that acknowledge and address the trauma of residents and their collective communities, including within health care services.

Post-Traumatic Growth

Post-traumatic growth (PTG) is when an individual finds the positives from a life altering experience and makes large shifts. "PTG reconceptualized trauma recovery by focusing on the beneficial cognitive and personality shifts resulting from grappling with traumatic events" (Ortega-Williams et al., 2021, p. 224; Tedeschi & Calhoun, 1996). In other words, when someone who has PTSD symptoms finds ways to make meaning out of the trauma. Post-traumatic growth exists within five domains of individual level functioning: 1) relating to others, 2) new possibilities, 3) personal strength, 4) spiritual change, and 5) appreciation for life (Tedeschi & Calhoun, 1996). The responses vary between individuals but examples would be finding God, starting charities, challenging oneself in new ways, and discovering a new talent (Tedeschi & Calhoun, 1996; Wu et al., 2019; Ortega-Williams et al., 2021). Post-traumatic growth has been distinguished as differing from resiliency. Resiliency is the positive manner in which someone rebounds from an adverse situation. PTG "defines a leap forward in functioning beyond the capabilities or inclinations observed in a person's personality prior to the traumatic event" (Tedeschi & Calhoun, 2004; Ortega-Williams et al., 2021). There also have to be symptoms of PTSD in order to have PTG.

When working on trauma recovery it can help social workers to know that "PTG focuses on the beneficial cognitive and personality shifts from grappling with traumatic events" (Tedeschi & Calhoun, 1996; Bloom, 1998; Ortega-Williams et al., 2021). One way to encourage this could be to work with survivors on creating new positive narratives for traumatic events. Since studies show that survivors need openness and extraversion among their characteristics in order to experience PTG, this is another area where work could be done—encouraging openness to new possibilities and desire for social connection (Tedeschi & Calhoun, 1996). These characteristics will help them transmute the trauma.

Historical Trauma Post-Traumatic Growth Framework

Bryant-Davis and Ocampo (2005) discovered that "racially targeted assaults on one's ethnic group have emotional and cognitive impacts that are salient at the individual and racial group level" (Ortega-Williams et al., 2021, p. 226). Inherent racism in a society, for example, can generate pervasive hyperarousal which impacts wellness. Therefore, interacting with a community that has experienced historical/systemic violence and discrimination based on racial and ethnic identity requires a framework that simultaneously addresses individual and mass group-level growth and healing (Oretga-Williams et al., 2021).

When focusing on community organizing and shared trauma, a framework is necessary that integrates 1) the reality of historical trauma for communities of color, and 2) the ability to grow from the harm, while also addressing mass group growth. Dr. Ortega-Williams and colleagues recognized there was alignment with historical trauma research and post-traumatic growth research. The Historical Trauma Post-Traumatic Growth (HT-PTG) framework combines HT's focus on historical collective trauma with PTG's mechanisms of growth to include group-level (collective) domains of growth and healing (Ortega-Williams et al., 2021). The five domains are inspired by Indigenous epistemologies that appreciate the interconnectedness of all aspects of creation to maintain balance. The domains include 1) collective strength, 2) collective spiritual change, 3) relating to ancestors and culture, 4) new possibilities for collective destiny, and 5) appreciation for our lives (Ortega-Williams et al., 2021). It follows that individual healing is dependent on group healing and vice versa. Growth, healing, transformation, and creativity are centered in this framework with "the multiple domains relating, imagining possibilities, and change processes interacting toward developing PTG" (Oretega-Williams et al., 2021, p. 228). The HT-PTG framework is a radical way to heal shared trauma in a community setting by centering healing and focusing on not just the individual but also on the mass group and its transformation.

Trauma-Informed Community Organizing

Trauma-informed care is "an approach to engaging people with histories of trauma that recognizes the presence of trauma symptoms and acknowledges the role that trauma has played in their lives" (Agency for Healthcare Research and Quality, 2016, para. 4). This holistic approach does not define a person solely by one part, but recognizes the whole person. For example, instead of saying "a homeless person," the language shifts to "a person who is unhoused." This shift in language then enables us to better recognize and support the assets and the potential one has instead of the deficits. Trauma-informed care is a term that originated from the health care field but is now being applied to a wide range of other professions and roles. Trauma-informed care has four goals, known as the four R's. These are:

> [it] realizes the widespread impact of trauma and understands potential paths for recovery; recognizes the signs and symptoms of trauma in clients, families, staff, and others involved with the system; and responds by fully integrating knowledge about trauma into policies, procedures, and practices, and seeks to actively resist re-traumatization.
> (SAMHSA, 2014, p. 9)

Trauma-informed mental health professionals and community organizers recognize the power different helping professions (i.e. social work) have had as historical institutions as well as the ways in which these professions have used and abused that power. They recognize the necessity of sharing power with the community. Consequently, they consider how to share power equitably, effectively, and intentionally. Instead of asking "What's wrong with you?" they ask "What has happened to you and what do you need?" Individuals have different responses to trauma. Symptoms and difficult behaviors, for instance, can be strategies developed to cope with trauma. We do not need to know why someone is reacting the way they are but we do need to understand that every person deserves empathy, compassion, and healing.

A trauma-informed approach to community organizing realizes that every choice we make, every interaction we have, every action we take, every policy we create, all have the potential to be retraumatizing or healing for our communities and for each other. In order to choose healing, we must be intentional about creating cultural shifts in ourselves, our work, our organizations, and our communities.

The Case for Radical Healing: Future Directions to Support Community Organizers—the TICB model

The Trauma-Informed Community Building (TICB) model, developed by BRIDGE Housing Corporation and Health Equity Institute, is an alternative to traditional community-building models because its principles and strategies recognize the everyday stresses in residents' lives and directly respond to the needs of residents traumatized by violence, generational poverty, and racism. It was created, in 2015 in San Francisco (SF), to capture the approach BRIDGE staff were using to engage with the community—adapting and building upon the trauma-informed service approach. They identified strategies for effectively engaging public housing communities affected by trauma and developed programming based around these strategies (Falkenburger et al., 2018). Available evidence from early implementation of the Trauma-Informed Community Building model in Potrero Hill, SF suggests that these initiatives may increase physical activity, connections among individuals from different cultures and generations, and feelings of safety among participants, while also improving mental health (Pinderhughes et al., 2015).

In 2017, The Health Equity Institute, with input from HOPE SF (a cross-sector initiative that seeks to transform San Francisco's most distressed public housing sites), collaborated with the Urban Institute to develop a new version of the TICB model, emphasizing that TICB must go hand in hand with promoting community strength and healing. Further, this new version places more emphasis on the structural harms that underlie community trauma and the need for accountability and transparency around these issues (Falkenburger et al., 2018). This approach means that the impact of the absence of social support agencies that may have come and gone from a community, because of legitimate funding constraints, are acknowledged. In addition, negative experiences community members may have had with the agency are openly recognized, providing space for open discussion with the community, and offering a new path forward.

This new path includes collaborative interventions that address these losses / community trauma and offers opportunities for healing, generating viable and sustainable community change through improved policies, programs, and institutional practices. Communities that have been historically oppressed and excluded live with the daily stressors of violence and poverty, which stem from historic and structural conditions of racism, disenfranchisement, and isolation. Part of this trauma is the result of an extensive history of broken promises made by those intervening in marginalized communities. Stakeholders need to acknowledge these community-level traumas. As they confront the trauma, communities can heal. Outlets for community members to express their collective trauma, efforts to reframe community narratives, peer support networks, and investment in community health and well-being are all opportunities for healing from trauma.

The Trauma-Informed Community Building and Engagement model strives to build communities with a "strong social fabric, positive health outcomes, meaningful community leadership, and vibrant community institutions" (Falkenburger et al., 2018, p. 5). It aims to achieve this goal by "acknowledging and addressing poverty and systemic racism, including opportunities for creative expression, recognizing the history of place and residents, implementing resident-driven programs, and emphasizing the sustainability and consistency of programming" (Falkenburger et al., 2018, p. 5). TICB is an example of an emerging practice to address trauma at the community level, yet few evolving frameworks exist for addressing and preventing it, especially among community organizers. Current strategies for treating and responding to trauma are limited due to a primary focus on the individual, "without integrating political, economic, social, or historical group traumas" (Ortega-Williams et al., 2021, p. 221).

Radical Healing as a Proactive and Responsive Framework for Community Organizers: Tending to Trauma in Ourselves

As community organizers and social workers, we are not immune to experiencing trauma ourselves. When our own experiences overlap or are affected by the people we encounter, we are even more vulnerable to shared trauma. In order to sustain ourselves as we commit to this work and minimize the risk of PTSD, we must prioritize taking care of our mental health and well-being by being proactive and strategic about creating self-care plans that work for us and meet our needs.

Ginwright (2015) states, "one of the greatest challenges facing social justice work is the growing sense of spiritual emptiness and burnout" (p. 37). The writers of this chapter have suffered from racial battle fatigue and shared trauma. We are intimately familiar with "weathering." It has been incredibly taxing and we have not been offered many ways to navigate this. As Black female organizers, we have often worked ourselves to the point of severe illness in order to combat systemic injustice. Constant advocacy and organizing has led to physiological and psychological strain. As such, we are aware of the need for strategies to keep community organizers moving forward—through despair and doubt, past anger and disappointment—when challenging inequality.

Derrick Bell brings critical race theory to life in his classic novel, *Faces at the Bottom of the Well*, which was re-published in 2018 with a new forward. In it, fellow critical race scholar Michelle Alexander states:

> What if Bell was right? What if justice for the dark faces at the "bottom of the well" can't actually be won in the United States? What if all "progress" towards racial justice is illusory, temporary and inevitably unstable? What if white supremacy will always rebound, finding new ways to reconstitute itself? What if racism is permanent? What if?
>
> (Alexander, in Bell, 2018, p. v)

Radical healing counters these questions and says instead; and if? If racism is in fact permanent, is that not even more of a reason to turn to more long-term methods of survival—methods that don't deplete and demand from us but instead revive our spirits? If we are to live alongside racism every day, we need long-term methods of survival, methods that can ensure we survive while attempting to thrive. Radical healing is therefore conceptualized as a way to deconstruct systems of oppression while simultaneously reconstructing systems of support that cultivate individual and community well-being. Radical healing as both pedagogy and praxis allows social justice advocates to build our capacity for hope, critical consciousness, and social change in the midst of oppression (Peterson, 2018).

Shawn Ginwright defines radical healing as a process for restoring the health and well-being of students who have been exposed to chronic poverty, racism, and violence. He conceptualizes radical healing as a way to develop critical consciousness of social oppression in order to counter hopelessness and confront racism and oppression. He argues that this framework has resulted in profound transformation (Ginwright, 2015). This version of radical healing is profoundly powerful. Ginwright (2015) believes that both organizing and healing are required for sustainable social change. He talks about healing justice or the ways in which activism can foster healing for Black individuals experiencing violence, crime, and poverty. He believes that social institutions and policies harm more than they help and attempts instead to build community practices that promote well-being (Ginwright, 2015).

Applying Yosso's (2002) description of a Critical Race Curriculum and synthesizing existing racial justice healing models, we propose that radical healing should: 1) honor multiple epistemologies (ways of knowing) and ontologies (ways of being); 2) center stories of individual and community resiliency in the face of systemic oppression; 3) identify and interrogate the ways in which racialized oppression undermines wellness and influences both individual and community healing; 4) utilize an interdisciplinary approach to capture the complexities of healing; 5) incorporate pedagogies for transformation; and 6) promote healing as an act of resistance. Radical healing is a nurturing framework that aims to promote and sustain individual and community well-being alongside social justice activism. Community organizers can apply this framework by using an iterative model centered around teaching to transform, incorporating pedagogies of healing, encouraging radical self-care, and promoting collective healing (Aloziem, 2022).

Radical healing urges that complete change is necessary and that we do not accommodate systemic oppression, but rather resist through growth and healing. Healing is the foundation and provides insight into how women of color fit into an overall dimension. It seeks to mitigate the impacts of shared trauma when organizing in the community. In response to shared trauma, radical healing attempts to foster shared resilience by combining the trauma-informed community-building framework and HT-PTG. The radical healing required is aimed at restoring and maintaining the health and well-being of individuals who face oppression and those wanting to combat it. We believe that centering radical healing builds the capacity for individuals to fight for social change.

We believe in radical healing as a practice of social justice. We envision a world where radical healing is a necessary part of social justice work for both 1) practitioners, and 2) clients, individuals, and communities.

> I have seen that we cannot fully create effective movements for social change if individuals struggling for that change are not also self-actualized or working towards that end. When wounded individuals come together in groups to make change our collective struggle is often undermined by all that has not been dealt with emotionally.
>
> (hooks, 1993, p. 5)

Implications

Black women are always in search of healing because we need it. As Malcolm X said, "The most disrespected woman in America is the Black woman. The most unprotected person in America is the Black woman. The most neglected person in America is the Black woman" (1962, as cited in Jones, 2020). Black women are always in search of healing—we have had to be due to oppression. Healing then becomes political—an act of resistance. Black women are still able to show up in profound ways and have historically caused massive change despite the harm that is inflicted on us. Examining these models of resistance and modeling them is therefore worthwhile. Because we have historically had to do this work we are also experts on how to do it while not only surviving but thriving. Radical healing is essentially a framework built around this premise.

Living in a patriarchal, racist society also undeniably and measurably erodes our physical and mental well-being. Lab-based, literature-based, and anecdotal studies clearly reveal the link between discrimination and poor mental and physical health (Brondolo et al., 2009). While this research is ongoing, it is time to now also develop ideas for preventing the slow damage of these stressors. We must create policy solutions and interventions. A framework like radical healing can be a solution to this current crisis. As demonstrated by our own lived experience, radical healing can concurrently promote the well-being of both communities and their community organizers and social workers. This can be fulfilled by centering collective healing, promoting radical self-care, creating space for emotional processing and truth sharing, and connecting individuals to culturally relevant mental wellness services.

An Example of Radical Self-Care from Ozy

Self-care is multidimensional—it is emotional health, physical health, relational health, spiritual health, intellectual health, financial health. Several years ago, I created a self-care tracker where I tracked certain habits. Each of the different habits pertains to one of those dimensions in order for me to look at the whole self. That holistic approach is so important to and for me. It's become an amazing guide and a way for me to reflect on my mental health and well-being. I can see the days where I have every box filled out and then other days where I have only a few. I do not criticize myself for that, I just look at it and remind myself that there is room to take better care of myself, that healing is never a linear journey. I remind myself that each habit tracked is proof of my decision to nourish myself and that this is worth celebrating. I also reflect and ask myself what was going on that day or during that week that got in the way of me taking care of myself. Then I use what I learn from that reflection and create new plans and new approaches to guide my future behaviors. An important thing about this tracker is that it is not a rule book, it is a guidebook.

During the first year of this practice, I sometimes felt like I HAD to do every single thing every single day otherwise I felt super stressed and that kind of undermined the point of the practice. I had to find a way to loosen my approach. These days, instead of planning for time to complete all of these things on my self-care list, I attempt to be intentional in how I approach the day so that the items naturally flow in. This approach has shifted the power of the practice. Instead of work, it becomes both proof and reminder. I am able to know and name which parts of my psyche need maintenance because of what it means to exist in this Black body, and am then able to create a way to nurture these parts—not individually piece by piece but all at once and all the time. And is that not radical self-care?

I have shared this practice with individuals organizing for justice in organizational spaces and on picket lines. Each person I have shared it with has followed up to let me know how helpful and necessary this tool is. They share how it helps them be proactive about prioritizing their well-being, that it makes them better leaders and shifts their relationship to their work. Each time I receive that feedback I feel so filled. In some ways, supporting others in taking care supports my well-being as well.

How JaLisa Creates Space for Collective Healing

We tend to focus on individual healing but collective healing is imperative for collective liberation. Healing circles are an excellent example of this. These are spaces for people to share their experiences, to build community, feel supported around struggles or issues (without being dismissed or negated or shut down), and get support for emotions and identities while establishing common ground with one another. Healing circles are facilitated group experiences where participants are guided through answering a series of questions that progressively go deeper and get more personal. They allow for participants to engage in deep listening, hearing the stories of people they might not otherwise connect with and have a heartfelt conversation. Healing circles offer ways for us to heal from the traumatic wounds of the past, to build mutually respectful relationships across lines of difference and to transform ourselves into a more connected community.

It honestly started out as a way to get back at an ex-partner that called me "uninspiring" and it evolved so beautifully over the years. In 2018, I started a community event called "Flowetry: Poetry in Motion." At this point I was already doing small-scale community workshops on self-care, journaling, and other mindfulness practices so I just wanted to elevate some of these lessons into a space for my people to have an experience. I contacted different POC poets and yogis in the city to see if they would be interested in trying this idea out with me: having the poet perform and the yogi flow to the words behind a well-lit curtain, creating a lovely shadow effect. I made sure we had POC vendors, and fundraised for a local non-profit. I wanted this to be an experience for the community to come together and heal with words, libations, vibrations. We packed the room from wall to wall with folks of color and allies wanting healing and goodness. We laughed, cried, danced, and spoke gratitudes for connecting in such an intimate way. After that, I did a few more Flowetrys with different themes and more people and more healing. It has been such an honor to facilitate such transformational spaces.

Conclusion

In order to work towards creating social justice, we must commit to the ongoing work of liberating ourselves. We must value our well-being as much as we value social justice. Research must consider investigating the empirical dimensions of healing in social justice settings as well as the harm caused to social workers of color engaged in activist or social justice efforts. Unless we find a way to persist and center well-being as we deconstruct, we will continue to damage and destroy our bodies and spirits.

The contribution of this chapter is twofold. It provides a theoretical framework for radical healing and enriches the current research and writing about shared trauma by applying it to community organizing. The chapter also details our lived experience as social workers and community organizers and explores coping strategies for shared trauma. Although existing shared trauma and shared trauma reality research commonly describes the consequences that can arise, coping strategies for community organizers have not previously been conceptualized (Dekel et al., 2016). For this reason, we used radical healing which necessitates we focus on collective healing alongside social justice work. "Systematic subjugation of a social group based on ethnic or racial identity requires more than individual coping mechanisms to maintain wellness" (Ortega-Williams et al., 2021, p. 221). The dominant discourse in professional trauma recovery centers on treating individuals (Edström & Dolan, 2019). A trauma-informed culturally responsive approach to community building prevents traumatizing/retraumatizing communities and ourselves. Radical healing specifically supports those most marginalized by centering their approaches to healing. This will help sustain the work, heal shared trauma and lead to growth. It also ultimately contributes to creating a just and equitable society

Radical healing should be considered a legitimate goal of community organizing, not simply a way to assist with anti-oppression efforts. We must consider work that incorporates healing as not only valuable but necessary. We must all value healing as a political path to freedom. We must develop new theories and ways of being that are anchored by our attempts at naming systematic oppression and practices by which we might collectively engage in resistance that transforms the world as we currently know it. We must merge ways of knowing with ways of being. As bell hooks (1993) urges "when we choose to heal, when we choose to love, we are choosing liberation. This is where all authentic activism begins" (p. 147).

References

Agency for Healthcare Research and Quality. (2016). *Trauma-informed care.* Retrieved from: www.ahrq.gov/ncepcr/tools/healthier-pregnancy/fact-sheets/trauma.html.

Baum, N. (2010). Shared traumatic reality in communal disasters: Toward a conceptualization. *Psychotherapy: Theory, Research, Practice, Training,* 47(2), 249.

Bell, D. (2018). *Faces at the bottom of the well: The permanence of racism.* Hachette UK.

Beltrán, R., Olsen, P., Ramey, A., Klawetter, S., & Walters, K. (2014). Digital tapestry: Weaving stories of empowerment with Indigenous youth. In P. McCardle & V. Berninger (Eds.), *Narrowing the achievement gap for Native American students: Paying the educational debt* (pp. 9–22). Routledge.

Bloom, S. L. (1998). By the crowd they have been broken, by the crowd they shall be healed: The social transformation of trauma. In R. G. Tedeschi, C. L. Park, & L. G. Calhoun (Eds.), *Posttraumatic growth: Positive changes in the aftermath of crisis* (pp. 179–213). Lawrence Erlbaum Associates Publishers.

Boulanger, G. (2013). Fearful symmetry: Shared trauma in New Orleans after Hurricane Katrina. *Psychoanalytic Dialogues,* 23, 31–44.

Brave Heart, M. (1998). The return to the sacred path: Healing the historical trauma and historical unresolved grief response among the Lakota through a psychoeducational group intervention. *Smith College Studies in Social Work,* 68(3), 288–305.

Brave Heart, M., & Horse, M. Y. (2000). Wakiksuyapi: Carrying the historical trauma of the Lakota. *Tulane Studies in Social Welfare,* 21(22), 245–266.

Brondolo, E., Ver Halen, N. B., Pencille, M., Beatty, D., & Contrada, R. J. (2009). Coping with racism: A selective review of the literature and a theoretical and methodological critique. *Journal of Behavioral Medicine,* 32(1), 64–88.

Bryant-Davis, T., & Ocampo, C. (2005). Racist incident-based trauma. *The Counseling Psychologist*, 33(4), 479–500.

Dashorst, P., Mooren, T. M., Kleber, R. J., De Jong, P. J., & Huntjens, R. J. (2019, August 30). *Intergenerational consequences of the Holocaust on offspring mental health: A systematic review of associated factors and mechanisms*. Retrieved from: www.ncbi.nlm.nih.gov/pmc/articles/PMC6720013/.

Dekel, R., & Baum, N. (2010). Intervention in a shared traumatic reality: A new challenge for social workers. *British Journal of Social Work*, 40(6), 1927–1944.

Dekel, R., Lavi, T., & Nuttman-Schwartz, O. (2016). Shared traumatic reality and boundary theory: How mental health professionals cope with the home/work conflict during continuous security threats. *Journal of Couple & Relationship Therapy*, 15(2), 121–134.

Designer, N. W. (2014). *Examining the theory of historical trauma among Native Americans*. Retrieved from: https://tpcjournal.nbcc.org/examining-the-theory-of-historical-trauma-among-native-americans/.

Duran, E. (2006). *Healing the soul wound: Counseling with American Indians and other Native peoples*. Teachers College Press.

Edström, J., & Dolan, C. (2019). Breaking the spell of silence: Collective healing as activism amongst refugee male survivors of sexual violence in Uganda. *Journal of Refugee Studies*, 32(2), 175–196.

Falkenburger, E., Arena, O., & Wolin, J. (2018). *Trauma-informed community building and engagement*. The Urban Institute.

Freedman, S., & Mashiach, R. T. (2018). Shared trauma reality in war: Mental health therapists' experience. *PLoS one*, 13(2), 1–13. https://doi.org/10.1371/journal.pone.0191949.

Garcia, M. A., Homan, P. A., García, C., & Brown, T. H. (2021). The color of COVID-19: Structural racism and the disproportionate impact of the pandemic on older black and Latinx adults. *The Journals of Gerontology: Series B*, 76(3), e75–e80. https://doi.org/10.1093/geronb/gbaa114.

Geronimus, A. T., Hicken, M., Keene, D., & Bound, J. (2006). "Weathering" and age patterns of allostatic load scores among blacks and whites in the United States. *American Journal of Public Health*, 96(5), 826–833.

Ginwright, S. A. (2015). Radically healing black lives: A love note to justice. *New Directions for Student Leadership*, 148, 33–44.

Goosby, B. J., & Heidbrink, C. (2013). The transgenerational consequences of discrimination on African-American health outcomes. *Sociology Compass*, 7(8), 630–643.

Helms, J. E., Nicolas, G., & Green, C. E. (2010). Racism and ethnoviolence as trauma: Enhancing professional training. *Traumatology*, 16(4), 53–62.

Hemphill, P. (2020). *Finding our way podcast*. Retrieved from: www.stitcher.com/show/finding-our-way.

Hicks, P. T. (2017). *Student development and social justice: Critical learning, radical healing, and community engagement*. Springer International Publishing. https://doi.org/10.1007/978-3-319-57457-8.

Hirschberger, G. (2018). Collective trauma and the social construction of meaning. *Frontiers in Psychology*, 9, 1411. https://link.gale.com/apps/doc/A549659036/HRCA?u=auraria_main&sid=summon&xid=41a7d1b0.

hooks, b. (1993). *Sisters of the yam: Black women and self-recovery.* South End Press.

Isobel, S., Goodyear, M., Furness, T., & Foster, K. (2019). Preventing intergenerational trauma transmission: A critical interpretive synthesis. *Journal of Clinical Nursing*, 28(7–8), 1100–1113. doi:10.1111/jocn.14735.

Jones, F. (2020, August 7). Malcolm X stood up for black women when few others would. *Medium.* Retrieved from: https://zora.medium.com/malcolm-x-stood-up-for-black-women-when-few-others-would-68e8b2ea2747.

Khazanchi, R., Evans, C. T., & Marcelin, J. R. (2020). Racism, not race, drives inequity across the COVID-19 continuum. *JAMA Network Open*, 3(9), e2019933–e2019933.

Lavi, T., Nuttman-Schwartz, O., & Dekel, R. (2015). Therapeutic intervention in a continuous shared traumatic reality: An example from the Israeli-Palestinian conflict. *British Journal of Social Work*, 1–17. doi:10.1093/bjsw/bev127.

Leavitt, R. A., Ertl, A., Sheats, K., Petrosky, E., Ivey-Stephenson, A., & Fowler, K. A. (2018). Suicides among American Indian/Alaska Natives: National violent death reporting system, 18 states, 2003–2014. *Morbidity and Mortality Weekly Report*, 67(8), 237.

Martinez, M., & Kawam, E. (2016). Historical trauma and social work: What you need to know. *The New Social Worker.* www.socialworker.com/feature-articles/practice/historical-trauma-and-social-work-what-you-need-to-know/.

Mohatt, N. V., Thompson, A. B., Thai, N. D., & Tebes, J. K. (2014). Historical trauma as public narrative: A conceptual review of how history impacts present day health. *Social Science Medicine*, 106, 128–136.

Office of the Surgeon General (US). (n.d.). *Mental health care for African Americans.* Retrieved from: www.ncbi.nlm.nih.gov/books/NBK44251/.

Ortega-Williams, A., Beltran, R., Schultz, K., Henderson, Z. R.-G., Colon, L., & Teyra, C. (2021). An integrated historical trauma and post-traumatic growth framework: A cross-cultural exploration. *Journal of Trauma & Dissociation*, 22(2), 220–240.

Parker, G. (2020). *Restorative yoga for ethnic and race based stress and trauma.* Jessica Kingsley Publisher.

Pennebaker, J. W. (2004). *Writing to heal: A guided journal for recovering from trauma and emotional upheaval.* New Harbinger Publications.

Pinderhughes, H., Davis, R., & Williams, M. (2015). *Adverse community experiences and resilience: A framework for addressing and preventing community trauma.* The Prevention Institute.

Rowlands, A. (2013). Disaster recovery management in Australia and the contribution of social work. *Journal of Social Work in Disability & Rehabilitation*, 12(1), 1–20.

Sánchez, R. (2006). On a critical realist theory of identity. In L. M. Alcoff, M. Hames-García, S. P. Mohanty, & P. M. L. Moya (Eds.), *Identity Politics Reconsidered* (pp. 31–52). Palgrave Macmillan US. https://doi.org/10.1057/9781403983398_3.

Saul, J. (2013). *Collective trauma, collective healing: Promoting community resilience in the aftermath of disaster.* ProQuest Ebook Central.

Siddiqui, H. Y. (1997). *Working with communities.* Hira Publications.

Simon, R. D. (1982). *Community organization for urban social change: A historical perspective* [Review of *Community organization for urban social change: A historical perspective*]. *The Journal of American History*, 69(3), 734–735. https://doi.org/10.2307/1903208.

Smith, W. A., Yosso, T. J., & Solórzano, D. G. (2011). Challenging racial battle fatigue on historically white campuses: A critical race examination of race-related stress. In R. D. Coates (Ed.), *Covert Racism*. Brill. https://doi.org/10.1163/ej.9789004203655.i-461.82.

Substance Abuse and Mental Health Services Administration. (2014). *SAMHSA's concept of trauma and guidance for a trauma-informed approach*. HHS Publication No. (SMA) 14–4884. SAMHSA.

Tedeschi, R. G., & Calhoun, L. G. (1996). The posttraumatic growth inventory: Measuring the positive legacy of trauma. *Journal of Traumatic Stress*, 9(3), 455–471.

Tedeschi, R. G., & Calhoun, L. G. (2004). Posttraumatic growth: Conceptual foundations and empirical evidence. *Psychological Inquiry*, 15(1), 1–18.

Tosone, C. (2012). Shared trauma. In C. Figley (Ed.), *Encyclopedia of Trauma*. Sage Publishers.

Tosone, C. (2021). *Shared trauma, shared resilience during a pandemic*. Springer. doi:10.1007/978-3-030-61442-3.

Tosone, C., Nuttman-Shwartz, O., & Stephens, T. (2012). Shared trauma: When the professional is personal. *Clinical Social Work Journal*, 40(2), 231–239.

Tosone, C., McTighe, J. P., & Bauwens, J. (2015). Shared traumatic stress among social workers in the aftermath of Hurricane Katrina. *British Journal of Social Work*, 45(4), 1313–1329.

Villarosa, L. (2018, April 11). Why America's black mothers and babies are in a life-or-death crisis. *The New York Times Magazine*, 11.

Watson, M. F., Bacigalupe, G., Daneshpour, M., Han, W. J., & Parra-Cardona, R. (2020). COVID-19 interconnectedness: Health inequity, the climate crisis, and collective trauma. *Family Process*, 59(3), 832–846.

Weinstein, E., Wolin, J., & Rose, S. (2014). *Trauma informed community building: A model for strengthening community in trauma affected neighborhoods*. BRIDGE Housing Corporation.

Wilson, S. (2008). *Research is ceremony: Indigenous research methods*. Fernwood Pub.

Wu, X., Kaminga, A. C., Dai, W., Deng, J., Wang, Z., Pan, X., & Liu, A. (2019). The prevalence of moderate-to-high posttraumatic growth: A systematic review and meta-analysis. *Journal of Affective Disorders*, 243, 408–415. https://doi.org/10.1016/j.jad.2018.09.023.

Yosso, T. J. (2002). Toward a critical race curriculum. *Equity & Excellence in Education*, 35(2), 93–107.

Chapter 10

In Conclusion
Lessons Learned Going Forward

Ann Goelitz

I stated in the introduction that there was a message of hope that entwined *Shared Mass Trauma in Social Work*, and this too is the thrust of this final chapter. I will not pretend it was always easy to read, but am glad to have read it and to have been a part of its making. It made me a better person—more aware of the world and its adversities and foibles. That was accomplished, at least in part, by the sincere, honest, and genuine approaches to a complex issue and also by the credibility of the messages of hope shared in each chapter. Rather than being standoffish, this book creeps into your being as you read, changing how you look at things. That to me is the mark of a good read and, more importantly, of a useful resource for those working in the midst of mass trauma.

Lessons Learned

There were many lessons learned throughout the book. To highlight a few: 1) mass trauma is not equally shared by all, 2) the impact of shared trauma is compounded by numerous factors such as the chronicity of mass trauma, 3) shared trauma exists not only with mental health practitioners, but also with a) other healthcare workers, b) domestic partners of healthcare workers, and c) in other social work modalities such as group work and community organizing.

For those familiar with trauma, the **second lesson learned**—that shared trauma's impact is compounded by other factors—is probably the easiest to discern. We know that when an individual is a trauma survivor and has other significant issues to deal with as well, they are more likely to be triggered by the trauma. Even having a broken bone increases vulnerability and vulnerability is a hallmark of trauma. The broken bone opens the door to that trauma vulnerability and there is the possibility we will be pulled in again to the feelings of being bullied growing up or sexually molested as an adult (Goelitz, 2021).

Compounding factors reported by the authors included changes to how we work with clients as a result of shared trauma. In Chapter 5, for

DOI: 10.4324/9781003176947-13

example, Knight and Gitterman pointed out that with the onset of the COVID-19 pandemic, working online rather than in person became the new reality for many social workers and necessitated unforeseen adjustments. As was true for many psychotherapists specializing in trauma, I did EMDR and hypnosis in person and wondered how these modalities would work online, if at all. In the beginning, just being able to connect and focus while online was difficult as I got used to reading cues I would normally get through body language or the feel of the client as they walked in and their energy permeated my office. Technical problems were another distraction that interrupted sessions and caused them to start late or end early. Adding to that, I have always been easily distracted when online, and found this to be a common experience for both patients and professionals.

Now, over a year and a half later, I have grown to love working online and have no problems doing either hypnosis or EMDR, even with those I have never met in person. I have found a laser focus online that I never had in person. All there is to focus on is each other and focus we do. I get to see the inside of their homes, meet their pets and domestic partners, see their prized possessions and mementos—things I was rarely able to share while working in person. It has been a gift. Of course all the changes to the way we work due to mass trauma may not feel like gifts and could be physical/emotional and personal/professional risk factors. Some may even be potentially life threatening to ourselves or others—such as entering a war zone in Israel to see clients, going home fearful of spreading the virus to family after treating COVID-19 patients without proper protection from contagion, entering the scene of a natural disaster that continues to unfold, and the list goes on.

Other professional risk factors that can compound the impact of shared trauma include inexperience—either due to being new to the field or to trauma—and lack of adequate assistance by way of training, supervision, or peer support (Nuttman-Shwartz, 2015). Personal matters, such as having young children, can also get in the way (Pagorek-Eshel & Finklestein, 2019). We might worry about our children related to the mass trauma we are experiencing or they may be distracting if we are trying to work online from home. There is also the problem of balancing work and family. A feat made more difficult as lines become more blurred during mass trauma and demands on time, energy, and psychic presence increase (Keinan-Kon, 1998; Kogan, 2004; Miller-Florsheim, 2002).

Chronicity plus issues related to the chronicity are also compounding factors when in the midst of mass trauma. This was illustrated by Nuttman-Shwartz in the chapter on war and terrorism, which centered on the ongoing Israeli/Palestinian conflict, and in the chapters on police brutality—by Jette and Sacks—and community organizing—by Aloziem and Williams—which addressed the chronic nature of racism and violence against Black people in the US. Repeated exposure to shared trauma over time increases its impact, as do other issues related to chronicity, such as relating deeply to aspects of the trauma, e.g. a Black widow's experience of a lifetime of racism and fear is compounded by the murder of her husband at the hands of the police; a mother's experience of war and terrorism is made worse because she fears for the life of her son, who is an Israeli soldier; and the experiences of COVID-19 for natives of the areas of the Palestinian, Black Lives Matter, or Ukraine conflicts are magnified by the two mass traumas they are living (Campbell et al., 2021; Freedman & Tuval-Mashiach, 2018).

Other trauma shared between practitioner and client—be it individual or mass trauma—is also a compounding factor, complicating the effects of shared trauma even more. If a practitioner, for instance, is Black, has lost a loved one to police violence and is working with a client with a similar trauma history, shared trauma intensifies and the work is impacted. This was illustrated in Chapter 1 with the example of a therapist and client both having a connection to the holocaust. Collective generational trauma like the Holocaust and slavery have particularly disturbing and confusing effects because of their egregiousness and historical longevity.

In the chapter on community organizing, Aloziem and Williams discuss another example of simultaneous mass traumas—the dual traumas of racism and COVID-19. This idea leads to the **first lesson learned**—that mass trauma is not equally shared by all (Tosone, 2012). Obvious differences are that 1) New Yorkers' experience of 9/11 was different than that of Americans not affected as directly or of those in other countries who may not have ever experienced terrorism, and 2) the Israeli/Palestine conflict affects those in the midst of the conflict in different ways than those on its outskirts. A perhaps less obvious example is that mass trauma is experienced very differently by those with social inequities so that individuals or groups of individuals without those inequities are not experiencing the same mass trauma as are those who are disadvantaged.

It follows that the inequity of racism and racial violence may be upsetting, especially since we have been trained to be sensitive and compassionate, but it is not a mass trauma for **us** unless **our** ancestors have been oppressed for years, dating back to the horrors of slavery. Similarly, we may not like the fact that many lack adequate resources, a situation which has worsened with each mass trauma and which is a mass trauma in and of itself, but we cannot experience this as a mass trauma either unless we have been deprived in the same way. Both racism and other inequities have been shown to increase with mass trauma, e.g. natural disaster (Zwi et al., 2018) and COVID-19 (Ramsari, 2020; WEF, 2021). Blacks have even been disproportionately affected by COVID-19 (Khazanchi et al., 2020), contributing to the dual pandemic/racism trauma concept purported by Aloziem and Williams.

This is an important concept since just as I cannot understand what it is like to have gone through the Holocaust and ensuing discrimination, I also cannot understand what it means to have gone through slavery and years of oppression since that time. If I assume I understand as I work with clients who have had these experiences, it will not be possible for me to be effective and authentically connected. This is true because our and our clients' positionality, which includes all of what makes us who we are—our view of the world, our economic/societal/cultural position, plus what we believe in—determines how we experience mass trauma. Therefore, in order to connect with who our clients are during mass trauma and allow them to intersect with who we are, we must follow the tenets of social work and trauma informed care (TIC)—both of which instruct us to go where the client is—as we also stay aware and connected to who and where we are from moment to moment (Goelitz, 2021).

The **third lesson learned** relates to the scope of shared trauma. The bulk of the research and publications on shared trauma focus on mental health and psychotherapy. This book addresses other areas, widening the scope and opening the way for more in-depth looks at the areas introduced and for learning even more about how shared trauma manifests and ways to work with it effectively. The pandemic chapter focuses on doctors and nurses treating COVID-19 patients. Siegel and Dekel found the existence of shared trauma between these healthcare workers and their domestic partners. The chapters on group work and community organizing also reported shared trauma in these modalities. In all three new areas of investigation, ways of working with the shared trauma were also discussed. It will be exciting to see how our knowledge base increases as the scope of shared trauma studies widens even more.

Opportunities for Growth

There are other reasons for excitement related to shared trauma, and among these are its inherent possibilities for growth, as illuminated by this book. It turns out that shared trauma is a double-edged sword of resilience versus vulnerability. The vulnerability is a mix of things that include 1) feeling off kilter because of the shared trauma, 2) unsure of how to work with clients from that off kilter place, and 3) other negative feelings/experiences the shared trauma invokes. The resilience is imbued with a hope for the future that lies beyond that off kilter place.

The off kilter feeling includes social workers being so aware of their own reactions to the shared trauma that they had difficulty focusing on client issues (Tosone et al., 2003) as they experienced things like: blurred boundaries between their personal and professional lives (Tosone et al., 2012), changes to their routines and roles (Shamai & Ron, 2009), and doubts about the appropriateness of their current work roles (Tosone et al., 2003). Aloziem and Williams, in the community organizing chapter, and Siegel and Dekel, in the pandemic chapter, also reported increased maladaptive responses to stress among those affected by shared trauma. As we know, these misguided attempts to cope tend to worsen the feeling of being off balance, further exacerbating the impact of collective trauma.

Many of the negative effects reported by practitioners were more professional than personal. These included blurred boundaries with clients (Cohen-Serrins, 2021) or rigid boundaries which increased distance between them and their clients (Baum, 2010), exacerbated countertransference (Tosone, 2019), organizational turnover (Willard-Grace et al., 2019), and organizational insecurity due to shared trauma dangers and concerns their organizations would not protect them or provide them with adequate support (Vallas & Christin, 2018; Fraizer et al., 2017), among others.

These reactions may sound intense and they certainly can be, but the positive effects reported in this book shine, in many cases dimming the negative effects. Even when negative effects were reported, positive ones were as well. Demonstrating this, in her 2008 shared trauma study, Seeley found that anxiety could be projected back and forth between therapists and clients but that, perhaps counteracting this, shared trauma also increased empathy in therapeutic relationships. Other authors found an increased tendency to disclose that could be mistakenly misused to clients' detriment but that could also increase intimacy when solidly focused on the clients' needs rather than the therapists' (Bauwens & Tosone, 2010; Tosone et al., 2012). Similarly, in Chapter 1, Tosone and Bloomberg noted that although shared trauma shook up the way social workers and clients worked together, it also allowed them to bond as they experienced that together.

These positive effects may be byproducts of the vulnerable and off kilter aspect of shared trauma noted at the beginning of this section. Brene Brown's (2013) research showed the importance of vulnerability and its role in increasing connection among individuals. It follows that we can have more intimacy with our clients if we are willing to be with the vulnerability and not run away in fear, because vulnerability can bring up fear. There is that double-edged shared trauma sword again. The sword that has negative aspects but enough positivity to hopefully balance and even transcend the negativity.

On another note, in the chapter on community organizing, Aloziem and Williams described being exhausted by the fight for justice in their chapter on community organizing but that this was what inspired them to promote attention to shared trauma effects and subsequent self-care. Others found that shared trauma encouraged other important activities: self-care, gratitude for their work as clinicians, learning new clinical skills, and building closer relationships with clients (Tosone et al., 2011; Bauwens & Tosone, 2010; Nuttman-Shwartz, 2014; Day et al., 2017).

All this positivity points toward the development of resilience as a result of experiencing shared trauma. This was shown by Knight and Gitterman in the group work chapter. They noted that symptoms, such as isolation, that developed as a result of COVID-19, lessoned as group members shared about them and learned that others experienced them as well (Baird & Alaggia, 2021; Huang & Wong, 2013). In the chapter on natural disaster, Tan similarly found that support groups helped with the recovery processes of communities (Huang et al., 2016) and thus their resilience. Others have observed that when both practitioners and clients experience these positive effects, it can increase practitioners' feelings of aplomb and their abilities to work with clients (Clemans, 2005), another plus for our profession.

Tips and Tricks—Self-care, Self-care, Self-care

Many tips were shared in each chapter of the book. What stood out and was at the basis of most of the tips was self-care, and lots of it. My own experience with COVID-19 taught me this as well. My partner and I both got COVID early on in the pandemic. I was sick and felt exhausted and hopeless as I tried to care for my much sicker partner and my clients, once I was well enough to work with them. I could not sleep because his symptoms increased at night. His temperature soared and he became delirious and had convulsions. His doctor was aware of this but warned us not to go to the hospital unless it was dire because at that time they were not equipped to handle the cases coming in. My niece's mother encouraged me to keep up my yoga even though I was sick because it would help my lymphatic system, so I did. As I got more hopeless and scared, I increased my exercise and meditation to an hour each a day. And I contacted a friend or got on a virtual conference call at least once a day. All that self-care saved me and my partner, because I was then able to be a better caregiver. It also improved my relationships with clients, allowing them to express their gratitude, for example. While I was out sick, one sent me a touching video, singing a song of appreciation for me. Another told the therapist who filled in for me how important I was to her. We discussed these gifts in therapy, magnifying them even more. I absolutely feel closer to my clients now than before COVID even though I haven't seen any of them in person for over a year and a half.

Another important component of the tips shared was following the principles of social work and of TIC. In the chapter on psychotherapy, Barry and Singer talk about one in particular, the "importance of human relationships." One of the six core values of social work (NASW, 2021), this principle emphasizes the importance of really being with and connected to clients, an area where we have seen some negative but what appear to be more positive effects from shared trauma. Shared trauma seems to have the potential to increase connection between social workers and their clients, potentially increasing our abilities to adhere to this principle and be with our clients where they are, another social work tenet.

In the chapter on community organizing, Aloziem and Williams discuss the importance of following the TIC principles. They remind us that all we do as social workers has the potential to inadvertently retraumitize clients or help them heal and that choosing the direction of healing requires close attention to culture—our personal culture, our work culture, and the cultures of communities we interact with. This is true because it is through culture that we learn about who we and others are. Making it our intention for culture to be a priority—one of the tenets of TIC—entails heightening our awareness and learning as much as we can about culture. In the group work chapter, Knight and Gitterman also discuss the importance of attention to culture, in this case the culture of the group. They point out that awareness in this area can assist social workers as they lead groups and as evidence of shared trauma surfaces, providing pointers on how you can then work with it.

Further reinforcing what we are learning about shared trauma during collective disasters, NASW's most recent revisions to the social work principles/code of ethics (at the time of writing this book) include the importance of cultural competence and self-care (2021). Self-care is key, but as much as we talk to our clients about it, we do not always do it ourselves. Here are some ways to incorporate it into your social work practice and your daily life. In the chapter on psychotherapy, Barry and Singer encourage the use of the accompaniment model when working with clients. It consists of working as partners, rather than hierarchically, and being a witness, as we stay focused on our positionality and hence on our culture (Whitmore & Warren, 1997). This requires awareness and knowledge of who we are, and not just who we are on the surface, but in all parts of ourselves. Tosone et al. suggest these ways of getting more in touch with our humanness: writing a trauma narrative, and radical self-care (2014). Aloziem and Williams, in Chapter 9, recommend yoga and the use of a self-care tracker to help awareness and motivation related to self-care.

Radical self-care includes having a network of support, as was found after Hurricane Katrina in the US (Tosone et al., 2014). Of course it is not enough to have a network of support, we also need to make good use of it. An example of how this kind of support can help is that Siegel and Dekel, as reported in the pandemic chapter, found that the partners of healthcare workers acted as containers, helping the healthcare workers cope as they cared for COVID-19 patients. Besides having a network of support, Dekel & Baum also recommend finding ways to express and release feelings (2010), another one of those things we tell our clients to do but do not always do ourselves.

In the chapter on community organizing, Aloziem and Williams get even more serious about self-care, suggesting we make self-care a priority, taking care of our mental health and our well-being and developing self-care plans that work for us. This is important because self-care is personal and can change over time. What works for you may not work for me and what works for me now may not work for me two years from now. Meditation, for example, means different things to different individuals. For you it may mean being in nature. Others may go to church and pray or sit and quietly sip a cup of tea and of course for some it is practicing traditional meditation models such as Buddhist and Transcendental Meditation. Part of self-care is discovering who we are and what we need. A recommendation that I find works well for me and my clients is 30 minutes a day of physical activity and 30 minutes of meditative activity—leaving the form of each activity up to the individual.

Self-care is also needed in organizations. This includes teamwork, multidisciplinary teams in particular, as Siegel and Dekel found during the pandemic; supervision; flexibility with scheduling and personal time; training, especially in the arena of trauma; and ample supplies of implements needed for work (Tosone & Cohen-Serrins, 2021). Since Siegel and Dekel found that those partners who had training in self-care techniques fared better during the pandemic, self-care training is also important and a means for finding what works for us in terms of self-care. Peer support, another means of self-care, is recommended as well (Duffy et al., 2019).

Perhaps most importantly, there is the need for self-care at the level of community. This is clear in the chapter on police brutality where Jette and Sacks describe the trauma experienced by Black Americans. These communities need healing as do many others. In the chapter on natural disasters, Tan describes some of the ways communities heal after traumas such as earthquakes, emphasizing the importance of having a strong sense of community and how this aids healing as community members convene and commiserate; holding each other up and building resilience as they do. Aloziem and Williams state the case for community healing in their chapter on community organizing. Their message is an urgent one that sees the creation of a culture that promotes the healing of communities as the antidote to what ails us when it comes to racism—and nothing could be more relevant today.

Future Directions

As shown throughout this book, understanding shared trauma is key to recovery from mass calamity. It is not always easy to clearly understand, as illustrated with the unequal effects of police brutality, and is therefore a concept that evolves as we learn more about it. What we do know is that it is prevalent. Since the COVID-19 outbreak began, populations around the world have been hit by new and ongoing terrorism, racism, hurricanes, wild fires, other natural disasters compounded by climate change, mass shootings, police brutality, mass poverty and starvation, and we have witnessed the unequal effects of these events on community members. There is evidence of prevalence throughout history as well, as Tosone and Cohen-Serrins reported in their chapter.

So where do we go from here? The book has taught us about shared trauma, how it is evolving, and ways to work with it, for both ourselves and our clients, but what else do we need to learn in order to help protect the world from the effects of shared trauma, so that we can become proactive where possible?

The recommendations from this book include those for additional research in a number of areas. Research has been done, for instance, on shared trauma experienced during catastrophes that include war and terrorism, religious/political strife, hurricane, and pandemic. We have the opportunity to learn more by studying other types of mass trauma and ascertaining the differential impacts of each. Racism and other types of marginalization play a role in all mass traumas since, as Tosone and Bloomberg pointed out, there is generally less access to resources for these individuals. This is an arena that deserves attention as do other traumas such as mass starvation and poverty. Tosone and Cohen-Serrins noted that disasters in parts of the world where shared trauma has not yet been studied bear consideration as well. These include wars in the Congo, the Middle East, and East Asia.

Research on shared trauma has also been primarily focused on the mental health field. There are other areas that could and should be studied, in particular the medical field. Siegel and Dekel's findings indicate more work should be done with doctors and nurses, for example, and there are other healthcare providers that could be studied as well. There are probably not many who are exempt from the impact from shared mass trauma, which underlines the importance of continued study.

In addition to looking at fields outside of mental health, other work modalities would be rich areas to explore. The chapters on group work and community organizing show the importance of studying shared trauma in those modalities. There are other social work modalities such as child welfare, eldercare, and work with the disabled that need attention as well since these are vulnerable populations and as such potentially more at risk. The arena of research practice could also be of interest as Tosone and Cohen-Serrins suggested. There are other modalities outside of the field of social work that can be examined as well.

Nuttman-Shwartz recommended another area of inquiry in her chapter on war and terrorism—our clients, or as they are called in the medical field, patients. We need more of an understanding of what is happening on their side of the fence, or their side of the virtual call in COVID-19 times. We can speculate and ask our clients about this as we work with them but research in this area would glean even more information. Other lay people could be studied as well, just as Siegel and Dekel did with their work related to the partners of doctors and nurses during the pandemic.

Last but definitely not least, we need to know why shared trauma for some evokes negative responses and for others either positive responses, or a mix of both positive and negative. In other words why do some have reactions comparable to PTSD or to PTG, and what promotes resilience in those who experience shared trauma? Tosone and Bloomberg, in Chapter 1, pointed to the role spirituality plays in shared trauma responses and resilience. We would benefit from learning more about this and other dynamics such as culture— ours, our clients', and those of the organizations and communities we work with. Knowing how culture impacts shared trauma could be key to understanding more about it and how to work with it. This also leads into studying the inequality of shared trauma experiences among those affected and also the inequality of resilience. My experience of the pandemic is different from that of a Black American who is also facing police brutality and racism or an Israeli who is also experiencing war and terrorism. We need to be aware of what these differences are so that we can be effective in our work and promote awareness, understanding, healing, and resilience at the individual, group, and community level. Why else study and learn about shared trauma? This to me is the ultimate purpose—to dissect this evolving concept of shared trauma and to put it under the microscope with hope for a better society and world.

References

Baird, S. L., & Alaggia, R. (2021). Trauma-informed groups: Recommendations for group workers. *Clinical Social Work Journal*, 49, 10–19.

Baum, N. (2010). Shared traumatic reality in communal disasters: Toward a conceptualization. *Psychotherapy: Theory, Research, Practice, Training*, 47(2), 249–259. https://doi.org/10.1037/a0019784.

Bauwens, J., & Tosone, C. (2010). Professional posttraumatic growth after a shared traumatic experience: Manhattan clinicians' perspectives on post-9/11 practice. *Journal of Loss and Trauma*, 15(6), 498–517. https://doi.org/10.1080/15325024.2010.519267.

Brown, B. (2013). *Daring greatly: How the courage to be vulnerable transforms the way we live, love, parent and lead*. Gotham Books.

Campbell, J., Duffy, J., Tosone, C., & Falls, D. (2021). "Just get on with it": A qualitative study of social workers' experiences during the political conflict in Northern Ireland. *The British Journal of Social Work*, 51(4), 1314–1331.

Clemans, S. E. (2005). Recognizing vicarious traumatization: A single session group model for trauma workers. *Social Work with Groups*, 27(2–3), 55–74.

Cohen-Serrins, J. (2021). How COVID-19 exposed an inadequate approach to burnout: Moving beyond self-care. In C. Tosone (Ed.), *Shared trauma, shared resilience during a pandemic: Social work in the time of COVID-19* (pp. 259–268). Springer.

Day, K. W., Lawson, G., & Burge, P. (2017). Clinicians' experiences of shared trauma after the shootings at Virginia Tech. *Journal of Counseling & Development*, 95(3), 269–278.

Duffy, J., Campbell, J., & Tosone, C. (2019). The Northern Irish study: Voices of social work through the Troubles. In J. Duffy, J. Campbell, & C. Tosone (Eds.), *International Perspectives on Social Work and Political Conflict* (pp. 38–49). Routledge.

Frazier, M. L., Fainshmidt, S., Klinger, R. L., Pezeshkan, A., & Vracheva, V. (2017). Psychological safety: A meta-analytic review and extension. *Personnel Psychology*, 70(1), 113–165.

Freedman, S. A., & Tuval-Mashiach, R. (2018). Shared trauma reality in war: Mental health therapists' experience. *PloS one*, 13(2), e0191949. https://doi.org/10.1371/journal.pone.0191949.

Goelitz, A. (2021). *From trauma to healing: A social worker's guide to working with survivors* (2nd edn). Routledge.

Huang, Y., & Wong, H. (2013). Effects of social group work with survivors of the Wenchuan earthquake in a transitional community. *Health and Social Care in the Community*, 21, 327–337.

Huang, Y. N., Tan, N. T., & Liu, J. Q. (2016). Support, sense of community, and psychological status in the survivors of the Yaan earthquake. *Journal of Community Psychology*, 44(7), 919–936. doi:10.1002/JCOP.21818.

Keinan-Kon, N. (1998). Internal reality, external reality, and denial in the Gulf War. *Journal of the American Academy of Psychoanalysis*, 26(3), 417–442.

Khazanchi, R., Evans, C. T., & Marcelin, J. R. (2020). Racism, not race, drives inequity across the COVID-19 continuum. *JAMA Network Open*, 3(9), e2019933–e2019933.

Kogan, I. (2004). The role of the analyst in the analytic cure during times of chronic crises. *Journal of the American Psychoanalytic Association*, 52(3), 735–757. https://doi.org/10.1177/00030651040520031201.

Miller-Florsheim, D. (2002). From containment to leakage, from the collective to the unique: Therapist and patient in shared national trauma. In C. Covington, P. Williams, J. Arundale, J. Knox, & J. Alderdice (Eds.), *Terrorism and war: Unconscious dynamics of political violence* (pp. 71–86). Routledge.

National Association of Social Workers. (2021). *NASW code of ethics*. Retrieved from: www.socialworkers.org/About/Ethics/Code-of-Ethics/Code-of-Ethics-English.

Nuttman-Shwartz, O. (2014). Shared resilience in a traumatic reality. *Trauma, Violence, & Abuse*, 16(4), 466–475. https://doi.org/10.1177/1524838014557287.

Nuttman-Shwartz, O. (2015). Post-traumatic stress in social work. In J. Wright (Ed.), *The international encyclopedia of social & behavioural sciences* (2nd edn, Vol. 18, pp. 707–713). Elsevier.

Pagorek-Eshel, S., & Finklestein, M. (2019). Family resilience among parent–adolescent dyads exposed to ongoing rocket fire. *Psychological Trauma: Theory, Research, Practice, and Policy*, 11(3), 283–291. https://doi.org/10.1037/tra0000397.

Ramsari, A. (2020). The rise of the COVID-19 pandemic and the decline of global citizenship. In J. M. Ryan (Ed.), *COVID-19: Global pandemic, societal responses, ideological solutions* (pp. 94–106). Routledge.

Seeley, K. M. (2008). *Therapy after terror: 9/11, psychotherapists, and mental health*. Cambridge University Press.

Shamai, M., & Ron, P. (2009). Helping direct and indirect victims of national terror: Experiences of Israeli social workers. *Qualitative Health Research*, 19(1), 42–54.

Tosone, C. (2011). The legacy of September 11: Shared trauma, therapeutic intimacy, and professional post-traumatic growth. *Traumatology*, 17(3), 25–29. doi:10.1177/1534765611421963.

Tosone, C. (2012). Shared trauma. In C. Figley (Ed.), *Encyclopedia of Trauma* (pp. 626–627). Sage Publishing.

Tosone, C. (2019). Shared trauma and social work practice in communal disasters. In J. Duffy, J. Campbell, & C. Tosone (Eds.), *International perspectives on social work and political conflict* (pp. 50–64). Routledge.

Tosone, C., & Cohen-Serrins, J. (2021). *COVID-19 quality of professional practice survey.* Unpublished research findings.

Tosone, C., Bialkin, L., Lee, M., Martinez, A., Campbell, M., et al. (2003). Shared trauma: Group reflections on the September 11th disaster. *Psychoanalytical Social Work*, 10(1), 57–77.

Tosone, C., Nuttman-Shwartz, O., & Stephens, T. (2012). Shared trauma: When the professional is personal. *Clinical Social Work Journal*, 40(2), 231–239. https://doi.org/10.1007/s10615-012-0395-0.

Tosone, C., McTighe, J. P., & Bauwens, J. (2014). Shared traumatic stress among social workers in the aftermath of Hurricane Katrina. *British Journal of Social Work*, 45(4), 1313–1329. https://doi.org/10.1093/bjsw/bct194.

Vallas, S. P., & Christin, A. (2018). Work and identity in an era of precarious employment: How workers respond to "personal branding" discourse. *Work and Occupations*, 45(1), 3–37.

WEF. (2021). *The global risks report 2021* (16th edn). Retrieved from: www3.weforum.org/docs/WEF_The_Global_Risks_Report_2021.pdf.

Whitmore, E., & Wilson, M. (1997). Accompanying the process: Social work and international development practice. *International Social Work*, 40(1), 57–74. https://doi.org/10.1177/002087289704000105.

Willard-Grace, R., Knox, M., Huang, B., Hammer, H., Kivlahan, C., & Grumbach, K. (2019). Burnout and health care workforce turnover. *The Annals of Family Medicine*, 17(1), 36–41.

Zwi, A. B., Spurway, K., Marincowitz, R., Ranmuthugala, G., Hobday, K., & Thompson, L. (2018). *Do CBDRM initiatives impact on the social and economic costs of disasters?*EPPI-Centre. Retrieved from: https://eppi.ioe.ac.uk/cms/Portals/0/PDF%20reviews%20and%20summaries/CBRDM%20final%20report.pdf?ver=2018-2011-22-120410-370.

Glossary

Accompaniment	therapeutic practice characterized by the process of the provider going with, supporting, and enhancing the therapeutic process for the client.
Adversarial/post-traumatic growth	ways in which individuals benefit from and grow as a result of exposure to trauma.
Allostatic load scores	measurement of stress-associated body chemicals and their cumulative effects on the body's system.
Beginning group work phase	second phase in which the worker helps members develop mutual agreement about group purpose, methods, and expectations.
Blurred boundaries	a frequent consequence of shared trauma in which workers' personal lives encroach on their professional lives and vice versa.
Capacity building	enhancing the strengths or developing the abilities of individuals, communities, or organizations in order to maximize performance.
Carceral social work	collaborating with police and other arms of the penal system while supporting coercive and damaging practices, in particular those that reinforce racist social control.
Climate change	shift in weather patterns due to global warming.
Cognitive behavior therapy (CBT)	therapeutic modality designed to target cognitive distortions, problematic behaviors that impact a client's level of functioning, and emotional regulation.
Community-based	approach in which communities actively participate in dealing with issues that concern them.
Community participation	involvement of people in a community with 1) identification and assessment of issues, 2) the process of decision making, and 3) problem solving.
Compassion fatigue	cumulative compassion stress resulting from the "cost of caring." Encompasses the concepts of burnout, emotional contagion, and secondary victimization.

DOI: 10.4324/9781003176947-14

Double exposure	workers are both directly impacted by a traumatic event and indirectly impacted through their work with clients.
Dual focus	need for group workers to attend to: interactions between members; between individual members and the worker; and between the group-as-a-whole and the worker and members' environment.
Disaster management	organization and management of resources for dealing with crises, emergencies, and disasters; including the development and implementation of preparedness, responsiveness, and recovery strategies.
Ecological system	interactive components of specific social-physical environments.
Emotional contagion	phenomenon that occurs in groups when intense affect spreads from one member to another.
Empowerment	process of becoming stronger and more resourceful in controlling one's life, making decisions, and exercising of one's rights.
Ending group work phase	final phase in which the worker helps members identify and manage feelings about ending and recognize gains achieved and future work.
Epistemology	philosophical study of our ways of knowing, including "how we know what we know," what knowledge is, and how it is produced and shared.
Frontline worker	employees within essential industries who must physically show up to their jobs.
Greenhouse effect	warming the earth's surface that occurs as the sun's energy is absorbed and re-radiated by greenhouse gases.
Group work	practice modality based in members' shared experiences that focuses on them helping one another to achieve shared agreed-upon goals.
Historical trauma	refers to the collective and cumulative emotional wounding across generations that results from cataclysmic events targeting a community.
Historical trauma post-traumatic growth (HT-PTG)	combines historical collective trauma with collective domains of growth and healing.
Indirect trauma	impact that working with trauma survivors has on those engaged in this work.
Middle/work group work phase	third phase in which the worker helps members help one another to deal with common life traumas and related stressors and improve the adaptive fit between the members and between the group as a whole and the wider environment.

Mutual aid	foundation of social work practice with groups which emphasizes the benefits of members helping one another.
Natural disasters	events resulting from processes of the earth such as floods, hurricanes, earthquakes, and tsunamis.
Neurodiverse	refers to variations in the human brain that can lead to atypical thought and learning patterns or behaviors—often applied to individuals who fall within the autism spectrum.
Obsessive compulsive disorder (OCD)	a mental health diagnosis characterized by recurring, unwanted thoughts (obsessions), eliciting the need to engage in repetitive behaviors or actions (compulsions).
Ontology	philosophical study of social reality and our ways of being that contends with what can be known and how, and one's conception of reality.
Pandemic	infectious disease that spreads globally or affects a large number of people.
Positionality	refers to how one is positioned in society and where one positions oneself based on various identities; it is where you stand in relation to your social and political contexts, and structural and relational determinants.
Preparatory group work phase	initial stage in which the worker identifies common client needs and concerns and develops a responsive group modality.
Preparedness	ability of governments, organizations, and communities to anticipate and respond effectively to impending or current hazards, calamities, or disasters.
Professional boundary	physical, psychological and mental line between social workers and their clients that protects them from inappropriate over involvement and/or loss of control such as invasion of privacy.
Radical healing	methodology for restoring the health and well-being to individuals who have been exposed to chronic poverty, racism, and violence.
Relational therapy	therapeutic modality that focuses on the power of the relationship between therapist and client to promote healing.
Resilience	ways in which individuals bounce back from adversity/trauma exposure.
Retraumatization	reminder of a traumatic event elicited by conditions, situations, or stressors similar to the environment or circumstance of the original trauma that could

	occur as a result of professional interventions that generate feelings and reactions associated with the original traumatic event.
Secondary trauma	can occur suddenly and is directly related to the client's experience of trauma, and not to occupational stress per se as with compassion fatigue. Symptoms mirror those of the client and involve anxiety, depression, avoidance, and hyperarousal.
Shared resilience	positive experiences that can be mutually derived by both practitioner and client as they work together during a shared trauma.
Shared trauma	refers to the affective, behavioral, cognitive, spiritual, and multimodal responses that mental health professionals experience as a result of primary and secondary exposure to the same collective trauma as their clients, and includes multimodal and common symptoms such as exhaustion, depletion of empathy, and identification with the client that are attributed to the dual nature of the trauma.
Shared traumatic exposure	circumstance in which social workers and clients are exposed to the same communal traumatic event(s).
Shared traumatic reality	similar to shared trauma, but encompasses the wider traumatic reality that clinicians and clients living and working in the affected community are exposed to on a daily basis, with the emphasis on the impact of chronic trauma on interpersonal, communal, and societal levels.
Social capital	network of relationships among individuals and organizations that connect them and enable them to function effectively in society.
Social cohesion	the social glue and trust that allows members of society to effectively work together toward survival and well-being.
Social resilience	ability to bounce back, cope, or adjust to adverse situations or environmental and societal threats.
Social solidarity	collaborative cohesiveness between individuals or groups, enabling them to work together and take collective action based on common values and beliefs.
Terror management theory (TMT)	theory postulating that when one is reminded of the inevitability of death, it induces death anxiety which is often managed by attempts to cling more closely to family members and other loved ones, cultural beliefs, and other belief systems that provide meaning and value.

Trauma-informed care	approach that recognizes the unique needs of trauma survivors and those who work with them by promoting safety, trust, choice, collaboration, and empowerment at all levels of an organization.
Trauma-informed practice	approach to professional intervention that recognizes that many clients have histories of trauma, and responds to their unique needs by promoting safety, trust, choice collaboration, and empowerment.
Trauma-informed supervision	approach to supervision that adopts principles of trauma-informed practice and care.
Truth sharing	act of sharing one's truth or description of one's subjective reality. There is power in telling your story and there is even more power in sharing it with the world. The stories we tell are both reflective of what occurred and of who we are now.
Vicarious post-traumatic growth	ways in which workers benefit and grow from working with trauma survivors.
Vicarious trauma	manifestation of indirect trauma that parallels the consequence of direct exposure and is reflected in changes in workers' core beliefs about self and others.
Weathering	long-term physical, emotional, mental, and psychological effects of racism and white supremacy.
Wounded-healer	a helper who is affected by trauma, crisis, or other adverse experience.

Appendix I: Sample Shared Mass Trauma Course Syllabus

Course Description

This course is designed to provide a framework for practice with individuals, families, organizations, and communities while experiencing shared mass trauma such as pandemic or war. The coursework presented will enhance the skills and knowledge base of students and will be particularly useful to students interested in working with survivors of trauma.

Shared trauma is surrounded by a complex set of issues that will be addressed, including treatment choices, multicultural perspectives on shared trauma, psychosocial challenges, and secondary stresses connected with this type of work. Social work skills vital to this work will be examined including crisis intervention, supportive care, psychoeducation, psychosocial intervention, advocacy, and community organizing. Values and ethics in practice will be discussed as they relate to the role of social workers in a rapidly changing environment in which awareness of the short- and long-term effects of shared trauma is increasing. When possible, guest speakers will present on their areas of expertise.

Course Objectives

By the end of this course, students should be able to:

- Understand concepts of shared trauma
- Understand tenets of trauma-informed care
- Comprehend how shared trauma, trauma-informed care, and social work principles interconnect and intersect
- Summarize research findings on shared trauma
- Develop effective skills for building social resilience during crisis responses
- Understand the importance of knowledge, supervision, and support for trauma workers before, during, and after they work "under fire"

- Comprehend how shared trauma operates during the mass crises discussed in the course
- Conceptualize how it would operate during other communal disasters
- Comprehend how shared trauma operates when utilizing the practice modalities discussed in the course
- Conceptualize how it would operate when utilizing other practice modalities
- Develop an understanding of the practice approaches presented in the course
- Envision how you would use them and the concepts of shared trauma in your own work

This course addresses the following Social Work Educational Policy and Accreditation Standards, outlined by the Council on Social Work Education:

- Competency 1: Demonstrate Ethical and Professional Behavior
- Competency 2: Engage Anti-Racism, Diversity, Equity, and Inclusion in Practice
- Competency 3: Advance Human Rights and Social, Economic, and Environmental Justice
- Competency 4: Engage in Practice-Informed Research and Research-Informed Practice
- Competency 6: Engage with Individuals, Families, Groups, Organizations, and Communities
- Competency 8: Intervene with Individuals, Families, Groups, and Organizations, and Communities

Student Evaluation

Since professional dialogue and reflection are important components of this course, regular and timely attendance at each class is essential. In addition to physical presence, students are expected to read assignments for each class and to be prepared to engage in thoughtful and critical discussions of these as well as related fieldwork experiences during class. An assessment of class participation will be incorporated into the student's final grade. Several written assignments are also required. These include:

- A three-page personal or professional experience with mass trauma, due week 2
- Two two-page responses to the readings in a journal format, due week 5
- An eight- to ten-page paper, due week 10
- An in-class group project presentation demonstrating a trauma intervention, due week 12

The first paper is intended to encourage students to reflect upon their own experiences with mass trauma. It also requires a brief analysis of how these experiences may impact their work with clients coping with the same traumatic event. The second and third papers offer students an opportunity to reflect on the readings in their own words with informal references included. At least eight readings should be mentioned in each. The final paper provides students with an opportunity to critically apply what they have learned from class materials (i.e., readings, presentations, discussions) to a specific "case" from their own practice. If no such case exists in a student's practice, an appropriate case will be provided. This paper should include an annotated bibliography with at least ten references. The final class group presentation provides students with an opportunity to apply what they have learned about the concepts of shared trauma to their work, presenting on an intervention of their choice.

Exemplary papers and presentations reflect not only students' abilities to utilize class materials to challenge themselves as practitioners, but also their willingness to contribute to the ongoing development of empirical knowledge and practice wisdom by sharing ideas and experiences.

Required Reading

The required readings are comprised of:
Readings from 1) a text on reserve in the library or available for purchase at Amazon.com and other mail order venues, and 2) other readings on reserve in the library or available online:

- Goelitz, A. (Ed.). (2022). *Shared mass trauma in social work: Implications and strategies for resilient practice.* Routledge
- Eleven chapters from the above text
- Other readings on reserve in the library

Session Outlines with Reading Lists

Week 1—Topic: Introduction

TOPICS TO BE COVERED

- Introductions

  - Instructor
  - Students
  - Include in introductions something about your relationship to trauma and in particular mass trauma

- Definition of shared trauma

  - Why awareness of the impact of mass trauma is crucial for social workers
  - Importance of self-care while going through course as material may be traumatizing

REQUIRED READINGS

Introduction—Goelitz, A. (Ed.). (2022). *Shared mass trauma in social work: Implications and strategies for resilient practice.* Routledge.

Nuttman-Shwartz, O., & Dekel, R. (2009). Challenges for students working in a shared traumatic reality. *British Journal of Social Work, 39,* 522–538. doi:10.1093/bjsw/bcm121.

OPTIONAL READINGS

Nuttman-Shwartz, O., & Dekel, R. (2008). Training students for a shared traumatic reality. *Social Work,* 53, 279–281. doi:10.1093/sw/53.3.279/.

Week 2—Topic: Conceptual Framework

TOPICS TO BE COVERED

- Impact on social workers of working with clients on trauma
- Shared trauma as one of the impacts of trauma
- Contextualization of shared trauma
- Understanding shared trauma
- Holding environments for social workers
- Positive outcomes as a result of shared trauma
- The importance of self-care for social workers working in shared trauma environments

REQUIRED READINGS

Chapter 1—Goelitz, A. (Ed.). (2022). *Shared mass trauma in social work: Implications and strategies for resilient practice.* Routledge.

Boulanger, G. (2013). Fearful symmetry: Shared trauma in New Orleans after Hurricane Katrina. *Psychoanalytic Dialogues,* 23(1), 31–44. https://doi.org/10.1080/10481885.2013.752700

OPTIONAL READINGS

Levenson, J. (2020). Translating trauma-informed principles into social work practice. *Social Work,* 65, 288–298.

Baum, N. (2014). Professionals' double exposure in the shared traumatic reality of wartime: Contributions to professional growth and stress. *The British Journal of Social Work*, 44(8), 2113–2134.

Week 3—Topic: Research Findings

TOPICS TO BE COVERED

- The reciprocal influence between our personal experiences with mass trauma and those of our clients
- What can occur as a result of that reciprocal influence including—

  - An increased tendency to self-disclose to clients about our experiences in general, and traumatic experiences in particular
  - An increased awareness of countertransference responses
  - An increased desire to make professional improvements that include—

    - Additional trauma training
    - Greater self-care

- Shared trauma assessment and measurement tools

REQUIRED READINGS

Chapter 2—Goelitz, A. (Ed.). (2022). *Shared mass trauma in social work: Implications and strategies for resilient practice*. Routledge.

Williams, D. S. (2021). Shared traumatic stress and the impact of COVID-19 on public child welfare workers. In C. Tosone (Ed.), *Shared trauma, shared resilience during a pandemic: Social work in the time of COVID-19*. Springer.

OPTIONAL READINGS

Tosone, C., Bauwens, J., & Glassman, M. (2016). The shared traumatic and professional posttraumatic growth inventory. *Research on Social Work Practice*, 26(3), 286–294.

Tosone, C., McTighe, J., Bauwens, J., & Naturale, A. (2011). Shared traumatic stress and the long-term impact of September 11th on Manhattan clinicians. *Journal of Traumatic Stress*, 24(5), 546–552.

Week 4—Topic: The Impact of Mass Trauma on Social Workers

TOPICS TO BE COVERED

- Mass trauma that can lead to shared trauma includes—

- Natural disasters compounded by global warming, including wild-fires, tornadoes, hurricanes, floods, tsunamis, avalanches, volcanoes, and more
- War, terrorism and religious/political strife
- Mass shootings
- Police brutality
- Pandemic
- Famine
- Mass poverty
- Racism

- Mass trauma differs from trauma that is not a result of widespread crisis
- Our reactions are different with mass trauma than with trauma that is not a result of widespread crisis
- Our clients' reactions are different with mass trauma than with trauma that is not a result of widespread crisis
- Reasons why the reactions are different

REQUIRED READINGS

Nuttman-Shwartz, O. (2015). Shared resilience in a traumatic reality: A new concept for trauma workers exposed personally and professionally to collective disaster. *Trauma, Violence and Abuse*, 16(4), 466–475. doi:10.1177/1524838014557287.

Tosone, C., Nuttman-Shwartz, O., & Stephens, T. (2012). Shared trauma: When the professional is personal. *Clinical Journal of Social Work*, 40(2), 231–239. doi:10.1007/s10615-012-0395-0.

Week 5—Topic: Pandemic

TOPICS TO BE COVERED

- Importance of screening for stress in order to provide tailored support
- Frontline workers in hospitals as an at-risk population

  - Due to stressors in general and specific pandemic-related stressors
  - Exposure to stressors at work and at home

- Shared trauma for spouses of professionals—unique aspects and challenges
- Family systems theory and its relationship to shared trauma
- Benefits of working with trauma-informed multidisciplinary teams

Related trauma-informed concepts—these apply to both us and our clients:

- Screening for trauma
- Minimizing distress and maximizing autonomy
- Increasing community, peer, and social support in times of crisis
- Renewing hope for the future and commitments towards relationships and life goals
- External vs. internal locus of control while navigating crisis
- Engaging in meaningful activities
- Treating oneself with a sense of support and compassion
- Prioritizing self-care

REQUIRED READINGS

Chapter 3—Goelitz, A. (Ed.). (2022). *Shared mass trauma in social work: Implications and strategies for resilient practice.* Routledge.

Dekel, R., Nuttman-Shwartz, O., & Lavi, T. (2016). Shared traumatic reality and boundary theory: How mental health professionals cope with the home/work conflict during continuous security threats, *Journal of Couple and Relationship Therapy*, 15(2), 121–134, doi:10.1080/15332691.2015.1068251.

OPTIONAL READINGS

Dekel, R. (2017). My personal and professional trauma resilience truisms. *Traumatology*, 23(1), 10.

Week 6—Topic: Police Brutality and Racism

TOPICS TO BE COVERED

- A historical review of discriminatory police practices in America
- Social work's relationship with discriminatory police practices in America
- Disenfranchised groups affected by discriminatory police
- Traumatic responses to discriminatory police
- Exploring the intersection of these traumatic responses and shared trauma
- Can racist police brutality be a shared trauma for social workers who are not members of disenfranchised groups and have thus not experienced this practice first hand?

REQUIRED READINGS

Chapter 4—Goelitz, A. (Ed.). (2022). *Shared mass trauma in social work: Implications and strategies for resilient practice.* Routledge.

Mesic, A., Franklin, L., Cansever, A., Potter, F., Sharma, A., Knopov, A., & Siegel, M. (2018). The relationship between structural racism and black-white disparities in fatal police shootings at the state level. *Journal of the National Medical Association*, 110(2), 106–116.

Pierson, E., Simoiu, C., Overgoor, J., Corbett-Davies, S., Jenson, D., et al. (2020). A large-scale analysis of racial disparities in police stops across the United States. *Nature Human Behaviour*, 4(7), 736–745.

DeVylder, J. E., Frey, J. J., Cogburn, C. D., Wilcox, H. C., Sharpe, T. L., et al. (2017). Elevated prevalence of suicide attempts among victims of police violence in the USA. *Journal of Urban Health*, 94(5), 629–636.

OPTIONAL READINGS

Increase your knowledge about police homicides and victimization:

1 Stolen Lives Project, Stolen Lives: Killed by Law Enforcement: www. stolenlives.org/
2 Fatal Encounters Database, started by Brian Burghart: www.fatalen counters.org
3 Killed by Police database: https://killedbypolice.net/kbp2020/
4 Mapping Police Violence Map: https://mappingpoliceviolence.org/
5 *The Washington Post*, The Police Shootings Database: https://tinyurl. com/sn3jtf7c
6 *The Guardian*, The Counted: https://tinyurl.com/sn3jtf7c

Week 7—Topic: Natural Disasters and Climate Change

TOPICS TO BE COVERED

Interpersonal resilience:

• Developing social supports and networks
• Utilizing social engagement and interpersonal skills
• Concepts of interpersonal resilience and social capital
• Social resilience as it relates to our response to mass trauma

Community and societal resilience:

• Concepts of community and societal resilience
• Community resilience, preparedness, crisis response and recovery
• Developing a sense of community
• Social solidarity and social cohesion
• Unity in diversity—recognizing and valuing difference, building trust and a common identity

REQUIRED READINGS

Chapter 5—Goelitz, A. (Ed.). (2022). *Shared mass trauma in social work: Implications and strategies for resilient practice.* Routledge.

Tosone, C., McTighe, J. P., & Bauwens, J. (2017). Shared traumatic stress among social workers in the aftermath of Hurricane Katrina. *The British Journal of Social Work*, 45(4), 1313–1329.

OPTIONAL READINGS

Rowlands, A. (2013). Disaster recovery management in Australia and the contribution of social work. *Journal of Social Work in Disability & Rehabilitation*, 12, 1–20, doi:10.1080/1536710X.2013.784173.

Week 8—Topic: War and Terrorism

TOPICS TO BE COVERED

- Aspects of loss and injury as a result of war and terror
- Shared trauma and shared resilience for professionals during war and terrorism—unique aspects and challenges
- Awareness of the shared nature of the mass trauma exposure—shared with family, community, and clients
- Impact on dyadic relations within the therapeutic setting
- Need for more support and recognition from family, peers, community, and society in times of crisis

Related concepts:

- The unremitting nature of war and terrorism
- Compassion fatigue, secondary trauma, and vicarious trauma as they relate to—

  - Compassion satisfaction, professional growth, and secondary growth/resilience

REQUIRED READINGS

Chapter 6—Goelitz, A. (Ed.). (2022). *Shared mass trauma in social work: Implications and strategies for resilient practice.* Routledge.

Nuttman-Shwartz, O. (2015). Shared resilience in a traumatic reality: A new concept for trauma workers exposed personally and professionally to collective disaster. *Trauma, Violence and Abuse*, 16(4), 466–475. doi:10.1177/1524838014557287.

OPTIONAL READINGS

Nuttman-Shwartz, O., & Sterenberg, R. (2017). Social work in the context of an ongoing security threat: Role description, personal experiences, and conceptualization. *British Journal of Social Work*, 47(3), 903–918.

Week 9—Topic: Psychotherapy

TOPICS TO BE COVERED

- The practice of accompaniment in social work practice
- Why switching from behavioral treatment to relational therapy can support clients' needs during times of mass trauma
- Principles of feminist relational approaches
- Concepts of Terror Management Theory as they relate to shared trauma
- How therapists and clients may tend to respond during mass trauma

    - Increased therapist self-disclosure and its effect on their relationship

REQUIRED READINGS

Chapter 7—Goelitz, A. (Ed.). (2022). *Shared mass trauma in social work: Implications and strategies for resilient practice.* Routledge.

Seeley, K. (2003). *The psychotherapy of trauma and the trauma of psychotherapy: Talking to therapists about 9–11.* www.coi.columbia.edu/pdf/seeley_pot.pdf

OPTIONAL READINGS

Day, K. W., Lawson, G., & Burge, P. (2017). Clinicians' experiences of shared trauma after the shootings at Virginia Tech. *Journal of Counseling & Development*, 95, 269–280.

Week 10—Topic: Group Work

TOPICS TO BE COVERED

The mutual aid model and the benefits of group work:

- Definition of mutual aid in groups
- Two-client paradigm with both group members and the group as a whole as clients
- Role, tasks, and skills of group work practice
- Benefits of group participation

Shared trauma and group work:

- Integration of trauma-informed care principles with group work practice
- Manifestations of shared trauma in groups—

  - Between members and between members and workers

- Group work skills that lessen the intrusive impact of shared trauma
- Group work skills that address manifestations of shared trauma in group

REQUIRED READINGS

Chapter 8—Goelitz, A. (Ed.). (2022). *Shared mass trauma in social work: Implications and strategies for resilient practice.* Routledge.

Maheshwari, N., Yadav, R., & Singh, N. (2010). Group counseling: A silver lining in the psychological management of disaster trauma. *Journal of Pharmacy & Bioallied Sciences*, 2, 267–274.

West-Olatunji, C., Henesy, R., & Varney, M. (2015). Group work during international disaster outreach projects: A model to advance cultural competence. *Journal for Specialists in Group Work*, 40(1), 38–54.

OPTIONAL READINGS

Baird, S. L., & Alaggia, R. (2021). Trauma-informed groups: Recommendations for group workers. *Clinical Social Work Journal*, 49, 10–19.

Knight, C. (2016). Tasks and skills of the group worker across phases of group development. In G. Greif & C. Knight (Eds.), *Group work and populations at risk*. Oxford University Press.

Phillips, S. B. (2013). From immersion to formulation and integration: The complicated journey of the trauma group leader. *Group*, 37, 31–39.

Week 11—Topic: Community Organizing

TOPICS TO BE COVERED

- Historical trauma
- Social justice burnout
- Post-traumatic growth
- Trauma-informed community engagement
- Collective healing
- Proactive self-care
- Racial battle fatigue
- Positionality

REQUIRED READINGS

Chapter 9—Goelitz, A. (Ed.). (2022). *Shared mass trauma in social work: Implications and strategies for resilient practice*. Routledge.

Ortega-Williams, A., Beltran, R., Schultz, K., Henderson, Z. R.-G., Colon, L., & Teyra, C. (2021). An integrated historical trauma and post-traumatic growth framework: A cross-cultural exploration. *Journal of Trauma & Dissociation*, 22(2), 220–240.

Week 12—Topic: Conclusion

(Group project presenting a shared trauma intervention due)

TOPICS TO BE COVERED

- Group project presentations
- Discussion of what students will take with them from the course

REQUIRED READINGS

Chapter 10—Goelitz, A. (Ed.). (2022). *Shared mass trauma in social work: Implications and strategies for resilient practice*. Routledge.

OPTIONAL READINGS

Knight, C. (2013). Indirect trauma: Implications for supervision, the organization, and the academic institution. *The Clinical Supervisor*, 32, 224–243.

Tullberg, E., & Boothe, G. (2019). Taking an organizational approach to addressing secondary trauma in child welfare settings. *Journal of Public Child Welfare*, 13, 345–367.

Appendix 2: Practice Exercises and Questions

Week 1: Introduction

Class discussion questions

- Why did you sign up for this class? Why is it important?
- Tune in to yourself and become conscious of how you have been affected by mass trauma. Write or share about it.

Small group discussion questions

- How do you take care of yourself? What are three things that you do for your own self-care?
- How do you place boundaries between your work and home life? How do you navigate these areas of your life as a professional? Spouse? Parent? Supervisor?

Class or small group discussion questions

- Who or what gives you support in your work? What is the importance of professional supervision in your work?

Week 2: Conceptual Framework

Class discussion questions

- How do you identify a shared trauma reality? How is it different from other traumatic situations?
- Share your professional and personal emotional responses when called to help during a shared trauma. If you do not have this experience, what do you think your responses would be?

- Identify and share the challenges you faced during encounters with clients during shared traumas. If you do not have this experience, what do you think your challenges would be?
- What are three things that you could do to prepare yourself for working in a shared trauma reality?

Week 3: Research Findings

Small group discussion questions

- Identify and share your ways of coping before, during, and after your shared trauma encounters. If you do not have this experience, what do you think your coping would be?
- How would you navigate between your own and your clients' needs, and between your professional and personal roles during shared trauma?
- How would you take care of yourself, your family members, and your staff during a shared trauma?
- Do you think there are benefits to being a social worker during shared reality situations?

Week 4: Impact of Mass Trauma on Social Workers

Class breaks into dyads for the following role play

- Choose roles with one student being the social worker and the other the client.
- Choose a scenario for the first meeting between social worker and client—modality, in person or virtual, reason for encounter, etc.
- Take a moment to tune in to yourself in your role.
- Role play that first short encounter, noting your reactions as you converse.
- Review the encounter afterwards, as students.
- If time allows, switch roles and go through the process again.
- Share about the experience with the class.

Week 5: Pandemic

Role play fishbowl style with class observing

- Review how the researcher in the chapter from *Shared Mass Trauma in Social Work* assigned for this week interviewed partners of frontline healthcare workers.

- Ask for two volunteers—a researcher and a partner of a frontline healthcare worker.
- Role play the interview using the questions outlined in the chapter.
- Remember what you have learned about tuning into yourself, preparing for encounters, and processing them after.
- Reflect on how being in a shared trauma together impacted the interview.

Week 6: Racism and Police Brutality

Case example with class discussion questions

- Review the case example of Khalon in the chapter from *Shared Mass Trauma in Social Work* assigned for this week.
- Tune in to yourself, considering your own interactions with the police as you prepare to meet with your client, Khalon.
- Class discussion about the case considering the following

  - Work with him to make an inoculation plan. Walk through potential police encounters with a series of what-if questions, acting as an authentic observer/advocate for him so he can process past, present, and future experiences.
  - Create a narrative therapy approach. If he could rewrite the story, how would it change?
  - Notice your own reactions as you work with him.

    - If you are Black, Indigenous, Latinx, LGBTQIA+, or disabled does it remind you of your own vulnerability with police, potentially leading to a shared trauma experience?
    - If you are not Black, Indigenous, Latinx, LGBTQIA+, or disabled, notice any implicit bias that may arise.

  - Consider all sides of the situation and everyone involved—including the police, friends, and family—when he is ready to process the trauma.

    - What messages must each individual have received as a young person to hold the feelings they express?
    - What was going on in each person's mind to react the way they did?
    - Consider what each person's implicit biases could be.

Week 7: Natural Disasters and Climate Change

Case examples with class discussion questions

Case 1: Therapeutic Group Work in Situation of Floods and Tsunami

Imagine you are a social worker, working with widows from a community that has experienced the trauma of a tsunami that wiped out the livelihoods of the entire village. You have also suffered loss of family members in the disaster. You have gathered women who have lost their husbands and children.

- How would you, knowing your own grief and loss experience, go about working with a therapeutic group as well as providing both emotional and economic support to the women?

The social worker in this case study gathered women of different faiths from the community and using available community resources provided both shelter and food. The women were able to support each other through sharing grief and coping experiences. In the process of economic recovery, they embarked on projects doing handicrafts and growing a therapeutic garden (with the help of the Ministry of Agriculture and Commerce). They were able to provide both social and psychological as well as financial support for each other and the community, thus demonstrating the use of community resilience, networks of support and building personal coping as aids for healing after disaster.

Case 2: Training of Volunteers and Mental Health Workers in Earthquake Zone

In the disaster recovery phase of the Sichuan earthquake, social workers provided training with local volunteers who experienced trauma themselves. Being aware of and owning their own experience was helpful in understanding boundaries and limits of care. They were thus able to work through their own trauma and gain understanding of the grief and loss process. This coupled with giving themselves "permission" to take breaks for self-care and to seek support allowed the workers to not only find ways of empowering themselves but also to help the villagers assert their independence and support each other.

- With this in mind, what would a mental health training and support for a community facing disaster look like?
- What are some ways the personal resilience of workers can be reinforced?

Week 8: War and Terrorism

Case example with class discussion questions

- Review the case example of balloons and kites exploding along the Gaza/Israel border in the chapter from *Shared Mass Trauma in Social Work* assigned for this week.
- Briefly discuss the impact of this example on the class.
- Break down into small groups.
- Discuss how something as innocent as a kite or balloon can cause terror and confusion, creating a shared traumatic reality that affects both therapist and client.
- Tune in to yourselves to see how you are impacted personally by the discussion.
- Share about this and process feelings as a group.
- Tune in to yourselves to imagine how you would be impacted professionally by the discussion.
- Share about this and process feelings as a group.
- Discuss ways to cope with the feelings as a group.

Week 9: Psychotherapy

Role play exercise:

- One person plays the therapist, another the client, and a third serves as observer or consultant.
- The purpose of the exercise it to practice hearing potentially upsetting feedback from clients about therapist self-disclosure and then processing it with them.
- The "therapist" shares with the "client" an emotional response they are comfortable with and an emotional response they are not comfortable with—like worry, sadness, or withdrawal.
- In this role play, the therapist self-discloses something personal in the therapy session.
- The client responds with an emotion that is either easy or hard for the therapist to address, letting the therapist know the self-disclosure didn't work for them.
- The therapist's job is to repair the relational rupture by validating the client's experience, exploring the connection between their self-disclosure and the client's emotional response, and letting the client know that their needs always come first in this therapeutic relationship.
- The client and therapist process the rupture.
- The observer or consultant talks with the client and therapist (still in character) about the self-disclosure and subsequent conversation to see how well the rupture has repaired.
- The therapist writes a short reflective essay to identify why they self-disclosed, what was easy or difficult about the client's response, and how they will think about this situation the next time it comes up.

Week 10: Group Work

Case example with class discussion questions

- Review the following case example.
- The social worker, a member of the LGBTQIA+ community, is employed in an outpatient behavioral health program that serves members of this community. At the recent Pride Day parade, which was sponsored in part by the social worker's agency, a motorist drove through the crowd, injuring multiple individuals and killing five. The worker had attended the parade, witnessed the crash, and knew one of the injured participants.
- Consider the following two scenarios:

One: The worker has been facilitating a 16-week support group for nine individuals who had recently come out. The group has been meeting for five weeks and addresses issues such as coming out to friends and family, members' concerns about their new identity and status, and establishing romantic and intimate relationships. Prior to the sixth session, the crash at the parade occurred. Two members of the group attended the parade. The worker is unsure whether any other members attended and, if so, whether they had seen the crash.

Two: In response to the parade tragedy, the agency will offer a six-session group to help members of the LGBTQIA+ community cope with their reactions to the event; the group will be led by the social worker. Ten individuals have signed up to participate in the group. All had attended the parade. While none knew any of the injured or murdered victims, most had witnessed the tragedy.

For scenarios one and two

- Put yourself in the shoes of the worker. As a member of the LGBTQIA+ community yourself, knowing one of the victims, and having witnessed the crash, how are you feeling about what happened?
- When you meet with the group, would/should you acknowledge your own experience at the parade? If yes, how would you do this? If no, why not?

For scenario one

- How would you approach your next meeting with the group?
- What group work skills would you need to employ to "recontract" with the group and provide members with the opportunity to discuss their reactions to the tragedy?

- What concerns and challenges might you encounter as you meet with members for this and subsequent sessions?

For scenario two

- In your first meeting with the group, how would you explain your role and purpose and the role and purpose of the group?
- What expectations do you think should guide members' interactions with one another
- What concerns and challenges might you encounter as this group begins?

Week 11: Community Organizing

Collective Racial Healing Circle

Objective: To exchange ideas, process conflict, vent needs, identify resources, and heal trauma in community.

1. Do a check-in activity to get everyone in the circle.
2. Create group guidelines together to assist in your group expectations.
3. Do a grounding exercise.
4. Integrate small group discussion, large group discussion, and activities to encourage examination of mindfulness, self-care, community engagement, white supremacy, etc.
5. End with community sharing.
6. Have resources to share / homework to do.
7. Do a grounding exercise to exit.

Positionality Pie Chart Exercise

Objective: Each student will create a positionality pie chart and write a positionality statement of no more than 750 words, which describes the potential impact of their race and intersectional identity on the research/ work they are involved in.

Self-Care Plan

Objective: To create space for students to proactively plan their self-care.
Process: Students will be encouraged to create a self-care plan. Following the completion of the plan, students will send themselves a letter to be received a year after the exercise.

Week 12: Conclusion: Lessons Learned

(Group projects presenting a shared trauma intervention)
  Class discussion questions:

- How has your idea of shared trauma changed as a result of this course?
- Name some ways what you've learned will affect your future work with clients.
- Which chapter had the most impact on you and why?
- Do you think most social workers would benefit from taking a similar course? Why or why not?
- What would you like to see added to the course?
- Did you find taking this course brought you together as a class?

Index

For Product Safety Concerns and Information please contact our EU
representative GPSR@taylorandfrancis.com
Taylor & Francis Verlag GmbH, Kaufingerstraße 24, 80331 München, Germany